CW00709087

Leprosy Mission
50 Portland Place
London W1N 3DG

Lupus UK
Queens Court
9–17 Eastern Road
Romford, Essex RM1 3NG
Tel: 0708 731 251
      0708 731 252

Marfan Association
6 Queens Road
Farnborough
Hampshire GU14 6DH
Tel: 0252 547 441

Naevus Support Group
58 Necton Road
Wheathampstead
Hertfordshire AL4 8AU
Tel: 058 283 2853

National Eczema Society
4 Tavistock Place
London WC1H 9RA
Tel: 071 388 4097

**Neurofibromatosis Association
(LINK)**
120 London Road
Kingston-upon-Thames
Surrey KT2 6QJ
Tel: 081 547 1636

The Psoriasis Association
7 Milton Street
Northampton NN2 7JG
Tel: 0604 711 129

**Raynaud's and Scleroderma
Association Trust**
112 Crewe Road
Alsager
Cheshire ST7 2JA
Tel: 0270 872 776

Scleroderma Society
61 Sandpits Lane
St Albans
Hertfordshire AL1 4EY
Tel: 0727 55054

Terrence Higgins Trust Ltd
(BM AIDS)
52–54 Gray's Inn Road
London WC1X 8JU
Tel: 071 831 0330

**Tuberose Sclerosis Association of
Great Britain**
Little Barnsley Farm
Catshill, Bromsgrove
Worcester B61 0NQ

The Vitiligo Group
PO Box 919
London SE21 8AW
Tel: 081 776 7022

**Women's F.
Rights Info**
52–54 Feath
London EC1Y oK1
Tel: 071 251 6580

**Hospitals where laser treatment is
available under the NHS**

Department of Plastic Surgery
St John's Hospital at Howden
West Livingstone
West Lothian EH54 6PP
Tel: 0506 419 666

Department of Dermatology
Leeds General Infirmary
Great George Street, Leeds LS1 3EX
Tel: 0532 437 188

Department of Dermatology
Bridgend General Hospital
Quarella Road, Bridgend
CF31 1JP
Tel: 0656 662 166

Department of Plastic Surgery
Bedford General Hospital (South
Wing)
Kempston Road, Bedford MK42 9DJ
Tel: 0234 355 122

Treatment in Dermatology

Barbara Leppard *Senior Lecturer, Department of Medicine,*
University of Southampton; Honorary Consultant Dermatologist,
Royal South Hants Hospital, Southampton, England

Richard Ashton *Consultant Dermatologist,*
Royal Naval Hospital, Haslar, Gosport; Honorary Consultant Dermatologist,
Royal South Hants Hospital, Southampton, England

RADCLIFFE MEDICAL PRESS • OXFORD

© 1993 Radcliffe Medical Press Ltd
15 Kings Meadow, Ferry Hinksey Road,
Oxford OX2 0DP

British Library Cataloguing in Publication Data

A Catalogue record for this book is available from the British Library

ISBN 1 870905 52 0

Typeset by Advance Typesetting Ltd, Oxfordshire
Printed and bound in Great Britain

Preface

This book has been written as a companion volume to *Differential Diagnosis in Dermatology*. Once you have made a diagnosis, this book will tell you what to do about it. For those who are not confident about treating skin conditions, the treatment options seem to lie between 0.1% betamethasone 17-valerate (Betnovate) ointment or cream, miconazole (Canestan) cream, calamine lotion and chlorpheniramine (Piriton) tablets. This book will enable you to be more rational in your approach and a lot more successful. It is written from the point of view of the patient, ie, if I were the patient, what I would want my doctor to know in order to treat me. By this we mean that if the cause is straightforward, and it is simply a matter of putting a certain ointment on the skin or taking a certain tablet, that is all the information supplied, but if you need to understand why the disease has occurred to explain to the patient why he needs a particular treatment, then that information is also given. Likewise, if a treatment has potential side effects or you need to take precautions in prescribing it, all you need to know to use it safely is provided.

The illustrations have been chosen to help you make the diagnosis (if there is no illustration of the condition in *Differential Diagnosis in Dermatology*), to show you how a treatment or procedure is carried out, or to illustrate a piece of equipment so that you can show the patient what to expect.

We would like to thank many of our colleagues for sharing their expertise so willingly with us: Dr Chris Baughan, Mr Anthony Chant, Mr John Carruth, Dr Virginia Hall, Dr Martin Keefe, Dr Arthur Laxton, Dr William Perkins, Mr Clive Porter, Mr Gavin Royle, Dr Sri Singha and Dr Derek Waller. We would especially like to thank Michael White and Tim Browne, the medical photographers at the Royal South Hants Hospital and Haslar Hospital, for patiently taking photographs of all the various treatments, and the graphics departments at Haslar Hospital and Southampton General Hospital for preparing the line drawings, particularly Alain Holcroft at Haslar.

Barbara Leppard
Richard Ashton

March 1993

FOR SANDRA, SIMON, JIM AND LOUISE

Contents

Part 1 General principles of treatment

INTRODUCTION

There is a widespread belief that skin disease either responds to topical steroids or it does not. The result of this belief is that many patients do not get better and they, and their families, face months of frustration without any benefit at all. This book is intended to show that by following a few simple rules, the correct treatment can be given from the beginning without resorting to guesswork or 'hoping for the best'!

GENERAL PRINCIPLES

1 Make a diagnosis before embarking on treatment. Never think of treating a patient without first making a diagnosis or putting in hand the necessary investigations so that a diagnosis can be reached.

2 Be realistic about what is possible. As skin disease is visible, the patient will often assume that it must be easy to cure. Generally speaking, skin disease can be put into three groups with regard to this.

(i)   Those diseases that have a specific cause and hence a specific treatment. Once this has been given correctly, this should be the end of the problem. Such conditions include:

- contact allergic eczema
- fungal and bacterial infections
- infestations such as scabies and lice
- skin tumours.

(ii)   Those diseases where no cure is possible, but spontaneous remissions and exacerbations occur. These may be helped considerably by treatment, but a cure is not possible and should not be sought. These include:

- atopic eczema
- dermatitis herpetiformis
- pemphigus and pemphigoid
- psoriasis
- rosacea.

(iii) Those diseases which persist for a limited period of time and then disappear on their own. This group may sometimes require symptomatic treatment, and the patient should be reassured of their benign nature. Examples of these are:

- alopecia areata
- erythema multiforme
- guttate psoriasis
- lichen planus
- pityriasis rosea.

The patient should be made aware of which of these categories their skin disease is in, so that they have a better idea of response to treatment and prognosis.

3 Look at the whole person and not just at their rash. Often the problem that presents itself is quite straightforward but at the same time there may be deeper needs requiring attention. Body language speaks louder than words. A forced smile, a grimace, a pained expression, tears, wringing of the hands or constant fidgeting may all be signs that there is more going on than was at first apparent. Believe what you see rather than what the textbook tells you is the cause of this particular rash.

Patients with widespread skin disease often feel dirty, ashamed or guilty, thinking that somehow it is their fault that they are ill. They may be afraid that it is contagious, or that they have cancer or AIDS; women with hirsutism may fear that they are changing into men. Patients may also be embarrassed about having a rash because of:

- the look of it, especially if it is on a part of the body that shows, such as the face or the hands. They will notice people looking at it and assume that they will think it is contagious. Patients will often wear clothes that will hide it and limit their activities so that others will not see it (eg not going swimming or to the beach on holiday)
- the shedding of scales making a mess (particularly in psoriasis)
- the smell (particularly in patients with ulcerated legs)
- the mess which the treatment makes. Grease on the clothes and bedding, and the smell and mess of tar preparations are not popular with patients or their families
- its presence on the genital area. It often interferes with sexual activity because of embarrassment and patients may be afraid that their partner will think that it is contagious (that they have VD or AIDS).

It is important that you understand how the patient feels about having a skin problem as well as what to do about it.

4 Listen to what the patient has to say. Lay people often equate skin disease with 'nerves'. The patient will be anxious that you do not think that is the cause. At the same time, patients often have a very good idea why they have a problem and if you will give them time they will tell you what it is. Once patients are faced with someone who will listen, they will readily talk about their concerns and difficulties. They may find that by being able to express it:

- they understand it better
- that it is not nearly as bad as they thought
- that the solution is obvious now they have faced it
- that they can cope knowing that there is someone else who understands (even if nothing can be done about it).

5 Understand that not everyone wants to get well. Some patients get a great deal of attention because of their illness which they do not want to give up by getting better. For others it is somehow respectable to have a rash (which will not go away) but it is not all right to own up to guilt about some person or event, a poor self image or conflict in the family. Using one ointment or pill after another will not resolve any of these and it is better for the patient to face up to reality sooner rather than later.

6 Treatment of acute rashes

- Resting the skin is important in any acute or extensive skin disease. Going to bed is a helpful treatment in its own right. It is the basis for most in-patient treatment but can often be done just as well at home (by this we mean actually going to bed and not just lying down on the sofa; the latter will not stop the patient from pottering about). Sedation with trimeprazine or promethazine will often be needed to keep the patient resting in bed.
- Localized acute rashes should also be rested. If the patient has an acute blistering rash on his feet, it will not get better unless he stops walking around. Going to bed for a few days is likely to do more good than using a more potent medicament. In the same way, a patient with an acute hand eczema is unlikely to get better while continuing to do the washing up.
- The more acute the rash, the more bland the treatment needs to be. Never use potent treatments like dithranol or tar on acutely erupting psoriasis. If in doubt, white soft paraffin is unlikely to do any harm and will keep the patient comfortable.

7 Explain to the patient what is going on. It is important to explain to the patient what is wrong with them, what the treatment is and how to use it. Time spent at the first consultation explaining the nature of the problem and the correct use of the treatment will be time well spent.

TOPICAL TREATMENT

Any applied agent contains two components:
1 the base or vehicle
2 the active ingredient.
Both are equally important, but often the right type of base is not taken into consideration when prescribing a treatment. The function of the base is to transport the active constituent into the skin so that it is delivered to where it is needed. Generally speaking, the base is determined by the hydration of the skin at the particular site, while the pathological process determines the active constituent.

The base

All bases are made up from one or more of the following:
- powders, eg zinc oxide, starch, calamine (zinc carbonate and ferric oxide)
- liquids, eg water, alcohol, propylene glycol
- oils and greases, eg liquid paraffin, yellow and white soft paraffin (these are low melting point hydrocarbons), lanolin (wool alcohols), polyethylene glycols (synthetic waxes).

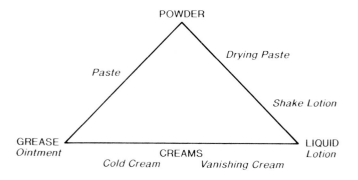

These may be mixed together to produce shake lotions, creams and pastes.

LOTIONS A lotion is any liquid. It may be a straightforward liquid such as normal saline or a solution of potassium permanganate, or a shake lotion consisting of a suspension of an insoluble powder in a liquid, eg:
- calamine lotion—calamine 15%, zinc oxide 5%, glycerine 5%, water 75%

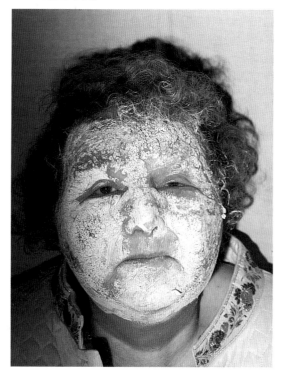

Figure 1 Calamine lotion applied to the face. It is contraindicated if there is a lot of exudate, as in this woman with an acute eczema, and it is very unsightly.

- increasing the proportion of powder results in what is termed a *drying paste*, eg zinc oxide 30%, talc 30%, glycerine 20%, water 20%.

Shake lotions, such as calamine lotion, have a cooling effect because the liquid evaporates leaving the inert powder on the skin. In practice these are hardly ever used except to cool sunburn; they are not very cosmetically acceptable when applied to parts of the body that show (Figure 1).

GELS Gels are transparent semi-solid emulsions of organic polymers (eg methylcellulose, agar or gelatine) in a liquid (eg water). They are solid (or semi-solid) in the cold and become liquid on warming up (like a jelly).

OINTMENTS Ointments contain little or no water and consist of organic hydrocarbons, alcohols and acids. Examples include:

- white soft paraffin (WSP) = Vaseline
- emulsifying ointment (emulsifying wax 30%, liquid paraffin 20%, white soft paraffin 50%) [emulsifying wax = cetostearyl alcohol, sodium lauryl sulphate and water]
- lanolin (fat derived from wool).

These are greasy and form an impermeable layer over the skin which prevents evaporation of water. Hydrocarbons are sub-divided by their melting points. Liquid paraffin is liquid at room temperature and is used in bath oils. White soft paraffin is semi-solid at room temperature, but melts at around body temperature, so rubs in easily. A mixture comprising equal parts of liquid paraffin and white soft paraffin is useful for covering large areas of the body with grease. Waxes have high melting points and are useful for stiffening up an ointment base. Some ointments may be water soluble, and consist of polyethylene glycols such as fatty acid propylene glycol (FAPG). These compounds are semi-solids similar to Vaseline, so they spread well on the skin and wash off with water.

CREAMS Creams are a mixture (emulsion) of an ointment with water. In order to prevent the two elements separating from one another, stabilizers and emulsifiers have to be added. There are two types of cream.

1 An emulsion of water in oil (like butter); these are the *cold creams*. They behave like oils in that they do not mix with any exudate from the skin. They are easier to apply than ointments, but more cosmetically acceptable, although they are greasier than the vanishing creams (*see* below). Many of them contain lanolin, which can cause a contact allergic eczema in some patients, eg oily cream (lanolin 50%, water 50%).

2 An emulsion of oil in water (like milk and cream); these are the *vanishing creams*. They rub into the skin easily and mix readily with water and are very popular with patients. Their main disadvantage is that they tend to make dry skin even drier because the water in them evaporates. If the skin is dry (eg in atopic eczema) a vanishing cream may make the condition worse; a cold cream or ointment will be better. A further disadvantage is that they must contain preservatives, such as parahydroxybenzoic acid esters (parabens), chlorocresol, propylene glycol or ethylene diamine, to prevent the cream from becoming infected. All the preservatives can act as sensitizers and cause a contact allergic eczema in some patients. Examples of oil in water creams are:

- aqueous cream (emulsifying ointment 30%, water 69.9%, and chlorocresol 0.1% [as preservative])
- cetomacrogol A cream which is used as a diluent for many steroid creams (cetomacrogol emulsifying ointment 39%, water 59.9%, chlorocresol 0.1% [as preservative]).

See also the table of moisturizers on page 92.

PASTES Pastes are mixtures of a powder in an ointment. They stay where you put them and do not spread away from that site as the skin warms up (like creams and ointments do). Lassar's paste is the one which is most commonly used. It contains 24% starch, 24% zinc oxide, 2% salicylic acid and 50% white soft paraffin.

Cooling pastes are preparations which contain a powder (zinc oxide), water (lime water) and an oil (arachis oil). They are called creams rather than pastes in the UK, eg Zinc Cream BP (zinc oxide 32 g, oleic acid 0.5 ml, arachis oil 32 ml, wool fat 8 g, calcium hydroxide 45 mg, water to 100 g).

When to use which base

Lotions are used on wet surfaces and hairy areas. They are used:

- on wet rashes, eg weeping eczema. Lotions containing potassium permanganate or aluminium acetate coagulate protein and help to dry up exudates

  If the rash is on the hands and/or the feet they can be soaked in a bowl containing the lotion for 10 minutes once or twice a day. If the whole body is affected, the lotion can be put in the bath and the patient allowed to soak in it. If the rash is on the face or a limb, wet dressings can be used—gauze dressings are soaked in the liquid and applied wet to the affected part; the dressings are either replaced frequently so that they are always wet, or further lotion is applied to the dressings to keep them wet.
- in the mouth, usually as a mouthwash
- on the scalp so that the hair is not dishevelled, and sometimes in the axillae or pubic area.

Gels are used as alternatives to lotions mainly on hairy parts of the body. For example, since all topical steroid lotions are in an alcoholic vehicle they are not suitable for applying to excoriated eczematous skin. A gel (which does not contain alcohol) containing a steroid can be rubbed into the scalp, it becomes liquid as it warms up and is therefore cosmetically acceptable (like a lotion) and does not sting.

Pastes are used when you want to apply a noxious chemical to a particular part of the skin without getting it onto the surrounding normal skin, eg dithranol in psoriasis. They are not used very much because they are unsightly. They have to be applied with a gloved hand or a spatula and be cleaned off with oil (eg arachis oil) rather than soap and water.

Ointments and creams are used most of the time. Which you use depends mainly on the patient's preference and the hydration of the skin. Start with a cream on normal or moist skin and an ointment on dry skin. Creams are much more cosmetically acceptable, particularly on the face (patients do not like walking around with a shiny face), in the flexures and when the medicament has to be applied all over (so that the clothes are not covered with grease), but may be too drying if the skin is itself dry (eg in patients with atopic eczema and ichthyosis). In general, ointments are more effective than creams, but you may have to try both to see which suits the patient best. As creams contain water, they must also contain preservatives to prevent contamination by bacteria and fungi, and these can cause a contact allergic eczema. In patients with acute eczema or contact allergic eczema where you do not know the cause, always use an ointment (which does not contain lanolin) rather than a cream until you have discovered the cause.

Active ingredients

STEROIDS Topical steroids are extremely useful in inflammatory conditions of the skin, particularly eczema, but they are not the treatment for everything (they are contraindicated in acne, rosacea, all infections [bacterial, viral and fungal] and infestations, and on leg ulcers). In topical steroids the basic steroid structure (Figure 2) has been modified in order to increase the potency (Figure 4). The three changes which have caused the structure to become more effective are:

- fluorination at C_9
- introduction of an unsaturated bond between C_1 and C_2
- changing the nature of the side chain at C_{21}.

Topical steroids are divided into four groups according to their potency (Table 1). There is a very large number to choose from and it is best to become familiar with a few (perhaps one or two from each group) rather than all of them. As a general rule, use the weakest possible steroid that will do the job. On the face do not use anything stronger than hydrocortisone; the only exception to this rule is in discoid lupus erythematosus (see page 41). Steroids in the very potent group should rarely be used; in most instances where you might be considering their use, systemic steroids would be safer. 50 g of 0.05% clobetasol propionate (Dermovate)/week will suppress the patient's adrenal glands. Hydrocortisone is 50 times weaker so is obviously a lot safer; in theory a patient could use up to 2.5 kg/week before suffering from the same side effects.

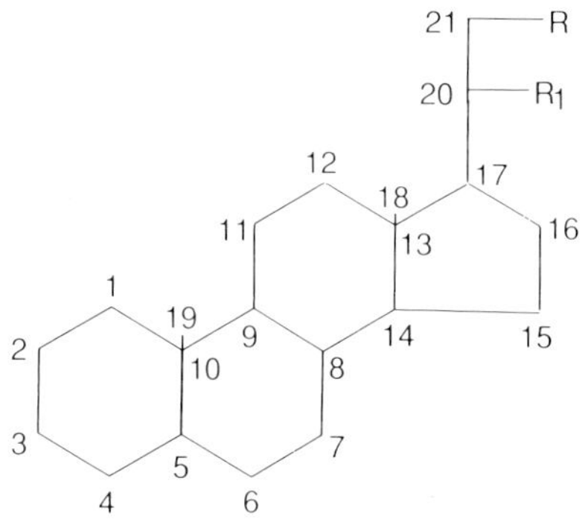

Figure 2 Basic steroid structure.

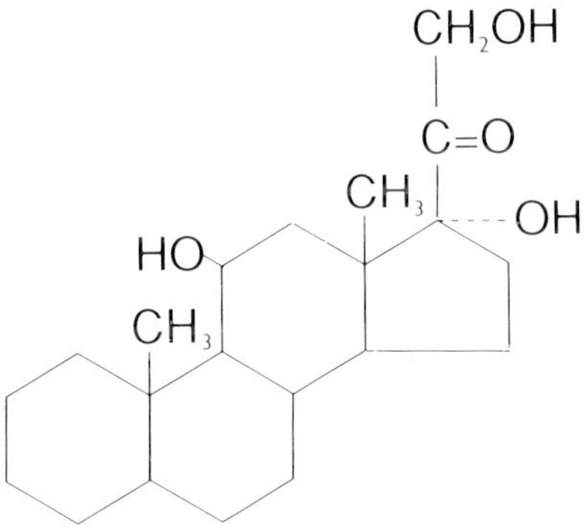

Figure 3 Hydrocortisone.

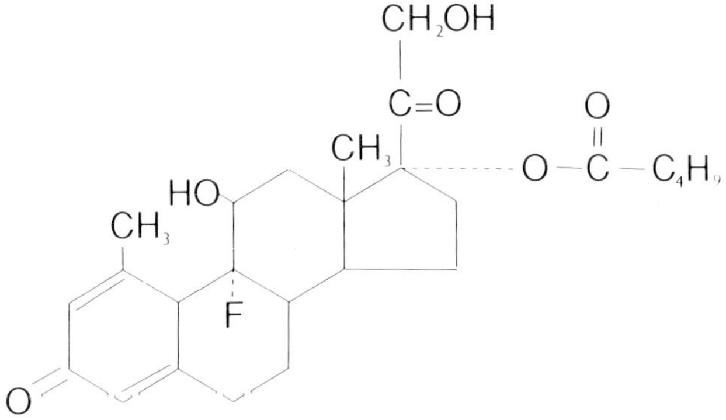

Figure 4 Betamethasone 17-valerate.

Table 1 Classification of different groups of topical steroids

Group 1 Mildly potent	Group 2 Moderately potent	Group 3 Potent	Group 4 Very potent
Alclometasone dipropionate 0.05% (Modrasone)	Betamethasone valerate 0.025% (Betnovate RD)	Beclomethasone dipropionate 0.025% (Propaderm)	Clobetasol propionate 0.05% (Dermovate)
Fluocinolone acetonide 0.0025% (Synalar 1:10)	Clobetasone butyrate 0.05% (Eumovate)	Betamethasone dipropionate 0.05% (Diprosone)	Diflucortolone valerate 0.3% (Nerisone forte)
Hydrocortisone 0.5–2.5% (Cobadex, Dioderm, Efcortelan, E45 HC, Hydrocortistab, Hydrocortisyl)	Desoxymethasone 0.05% (Stiedex LP)	Betamethasone valerate 0.1% (Betnovate)	Halcinonide 0.1% (Halciderm)
	Fluocinolone acetonide 0.00625% (Synalar 1:4)	Desoxymethasone 0.25% (Stiedex)	
	Flurandrenolone 0.0125% (Haelan)	Diflucortolone valerate 0.1% (Nerisone)	
		Fluocinolone acetonide 0.025% (Synalar)	
		Fluocinonide 0.05% (Metosyn)	
		Hydrocortisone 17-butyrate 0.1% (Locoid)	
		Mometasone furoate 0.1% (Elocon)	
		Triamcinolone acetonide 0.1% (Adcortyl, Ledercort)	

Relative potencies of the different groups compared with the potency of 1% hydrocortisone:

   Group 2—2.5 × stronger
   Group 3—10 × stronger
   Group 4—50 × stronger

We would recommend that you only use 1% hydrocortisone (or equivalent Group 1 steroid) on the face, and start with this elsewhere, and only use something stronger if it does not work. Remember that in the flexures absorption of the steroid will be increased because of occlusion. In practice we rarely find it necessary to use anything stronger than the potent group diluted 1:4 (eg 0.025% betamethasone 17-valerate [Betnovate RD], 0.00625% fluocinolone acetonide [Synalar 1:4] or 0.00625% beclomethasone dipropionate [Propaderm 1:4]).

Side effects of topical steroids

- Skin atrophy and striae from loss of dermal collagen (Figures 45 and 46, pages 59 and 61).
- Tearing of the skin leading to odd shaped scars (stellate scars) due to loss of dermal collagen.

- Easy bruising due to loss of collagen support of the blood vessels in the dermis.
- Perioral dermatitis when steroids from Groups 2, 3 and 4 are applied to the face of young adults.
- Telangiectasia on the face when steroids from Groups 2, 3 and 4 are applied to the face in middle and old age (Figure 5).
- Rebound phenomenon causing worsening of the skin condition when the steroid is stopped, especially in psoriasis.
- Susceptibility to infection.
- Tachyphylaxis, whereby repeated use of the steroid results in loss of effect. This can be avoided if the patient only uses emollients on two days of every week of treatment.
- Contact allergic eczema. About 2% of patients being treated with topical steroids become sensitized to the steroid (rather than the base).
- Cushing's syndrome when large amounts of potent or very potent steroids are used (Figure 33, page 49). This includes the moon face and buffalo hump and all the systemic effects that you get with oral steroids (*see* page 13).
- Pituitary axis depression when large amounts of steroid are being used, especially in young children if steroids stronger than 1% hydrocortisone are used.

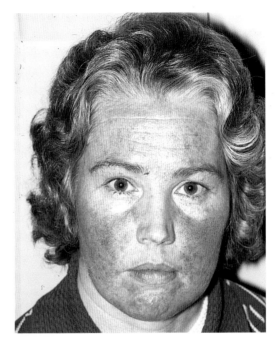

Figure 5 Steroid facies. After the age of about 25, the application of topical steroids stronger than hydrocortisone to the face will result in telangiectasia. If they have only been used for a short time (weeks—months), the changes will be reversible.

TAR Tar is not used very much these days because it is brown and smelly and patients do not like it. It can occasionally be used in eczema and psoriasis. There are basically three types of tar available.

1 Wood tars which are produced by the destructive distillation of beech, birch, pine or juniper. In the UK the only one which is used therapeutically is Oil of Cade which can be used to treat psoriasis of the scalp (*see* page 177).

2 Bituminous tars originally obtained from the distillation of shale deposits containing fossilized fish, hence ichthyol. Today they are mainly used in paste bandages (eg ichthammol bandages) to soothe chronic eczema (*see* page 55).

3 Coal tars are mixtures of 10,000 or so different compounds, mainly aromatic hydrocarbons (eg benzol, naphthalene and anthracene). Crude coal tar is what remains when coal is heated without air, originally done to produce coal gas. Which compounds in tar actually work is not known. They reduce DNA synthesis and therefore epidermal proliferation and are useful for stopping itching. Crude coal tar can be further refined by boiling and then alcoholic extraction to produce coal tar solution.

Crude coal tar is used in the treatment of both psoriasis and eczema. **In psoriasis:** It should not be used in acute erupting psoriasis, erythrodermic psoriasis or generalized pustular psoriasis because it will make them worse. It should also be avoided in the flexures because it will make the patient sore. It can be used on:

- stable plaque type psoriasis. 2%, 5% or 10% crude coal tar in WSP or Unguentum Merck can be applied once or twice a day; it is very messy (*see* Figure 119, page 157).
- the scalp. Mixed with salicylic acid and coconut oil (Ung. cocois co.) at night (*see* page 176).
- pustular psoriasis of the palms and soles. 2%, 5% or 10% crude coal tar (in increasing strengths) in WSP or Lassar's paste, or mixed with salicylic acid (coal tar and salicylic acid ointment BP) applied at night under gloves or socks to keep it off the bedding (*see* page 178).

In eczema: crude coal tar should not be used in an acute weeping eczema but it is very useful in discoid eczema (*see* page 64) or in lichen simplex (*see* page 111). It is usually prescribed in 2–5% strengths in WSP or Lassar's paste. It can also be used in paste bandages (Coltapaste or Tarband) if the eczema is confined to the limbs (Figure 42, page 56). These work by not only helping the itching but also by preventing the patient getting at the skin to scratch it.

Coal tar solution (liquor picis carbonis [LPC]) is mainly used in bath water by patients with psoriasis. It can also be used in a weak concentration (2–3%) in cream base for guttate psoriasis and acutely erupting psoriasis (*see* page 174).

Side effects of tar and problems with using it

- Tar is brown and smelly. Most patients do not like the look or smell of it (Figure 119, page 157) and it will stain clothes and bedding.

- It can cause an irritant reaction on the skin.
- Occasionally it causes a contact allergic eczema.
- It may cause a photosensitivity reaction.
- It will cause a folliculitis on hairy areas and is best avoided in patients who are very hairy.

DITHRANOL This is a synthetic anthracene derivative which is very effective in the treatment of psoriasis (*see* page 154). It is used mainly as a cream (0.1% gradually increasing to 0.25%, 0.5%, 1% and 2%) for short periods of time (short contact therapy, *see* page 155) or in Lassar's paste as a hospital treatment (*see* page 159). Its main disadvantages are that it burns normal skin (so the patient needs to take great care to put it only on the plaques of psoriasis) and stains the clothes (and bedding) an indelible mauve colour. It should not be used in acute eruptive psoriasis, erythrodermic psoriasis or generalized pustular psoriasis or the rash will get worse rather than better. **It should be used only in stable plaque type psoriasis.**

KERATOLYTIC AGENTS These are used to remove hyper-keratosis in a whole variety of skin conditions including warts, hyperkeratotic eczema on the palms and soles, psoriasis and tylosis. The ones most commonly used include:

- α-hydroxy acids (salicylic, lactic and benzoic acids). 2% or 5% salicylic acid ointment, applied twice a day, is useful for treating hyperkeratosis of the palms and soles or plane warts. It can be mixed with coal tar (coal tar and salicylic acid ointment BP) for treating psoriasis (*see* page 158), or with a topical steroid ointment for treating hyperkeratotic eczema (*see* page 65). Lactic acid is combined with salicylic acid in proprietary wart paints (*see* page 252), and benzoic acid is combined with salicylic acid (in Whitfield's ointment) for treating fungal infections of the skin (*see* page 209).

- propylene glycol. 50% propylene glycol in water is used under polythene occlusion at night to reduce the keratin in hyperkeratotic eczema on the palms and soles (*see* page 66). Normally a topical steroid ointment will be used in the daytime.
- urea. A 40% solution of urea can be used as a soak for treating patients with hyperkeratotic eczema on the hands and feet (*see* page 66) or tylosis. It is an alternative to propylene glycol but is more expensive because such large amounts are needed to fill a bowl.

ANTIBIOTICS As a general rule, topical antibiotics should not be used on the skin because most of them are potent skin sensitizers and will cause a contact allergic eczema. You do not want to sensitize someone to a drug which may in the future be life saving; it is much easier to become allergic to an antibiotic applied to the skin than to one taken by mouth or parenterally. Virtually everyone will become sensitized to penicillin if it is applied to the skin so this should never be used topically. Tetracyclines rarely cause problems and would be safe to use, but in practice they are not useful because the common skin pathogens, *Staphylococcus aureus* and *Streptococcus pyogenes* are not sensitive to tetracycline.

Topical antibiotics should only be used in very superficial infections which will clear up in a matter of days, eg impetigo. They should not be used in infected eczema (because that is likely to be a recurrent problem and the patient may well become sensitized after using it several times) or on infected looking leg ulcers (almost all patients with chronic venous ulceration are allergic to a number of antibiotics on patch testing because they have been used inappropriately in the past). Neomycin is useful since it is rarely used systemically and most staphylococci are sensitive to it. Mupirocin

(Bactroban) or fucidic acid (Fucidin) are alternatives which rarely cause problems (*see* page 94). Do not be tempted to use steroid-antibiotic mixtures because if the patient becomes allergic to the antibiotic in the mixture, the topical steroid will damp down the local reaction and you will only realize what has happened when the patient develops a widespread eczema. Most bacterial infections of the skin are more appropriately treated with systemic antibiotics.

ANTIFUNGAL AGENTS These can be divided into two groups: **(i) Those which are active against dermatophyte fungi** (which cause tinea). These work by inhibiting various enzymes needed for sterol synthesis in the fungal cell membrane (*see* Figures 172 and 173, page 210). Since these same enzymes are present in human cells, it is important that the drugs interfere with the fungal enzymes preferentially. All of these drugs have a broad spectrum of action against dermatophytes, yeasts, erythrasma and gram positive cocci. Because of this there is a temptation is to use them in any rash in the flexures or in the toewebs without first making a definite diagnosis. There is no harm in this if you have first taken scrapings for mycology culture. Then, if the patient does not get better with the treatment, you will have the answer from the laboratory as to whether fungus was present or not.

There are six groups of topical antifungal agents.

1 Keratolytic agents act differently to all the others. They remove the keratin on which the fungus lives rather than by destroying the fungus itself. The one most commonly used is Whitfield's ointment, a mixture of benzoic acid and salicylic acid in emulsifying ointment (*see* page 209).

2 Undecanoate as the acid zinc salt in Mycota powder. This is available for patients to buy without prescription.

3 Thiocarbamates (tolnaftate) are fungistatic (*see* page 212).

4   Morpholines (amorolfine) are fungistatic (*see* page 212).

5   Imidazoles. There are many drugs in this group (*see* pages 209 and 211). They are all fungistatic rather than fungicidal and of more or less equal efficacy; you can use whichever is the cheapest. A number of imidazole-hydrocortisone mixtures are also made; these are generally not as useful because they encourage treatment without first making a diagnosis. The mistaken belief is that they will work for both fungal infections and eczema. In practice, the imidazole alone will be much more effective for treating fungal infections.

6   Allylamines (terbinafine) are fungicidal and more effective than any of the other topical antifungal agents (*see* page 211).

(ii) Those which are active against yeasts such as *Candida* and *Pityrosporum* species (*see* pages 31 and 144).

- Imidazoles are broad spectrum antifungal agents and work for yeasts as well as dermatophytes (*see* page 32).
- Polyenes. Nystatin (named after the New York State Department of Health) is only effective against *Candida*. It is cheaper than the imidazoles but has the disadvantage that it stains yellow everything it comes into contact with. Amphotericin B is a broad spectrum polyene antifungal agent; it is mainly used as lozenges for treating infections in the mouth.
- Clioquinol (Vioform) is effective against *Candida* and various bacteria but not against dermatophytes. It also stains the skin and clothing yellow.
- Rosaniline dyes. Gentian violet is effective against yeasts and gram positive organisms. It is used as a 0.5% aqueous solution which is extremely messy (staining everything it comes into contact with purple—*see* Figure 17, page 31) but very useful in wet areas, eg *Candida* infections under the breasts.

SYSTEMIC TREATMENT

Antibiotics

Systemic antibiotics are used for the following.

1   **Staphylococcal infections** in the skin, eg boils, carbuncles, ecthyma, staphylococcal scalded skin syndrome, sycosis barbae, and infected eczema and scabies. Flucloxacillin 250 mg every 6 hours (double this for severe infections) is the drug of choice. For patients who are allergic to penicillin, erythromycin 500 mg every 6 hours is an alternative. With this dose, gastrointestinal upsets occur in about 20% of patients. The cephalosporins are not as good as flucloxacillin against *Staphylococcus aureus* so should not be used as the first line of treatment.

2   **Streptococcal infections** in the skin, eg erysipelas and cellulitis. Streptococci are always sensitive to penicillin so intravenous benzyl penicillin, 1200 mg every 6 hours, is the drug of choice. Erythromycin 500 mg every 6 hours orally is not as effective but is useful in patients who are allergic to penicillin. Streptococcal ecthyma, or eczema and scabies which are secondarily infected with *Streptococcus pyogenes* can be treated with phenoxymethylpenicillin 250 mg every 6 hours.

3   **Acne, perioral dermatitis and rosacea.** These are not due to infection with bacteria but nevertheless respond well to low doses of oxytetracycline, 250 mg twice a day. How they work is not fully understood (*see* pages 19, 134 and 188).

Antifungal agents

Normally fungal infections of the skin are treated with topical antifungal agents. The exceptions are if the hair and nails are involved, when it is not possible to get the antifungal agent to the site at which it is required. Four groups of antifungal agents are available for systemic use.

1   **Antibiotics (griseofulvin).** This is the cheapest of the options and works well for tinea capitis (*see* page 213), but is not very

effective for nail infections (*see* page 215). It is long acting so only has to be given once a day, but it has to be taken with food because it is absorbed with fat.

2 **Allylamines (terbinafine).** This is a fungicidal drug which is much more effective than griseofulvin and also much more expensive. It works well for any kind of dermatophyte infection but is particularly useful when the nails are involved. It is taken once a day for 3 months for nail infections (*see* page 215) or for 2 weeks for infections on the skin (*see* page 214).

3 **Imidazoles (ketoconazole).** This is very effective for treating pityriasis versicolor where it is given for just 1 week. It should not be used for longer periods of time because there is a small risk of liver toxicity (*see* page 145). It can also interact with terfenadine (Triludan) causing the latter to become more toxic (*see* page 246).

4 **Triazoles (fluconazole and itraconazole).** These are much more expensive than topical treatment for *Candida* so should only be used if topical agents have not worked (*see* page 32). They are used for infections with *Candida albicans* in patients who are immunosuppressed and who have not responded to topical treatment (those with malignant disease, AIDS or those on cytotoxic drugs).

Nystatin is not absorbed when given by mouth so the only reason for using it is if you want to clear the gut of *Candida albicans* (*see* page 34).

Antiviral agents

Acyclovir is the only systemic antiviral agent in current use. It is used for the following.

1 Herpes simplex—it is not used systemically for ordinary herpes simplex infections unless they are very severe, recur frequently or cause recurrent erythema multiforme (*see* pages 79 and 81).

2 Herpes zoster—800 mg orally five times a day for 7 days (*see* page 83).

3 Eczema herpeticum—5 mg/kg body weight intravenously every 8 hours for 5 days (*see* page 80).

Antihistamines

Non-sedative antihistamines are the most useful drugs in urticaria and angio-oedema. Terfenadine, astemizole and cetirizine are the ones most commonly used (*see* page 245).

Sedative antihistamines are useful in children with atopic eczema to ensure that they and their parents get a good night's sleep; it is essential to give a big enough dose (*see* page 51). They are also useful for adults with very widespread rashes who need to rest the skin, eg patients with erythrodermic eczema or psoriasis, and patients with acute blistering conditions on the feet who would otherwise find it difficult to rest in bed. Trimeprazine and promethazine are the most useful.

Steroids

Systemic steroids have a very limited use in the treatment of skin disease and are best restricted to use by a dermatologist. They should not be used in eczema or urticaria because, although the response may initially be dramatic, the disease is likely to flare badly when the tablets are stopped and it is then very difficult to get the patient off them. It is better to refer such a patient for an urgent dermatological opinion rather than start them on prednisone.

Systemic steroids are essential and may be life saving in:
- pemphigus (*see* page 133)
- pemphigoid (*see* page 131)

- systemic lupus erythematosus (*see* page 205)
- dermatomyositis (*see* page 41).

High doses are needed in all of these conditions and the risk of side effects is considerable. Interestingly such patients often do not show the typical steroid facies until the disease comes under control. For example, a patient can be on 60 mg prednisolone for several weeks without any evidence of a moon face, but as soon as the disease comes under control the face fattens up.

Equivalent doses of different systemic steroids	
Cortisone	100 mg
Hydrocortisone	80 mg
Prednisone or prednisolone	20 mg
Dexamethasone	2–4 mg

Side effects of systemic steroids
- Increased fat deposition on the face, shoulders and abdomen causing the moon face, buffalo hump and enlarged abdomen.
- Acne and hirsutism.
- Easy bruising and tearing of the skin.
- Striae.
- Delayed tissue healing.
- Increased susceptibility to infections (bacterial, fungal and viral).
- Salt and water retention leading to oedema, hypertension and congestive cardiac failure.
- Diabetes.
- Peptic ulceration leading to bleeding and perforation.
- Proximal muscle weakness.

- Osteoporosis leading to fractures particularly of the vertebrae and ribs.
- Aseptic necrosis of the femoral head.
- Cataracts and glaucoma.
- Depression or euphoria (steroid psychosis).
- Growth retardation in young children; this is not usually a problem unless steroids are given for more than 6 months.
- Suppression of the pituitary-adrenal axis leading to adrenal insufficiency on withdrawal or if the patient has some intercurrent illness or needs surgery.

Patients will need regular checking of:
- weight—to pick up fluid gain (weekly)
- blood pressure—looking for hypertension (monthly)
- urinalysis—looking for glycosuria (monthly)
- X-ray of spine—looking for osteoporosis (6 monthly)
- chest X-ray—looking for re-activation of TB (yearly).

If patients are on systemic steroids they must carry a steroid card or Medic alert tag with them at all times so that if they are involved in an accident or have some other illness extra steroids can be given to prevent an Addisonian crisis. Treatment with steroids must not therefore be undertaken lightly.

Immunosuppressive agents

A number of different immunosuppressive agents are used for severe skin disease, either in their own right or as steroid-sparing agents. They are all potentially dangerous and should only be initiated by a dermatologist. The most important ones are as follows.

1 Methotrexate is used for psoriasis (*see* page 161), Hailey-Hailey disease (chronic benign familial pemphigus, *see* page 78) and

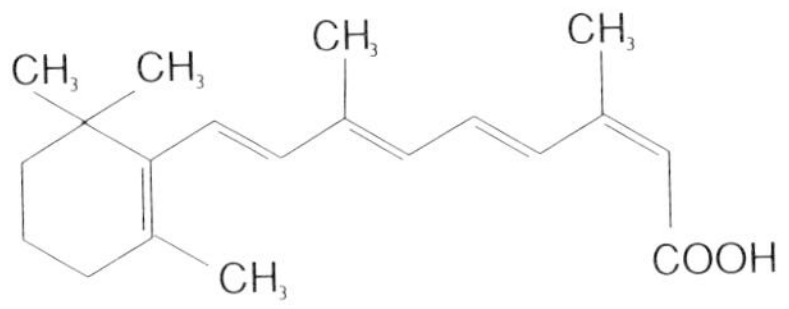

Figure 6 Isotretinoin.

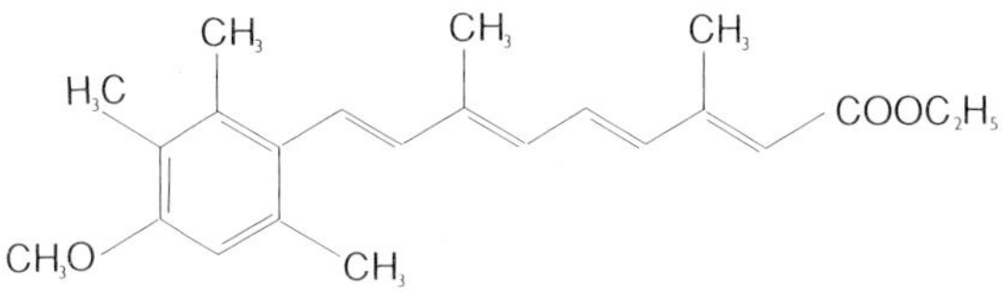

Figure 7 Etretinate.

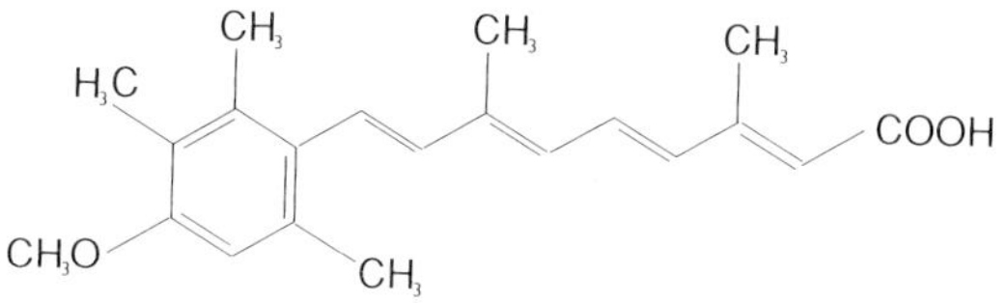

Figure 8 Acetretin.

dermatomyositis (*see* page 41). It works quickly, within about 48 hours, and is therefore very useful in a life-threatening situation such as generalized pustular psoriasis. Patients on this drug will need to have a full blood count measured regularly (once a week for the first 4 weeks and then every 2 months), and a liver biopsy once a year. They must not drink alcohol whilst taking the drug because liver damage is more likely to occur if they do.

2 Azathioprine is used for psoriasis (*see* page 163), atopic and photosensitive eczema (*see* pages 60 and 140), and as a steroid-sparing drug in pemphigus (*see* page 133), pemphigoid (*see* page 131), dermatomyositis (*see* page 41) and SLE (*see* page 205). It takes 6–8 weeks before there is any effect so it is inappropriate as a first line treatment in patients with pemphigus and pemphigoid. If there is any contraindication to treatment with systemic steroids the patient is often started on azathioprine as well as the steroids; after 6–8 weeks, when the azathioprine will have begun to work, the steroid dosage is gradually reduced. Most patients have no side effects with azathioprine but a few get severe gastrointestinal upsets (particularly the elderly), and there is an increased risk of lymphoma in the long term. A full blood count should be measured regularly (once a week for the first month and then every 2 months).

3 Hydroxyurea is used for psoriasis in patients who have not responded to methotrexate and azathioprine (*see* page 164) but it

takes 8–12 weeks to work. Patients on it will need a full blood count measured regularly (once a week for the first month and then every 2 months).

4 Cyclophosphamide is used in mucous membrane pemphigoid where it is the first drug of choice (*see* page 120). It takes 6–8 weeks to work and may cause a profound neutropenia or pancytopenia. The patient should have a full blood count measured regularly (once a week for the first month and then every 2 months).

5 Cyclosporin A is a drug which is mainly used to prevent rejection of organ transplants. It can be used in psoriasis (*see* page 170) and bad atopic eczema (*see* page 60). Its disadvantages are its cost (which is exorbitant) and its nephrotoxic effect. Patients taking this drug need to have their blood pressure checked every month (if it is raised above 160/95, nifedipine should be given to reduce it) and their blood urea and creatinine checked every 2 months (if the creatinine rises by 30% over the baseline level, the dose of cyclosporin A must be reduced).

Retinoids

Retinoids are derivatives of vitamin A (Figures 6–8). Their exact mode of action is unknown but they have many effects including:

- induction of differentiation in epidermal cells, which may be their effect in psoriasis, solar keratosis and Bowen's disease

They also suppress the development of epithelial tumours, such as basal and squamous cell carcinomas, but are not effective against fully established tumours

- shrinking of sebaceous glands causing decreased production of sebum
- anti-inflammatory effects probably by reducing prostaglandins and leukotrienes
- modulation of the immune response by enhancing T-helper cells and stimulating interleukin 1.

Retinoids are used for treating psoriasis (*see* page 168), acne (*see* page 21), ichthyosis (*see* page 94), Darier's disease (*see* page 40), pityriasis rubra pilaris (PRP, *see* page 144) and to prevent the development of epithelial tumours in patients who are immunosuppressed, especially those who have had renal transplants.

The retinoids in current use are as follows.

1 Isotretinoin, the 13-*cis* isomer of retinoic acid (Roaccutane), is used for the treatment of severe acne (*see* page 21).

2 Etretinate (Tigason) is an aromatic retinoid which is useful in diseases where there is abnormal keratinization (psoriasis, PRP and Darier's disease). In psoriasis it is a useful treatment when there are numerous small plaques which would make topical treatment difficult or tedious, or if the patient has erythrodermic psoriasis or pustular psoriasis of the palms and soles (*see* page 168). It can also be used in conjunction with PUVA (RePUVA) to decrease the amount of ultraviolet light that the patient is exposed to (*see* page 170). Its main disadvantage is that it is teratogenic and has a very long half life; women taking it must not become pregnant whilst taking it or for 2 years after stopping using it.

3 Acitretin (Neotigason) is a synthetic aromatic derivative of retinoic acid which has exactly the same uses as etretinate. It has a much shorter half life than etretinate and should therefore be safer for use in women. Unfortunately it may be converted to etretinate (which has been detected in the plasma of some patients taking acetretin), so at present it is still recommended that female patients do not get pregnant whilst taking it or for 2 years after stopping using it.

4 Arotinoids are very potent retinoids which are currently under investigation. They are not yet available clinically because their therapeutic potency is matched by equivalent side effects, but they may be of use in the future.

Side effects of retinoids
- Dryness of the lips, nose, eyes and face (*see* Figure 13, page 21).
- Scaling of the skin, especially the palms and soles leading to softness and/or soreness; the hands in particular often feel clammy (*see* Figure 132b, page 169).
- Soft nails and ingrowing toenails (*see* Figure 132d, page 169).
- Hair loss (*see* Figure 132c, page 169).
- Headaches and aches and pains in the joints and muscles.
- Rise in serum triglycerides and liver enzymes.
- Teratogenic (no effect on sperm).

All of these side effects are reversible when the treatment is stopped.

Part 2 Treatment of individual diseases

ACANTHOSIS NIGRICANS

There is no specific treatment. For the benign variety, pseudo-acanthosis nigricans, weight loss is often useful. In the malignant variety, indicated by extensive skin lesions and marked itching, removal of the underlying tumour is the only thing that is likely to help.

ACNE

Patients with acne should always be taken seriously. Modern treatment is very effective, so telling someone that they will grow out of it with time is not an acceptable approach. There is no need to restrict the diet in any way since acne is not due to eating too many chocolates, crisps, etc.

There are three factors which are important in the aetiology of acne and whichever treatment you choose will interfere with one or other of these (*see* Table below).

Treatment of an individual patient does not depend on how many spots he has, but on what kinds of spots are present.

Comedones only

Keratolytic agents should be used. These remove the surface keratin and unplug the follicular openings. Examples include:
- benzoyl peroxide (2.5%, 5%, 10%) as cream, lotion or gel
- retinoic acid 0.01% and 0.025% gel, 0.025% and 0.05% cream, and 0.025% lotion
- isotretinoin 0.05% gel
- azaleic acid cream
- sulphur and allantoin lotion
- sulphur and resorcinol cream.

Ultraviolet light has a similar effect to topical keratolytics, but cannot be purchased in a tube! The development of a suntan also masks the acne spots.

Instructions for use of keratolytic agents

The patient should wash the skin as normal with soap and water (medicated washes are not more effective). Start with 5% benzoyl peroxide applied at night (unless the patient has a very fair skin,

	Aetiology of acne	Treatments which interfere with this process
	Hyperkeratosis at the mouth of the hair follicle	Keratolytic agents Ultraviolet light Isotretinoin
	Sebum production	Anti-androgens Isotretinoin
	Propionibacterium acnes	Topical and systemic antibiotics Benzoyl peroxide Azaleic acid

in which case you start with 2.5%). All peeling agents tend to dry the skin and make it sore. If the skin becomes too sore, stop the treatment for a few days until it is comfortable again. Then restart benzoyl peroxide at the 2.5% strength, or continue the 5% strength but only use it every other night. If benzoyl peroxide does not work, try retinoic acid or isotretinoin instead; these too should be applied only once a day (at night before the patient goes to bed). Female patients can wear make up to cover their spots during the day but they must wash it off carefully at night so that the follicles do not get blocked (causing more comedones).

Do not apply topical steroids or mixtures containing topical steroids to acne because, although they reduce inflammation, they increase hyperkeratosis at the mouth of the hair follicle and thus produce more comedones.

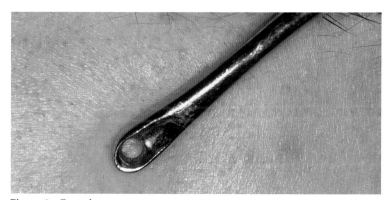

Figure 9 Comedone extractor.

If there are only a very few comedones present, a comedone extractor can be used (Figure 9). These are like small curettes with a hole in the middle. When they are pressed firmly over a blackhead, the contents are expressed through the hole. Squeezing

with the fingers should be avoided, since this can convert a comedone into an inflammatory papule.

There are a few patients with large numbers of closed comedones (whiteheads) which do not respond to treatment. Cauterizing each one under local anaesthetic (EMLA cream under polythene occlusion for 90 minutes beforehand), may be the only way to get rid of them. To avoid scarring, this is best done by a dermatologist who has some experience with this technique (Figures 10–12).

Inflammatory lesions—papules, pustules or nodules

These patients need systemic therapy. The options are as follows.
1 Long-term, low-dose antibiotics.
2 Anti-androgens (females only).
3 Isotretinoin (13-*cis*-retinoic acid).

1 Antibiotics. Oxytetracycline 250 mg twice daily is cheap and effective. It must be given on an empty stomach (half an hour before a meal or 2 hours after) as it chelates with calcium in milk and food, and with iron and antacids. Improvement of the acne is slow and usually not apparent for at least 2–3 months. If the tablets are continued, gradual improvement occurs for 6–12 months. Maintenance treatment must be continued until the acne gets better spontaneously, however long that is.

Tetracyclines are contraindicated if:
- the patient is under 12 years of age because it will cause staining of the teeth
- the patient is pregnant or trying to get pregnant, because it will cause staining of the teeth of the fetus
- the patient is lactating
- there is impaired renal function.

Side effects of oxytetracycline are few. Diarrhoea and vaginal candidiasis can cause problems; at this dosage it does not interfere with the absorption of the contraceptive pill. Very rarely it can produce benign intracranial hypertension.

If oxytetracycline does not work, check that the patient has been taking it regularly and on an empty stomach. If compliance has been good, the dose could be increased to 500 mg twice daily or the antibiotic changed to one of the following:

(i) erythromycin 250 mg twice daily (this can be taken with food).

(ii) minocycline 50 mg twice daily (highly fat soluble, so it can be taken with food and drink). It has been shown to be effective in patients who have failed to respond to, or could not tolerate, oxytetracycline. It should not be used as the first line of treatment however because it is *much* more expensive and may cause blue or bluish−grey discolouration of the skin and teeth (*see* Figure 31, page 47). It is also available as 100 mg sustained release capsules (Minocin MR) which only have to be taken once a day.

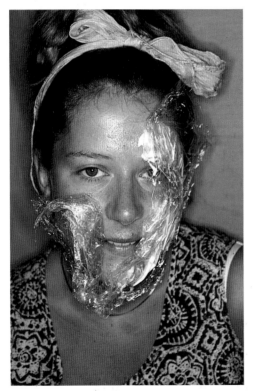

Figure 10 Applying EMLA cream under polythene occlusion.

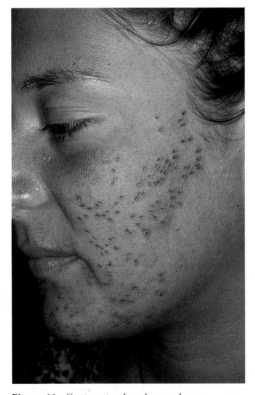

Figure 11 Cautery to closed comedones.

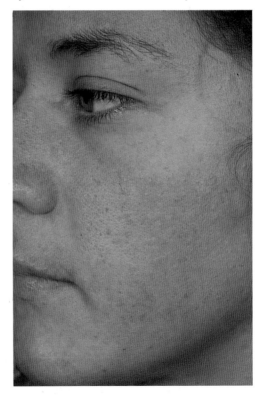

Figure 12 Result 6 months later.

(iii) Doxycycline 50 mg once daily is an alternative to minocycline.

Topical antibiotics work nearly as well as systemic antibiotics but have the theoretical disadvantages of causing resistant bacteria on the skin surface and contact allergic eczema. In practice, topical clindamycin (Dalacin T), erythromycin (Stiemycin and Zineryt [contains zinc as well as erythromycin which may help reduce bacterial resistance and make it more effective]) and tetracycline (Topicycline) are available commercially and can be applied once a day (usually at night). They are much more expensive than oral antibiotics, but are useful in pregnancy since there is negligible systemic absorption.

2 Anti-androgens. These are useful in female patients if antibiotics have not worked, or if they are already on a contraceptive pill and wish to continue on it. They should be avoided in women who smoke, who are over 35 years of age, or who are hypertensive, because of the increased risk of cardiovascular and thromboembolic disease. Cyproterone acetate may be given in high dosage (100 mg on days 5–14 of menstrual cycle with ethinyl oestradiol 50 μg on days 5–25 of cycle) or low dosage (2 mg) as an oral contraceptive pill, Dianette (this contains only 35 μg of oestrogen). Like antibiotics the maximum effect does not occur for 2–3 months, and treatment needs to be continued long term until the patient has grown out of her acne (however long that is, not just for 6 months which the packet recommends). It costs more than oxytetracycline or a normal oral contraceptive, so is not usually the first line of treatment.

3 Isotretinoin (13-*cis*-retinoic acid). This is only available in hospitals, but is the most effective treatment available. It should be used in patients with bad acne who have responded poorly to 6 months of systemic antibiotics. It is given as a single daily dose

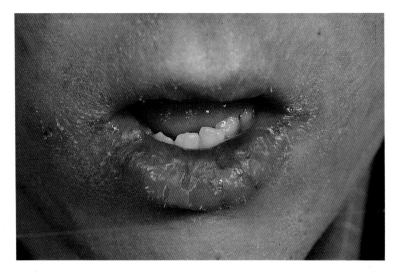

Figure 13 Dry lips and dryness of the skin around the lips due to isotretinoin.

(0.5–1.0 mg/kg body weight) with food for 4 months. Long-term remission is produced (several months to permanent).

It has numerous possible side effects which, if the patient is warned about them, are usually well tolerated. All are completely reversible when treatment is stopped. Side effects include:

- dryness and splitting of the lips (Figure 13). All patients get this and will need to use Vaseline or a lip salve regularly
- dry eyes. Wearing contact lenses is not necessarily a contra-indication to treatment. Hypromellose eye drops are occasionally needed
- nose bleeds secondary to dryness of the nasal mucous membranes
- muscle aches and pains especially after exercise
- irregularities of, or cessation of, periods in women

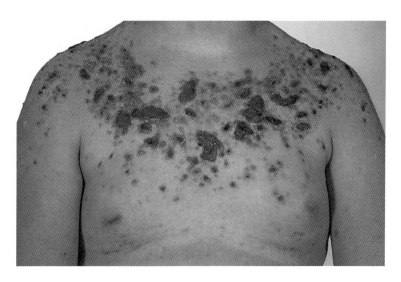

Figure 14 Apparent worsening of acne after 2 months' treatment with isotretinoin. Very extensive pyogenic granuloma-like lesions.

- rise in serum lipids
- rise in liver enzymes
- apparent worsening of the acne for the first few weeks with multiple pyogenic granuloma-like nodules (Figure 14).

It is teratogenic, so women should not become pregnant while on it or for 1 month afterwards.

Isotretinoin is also useful in women who go on getting acne into their 30s and 40s even if it is not very severe, since otherwise they are often totally demoralized.

On the rare occasions isotretinoin is not effective, it can be combined with minocycline 50 mg twice a day for 4 months. This combination seems to work when everything else has failed.

Comedones and inflammatory lesions

Patients should use both topical and systemic therapy.

The following drugs may make acne worse and should be avoided:

   systemic steroids or ACTH
   androgens and anabolic steroids in women
   iodides and bromides
   isoniazid
   lithium
   barbiturates and phenytoin

SPECIAL KINDS OF ACNE

Acné excorié

Patients should be told why they have the spots and be discouraged from picking them. Systemic tetracyclines or very low-dose 13-*cis*-retinoic acid (10–20 mg/day) may be helpful.

Infantile acne

Systemic antibiotics for many months are usually needed. Tetracycline in any form cannot be used because of staining of the teeth. Septrin paediatric suspension 240 mg twice daily is the easiest to use as it does not need replacing each week. Erythromycin 125 mg twice daily is an alternative. If there are only comedones present, a mild keratolytic agent can be used instead.

ALOPECIA AREATA

- Reassure the patient that the hair will regrow spontaneously, usually in about 3–6 months.
- Warn the patient that the hair may regrow white or blond until it is about 1.5 cm long, but that it will go back to its normal colour after that.
- A wig may be needed temporarily if the hair loss is extensive.
- In a small minority of patients the hair will not regrow.

It is worth checking the urine for sugar and doing the autoimmune profile because some patients may have diabetes, pernicious anaemia or thyroid disease.

Treatment available by dermatologists is unsatisfactory but includes:

1 Intralesional injection of triamcinolone (10 mg/ml). This will cause temporary regrowth of hair, but may cause atrophy of the skin.

2 Application of potent skin sensitizers to the bald areas, eg dinitrochlorobenzene, diphencyprone or primula obconica leaves. These cause an acute contact allergic eczema and sometimes regrowth of hair. Usually the eczema is too unpleasant for the patient to tolerate, and if the hair does regrow, it may fall out again when treatment is stopped.

Diphencyprone is the drug most commonly used but only about 20% of patients do well with it, usually those whose hair loss has been present for less than 2 years. If it works, it has to go on being painted on the bald areas once a week until regrowth of hair is well established. Diphencyprone is degraded by light so patients have to keep their heads covered for 24 hours after treatment.

3 PUVA twice or three times a week. The patient enters the UVA cabinet fully clothed, with a titanium dioxide sunscreen on any exposed parts (face, hands, etc) so that only the scalp (± eyebrows/beard) is treated (for details of the treatment schedules *see* page 165).

This often produces good regrowth of hair initially, but once the hair gets to be about 1.5 cm long, the UVA can no longer get to the scalp skin to produce its effect, and the hair will then fall out again.

There is a patient self-help group for alopecia areata and other types of hair loss:

HAIRLINE INTERNATIONAL
39 St John's Close
Knowle
Solihull
West Midlands B93 0NN
Tel: 0564 775 281 (Weekdays 9–3)

ALOPECIA—MALE PATTERN

For most men, no treatment is needed or sought since this is a normal physiological process. For a few who cannot come to terms with their baldness, the following are available:

1 2% minoxidil solution applied to the bald scalp twice daily. This does not produce regrowth of normal terminal hair, but long vellus hair in about a third of those who use it. If treatment is left off, the longer hair will fall out, so once started it will need to be continued indefinitely.

2 Hair transplants. Small punch biopsies are taken from the occipital area or sides of the scalp and are transplanted into the bald area (Figure 15).

3 Hair weaving. In this process, terminal hair is twisted onto the short vellus hairs which are present in male pattern alopecia. Since the hair cycle of vellus hairs is short (5 months), it will need to be repeated frequently.

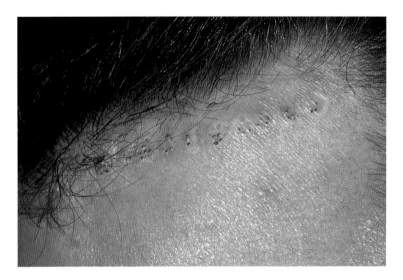

Figure 15 Hair transplants 10 days after the procedure—the grafts have taken well.

4 A wig. Generally speaking, wigs for men are not very cosmetically acceptable.

None of these options is currently available under the NHS.

ALOPECIA—FEMALE PATTERN

For minor degrees of this, no treatment is needed, but if it is noticeable, the following options can be considered:

1 Anti-androgens. Small doses of cyproterone acetate as in Dianette do not work. To be effective, 50–100 mg daily is required. For women of child-bearing age, it should be combined with an oestrogen as in acne, to prevent conception since it can cause feminization of a male fetus. The usual regime is cyproterone acetate 100 mg on days 5–14 of the menstrual cycle, together with ethinyl oestradiol 50 µg on days 5–25 of the cycle. For post menopausal women, it can be given alone on a daily basis, either 50 mg or 100 mg once a day. Side effects include weight gain, nausea, depression and headaches.

2 Spironolactone 100 mg twice daily. It is worth trying this for 6 months, particularly in older women. It may cause menstrual irregularities.

3 Topical minoxidil, as for male pattern baldness.

4 A wig.

ANGIO OEDEMA

Generally the treatment is the same as for urticaria. In an acute attack, provided there is no laryngeal oedema, a short-acting antihistamine such as chlorpheniramine (Piriton), 4 mg every 4 hours can be given until it settles. In recurrent episodes over a period of weeks or months, it is better to give a non-sedative antihistamine like terfenadine, 60–120 mg twice daily. In a life-threatening situation with swelling of the larynx or tongue, inject 0.5 ml of 1:1000 adrenaline solution intramuscularly.

ANGULAR CHEILITIS

This is usually due to a *Candida* infection under the patient's top denture. First scrape the underside of the denture and examine for spores and hyphae or send for culture. Tell the patient to clean his dentures after every meal with a hard toothbrush and soap. Treatment with nystatin is not usually necessary.

ANNULAR ERYTHEMA

If there is any scaling present, particularly if the rash is asymmetrical, the first thing to do is scrape it to make sure the diagnosis is not a fungal infection. If you are sure it is not, reassure the patient that it is nothing serious and that no treatment is necessary.

Check that it is not a single lesion which is growing, which would suggest a diagnosis of Lyme disease (*see* page 71).

APHTHOUS ULCERS

This is a self-limiting condition which often needs no treatment. Most patients will use things like Bonjela (choline salicylate and cetalkonium chloride) for symptomatic relief. For more trouble-some ulcers consider one of the following:

1 **2% sodium cromoglycate spray** (Rynacrom) sprayed directly onto the ulcers three times a day. About 50% of patients find this extremely helpful. It is not known how it works.

2 **Tetracycline mouthwash,** 250 mg/5 ml, held in the mouth and swished around for about five minutes 4–5 times a day.

3 **0.1% triamcinolone acetonide** (Adcortyl) **in orobase** applied to the ulcers three times a day.

4 **10% hydrocortisone in equal parts of glycerine and water** as a mouthwash three times a day. The patient must spit it out after use rather than swallow it, to make sure that not too much steroid is absorbed.

5 **2.5% hydrocortisone sodium succinate** (Corlan) **pellet**, held against the ulcer(s) until the pellet dissolves, twice daily.

If the patient is getting very frequent ulcers, check that he does not have Crohn's disease, ulcerative colitis or coeliac disease.

APLASIA CUTIS

If the defect is large, surgery may be required, otherwise the scalp hair will usually cover it.

ARBORIZING TELANGIECTASIA/THREAD VEINS

There is no easy solution to this problem. If there are lots of veins cosmetic camouflage will probably be needed. Small areas can be injected with a weak sclerosant such as 0.5% polidocanol (Sclerovein). Place a fine gauge (29 G) needle into the major feeding venule and inject a small amount of the solution; immediately the whole network blanches. In skilled hands this technique is effective and safe.

BALANITIS

The first thing is to examine the rest of the patient's skin to see if there is a rash elsewhere since inflammation of the glans may occur in many dermatological conditions, eg eczema, psoriasis, lichen planus and scabies. If the rest of the skin is normal:

1 Check the hygiene of the area.
2 Take a swab for bacteriology culture and *Candida*.
3 Check the urine for sugar.

If *Candida* is not present and the patient is not diabetic, soaking the penis in normal saline (1 tablespoon of salt in 1 pint of water) for 10 minutes twice a day for a week will clear the problem in 80–90% of patients. If it recurs this can be repeated.

If the patient is diabetic or *Candida* is present, after soaking in saline, the patient should apply topical nystatin cream or ointment or one of the imidazole creams (eg miconazole cream) two or three times a day until it clears.

If neither of these measures work, a urethral swab should be taken looking for anaerobes. If they are not found, the patient's sexual partner should also be examined. If anaerobes are found in the patient or his sexual partner, treatment is with oral metronidazole 400 mg three times a day for 10 days.

If none of the above methods help, 1% hydrocortisone cream can be tried. In some patients the cause is never found.

Circinate balanitis

This is part of Reiter's disease and should not be dealt with in isolation. For the balanitis, saline soaks (as above) are often helpful. For the urethritis, oxytetracycline 500 mg twice a day is given for 1–3 weeks depending on the response.

Erythroplasia of Queryat

5% 5-fluorouracil cream should be applied to the affected area twice daily for 8–12 weeks. If the meatus is involved amputation may be necessary.

Lichen sclerosis et atrophicus

If the man has not been circumcised, circumcision is probably the treatment of choice. If the problem is itching or soreness, a topical steroid in the form of 1% hydrocortisone cream applied twice daily is all that is needed. If that does not work, or if there is a problem with urethral stenosis, a much more potent topical steroid will be required. 0.5% clobetasol propionate (Dermovate) applied twice a day to the affected area and to the urethra if necessary will produce a very rapid and dramatic improvement. This should not be continued for more than 2–3 weeks. Once the disease is under control, a weaker topical steroid will usually work just as well.

Zoon's balanitis

A moderately potent topical steroid such as 0.025% betamethasone valerate (Betnovate RD) ointment applied twice a day is usually needed. A more potent steroid, like 0.1% betamethasone valerate (Betnovate) ointment, can be used for short periods of time if necessary.

BARTHOLIN CYST

No treatment is needed unless recurrent infections occur. Once the infection has been cleared with a systemic antibiotic marsupialization of the cyst lining to the skin is the treatment of choice. These cysts should not be excised because otherwise their secretions, which are important for lubricating the vagina during sexual intercourse, are lost.

BASAL CELL CARCINOMA (BCC)

Local excision or radiotherapy are the treatments of choice, each giving a 95% cure rate. Which is used depends on which will give the best cosmetic result at the particular site involved and which treatment is actually feasible to do in the patient (eg does the patient live near a centre where radiotherapy is carried out? Does he have transport? Is he working? etc).

Local excision

These tumours are not aggressively invasive, so removal of an ellipse of skin including the tumour with 1–2 mm of normal skin around the edge is sufficient. If it is not possible to remove the tumour and get the skin back together again, a full thickness skin graft or a skin flap may be needed. These are normally best done by a dermatologist or a plastic surgeon.

Radiotherapy

Before treatment is begun a biopsy should be done to confirm the diagnosis. To get a good cosmetic result and to lessen the local reaction, radiotherapy treatment is fractionated. Five daily fractions of 6.5 Gy are given for tumours less than 1 cm in diameter; 10 daily fractions of 3.75 Gy for tumours 2 cm across. If the patient is very frail, the time between fractions can be increased, so that 10 fractions are given over 10 weeks. This will cause virtually no local reaction and will be much more pleasant for the patient.

How to manage the local reaction after treatment

Nearly all patients will get some local reaction on the skin after radiotherapy treatment, but they should not get any systemic upset. Depending on the technique used, erythema, scaling, weeping, and the formation of a scab, will begin towards the end of treatment or shortly afterwards. It lasts for a variable time, but generally for up to 3–4 weeks.

Most patients do not need any treatment for the reaction. The area should be left open because covering it increases the risk of secondary infection. If it becomes wet, it can be bathed twice a day with bicarbonate of soda (a pinch of bicarbonate of soda in a tumbler of water), or with potassium permanganate (made up to a pale pink solution, *see* Figure 47, page 62).

Some people use 1% hydrocortisone ointment topically twice a day, but most reactions settle without this.

Radiotherapy is suitable for large tumours in the elderly which would otherwise need a skin graft.

Radiotherapy is not a suitable treatment in young people because the local damage is progressive, and they may run into problems of skin atrophy later. If a tumour is going to recur, most will do so in the first 2 years. Skin changes later than that will almost certainly be due to radiation damage.

Electrons rather than standard X-rays are very useful on the nose and ears, where they are less likely to damage cartilage. Here treatment will probably be given daily for 2–3 weeks.

Other possible treatments include:

1 Curettage and cautery. In some circumstances, this is the treatment of choice even though the recurrence rate is higher than with surgery or radiotherapy. It is a very simple procedure and much quicker than surgical excision, but should be done by someone who is skilled at it (usually a dermatologist). It is most useful in the following situations:

- patients who are very elderly
- patients with numerous small lesions

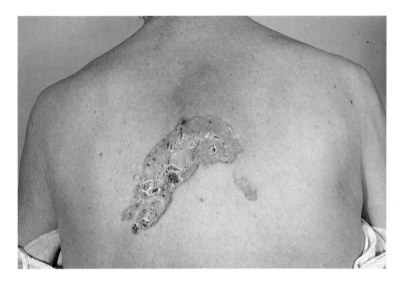

Figure 16 Large superficial BCC on the back of an 84-year-old woman. This would be suitable for treatment by curettage and cautery.

- patients who have taken arsenic in the past and who have multiple tumours. If these patients are seen regularly every 3–6 months, any new BCCs can be curetted off while they are still small
- single large tumours on the trunk or limbs.

Curettage should be avoided in younger patients, where the possibility of recurrence may make subsequent surgery difficult. This is particularly true where the tumour is in the naso-labial fold, the inner canthus of the eye or on the lower eyelid.

2 Cryotherapy using liquid nitrogen should only be used in patients who cannot get to the hospital or surgery for more orthodox treatment. The recurrence rate is about 30% after one year, so it should be reserved for the house bound elderly patient. The tumour is frozen for 30 seconds, allowed to thaw (which should take at least 90 seconds) and then frozen for a further 30 seconds. The idea of this mode of therapy is to produce necrosis of all tumour cells. This procedure is fairly unpleasant and some patients will prefer to have an injection of local anaesthetic beforehand. They should be warned that a blister will form, that it may weep and that an ulcer will form. The wound will normally take about a month to heal and can be dealt with the same as a radiotherapy reaction (*see* page 27).

All patients who have had a basal cell carcinoma should be advised about sun protection for the future. They should use a high protective factor sun screen (Factor 15 or above) when they are out of doors in the summer and whenever they go abroad (*see* Table 13, page 141) and wear a hat and long-sleeved shirt or blouse.

BASAL CELL PAPILLOMA (SEBORRHOEIC WART)

Most of these need no treatment. If they are very unsightly or catch in the patient's clothes, they can be removed either by freezing with liquid nitrogen (as for warts, *see* page 253) or by curettage and cautery under local anaesthetic. If they are curetted off, they should scrape off easily; if they do not, the diagnosis is wrong.

BECKER'S NAEVUS

Nothing can be done for these. The patient should be reassured that they are not premalignant.

BEHÇET'S DISEASE

This condition is not common. Its cause is not known and treatment is empirical and unsatisfactory. Patients should therefore be under the care of a dermatologist, a general physician or a rheumatologist with some experience in managing it.

The most commonly used drugs are:
- **Colchicine**, 500 µg twice daily, or
- **Azathioprine**, 2 mg/kg body weight/day (average dose = 50 mg three times a day).

For the mouth ulcers it is worth the patient trying:

1 **10% hydrocortisone** in equal parts of glycerine and water used as a mouthwash after each meal, but the patient should be warned that it has a very bitter taste. It should be spat out after use so that not too much steroid is absorbed.

2 **Steroid inhaler.** Beclomethasone dipropionate, 50 µg/puff, (Becotide 50) is usually used for asthma, but instead of inhaling it, the patient sprays it on the ulcers several times a day until the ulcers heal.

For patients who want to get in touch with other sufferers, there is a self-help group:

BEHÇET'S SYNDROME SOCIETY
3 Church Close
Lambourn
Newbury
Berkshire RG16 7PU
Telephone help lines: 0488 71116
0533 740 278
0904 626 602

BLACK HAIRY TONGUE

Brush the affected part of the tongue with Close Up or the red striped variety of Signal toothpaste on a soft toothbrush once a day, or

Apply 0.025% tretinoin gel (Retin-A) and brush it off with a soft toothbrush 5 minutes later. This is repeated daily until it clears (about 2 weeks).

BLACK HEEL

Explain to the patient that this is due to bleeding into the skin from rubbing by his shoes. He should wear proper fitting shoes, trainers or football boots.

BLUE NAEVUS

These are perfectly harmless and can be left alone. If they are particularly unsightly they can be excised under a local anaesthetic.

BOIL (and CARBUNCLE)

First check the patient's urine for sugar, since boils may be the presenting symptom of diabetes. If the boil is already pointing, it can be lanced to let the pus out. If there is no obvious pus, treat with oral flucloxacillin 250 mg four times daily for 7 days. Before starting antibiotics, take bacteriology swabs from the boil, the anterior nares, the perianal skin and any rash that the patient has because the causative organism, *Staphylococcus aureus*, usually comes from the patient himself. The carriage site should be treated with topical neomycin, mupirocin or fucidic acid ointment four times a day for 2 weeks to prevent recurrent infections.

If recurrent boils occur and the carriage site has been treated, check the rest of the family (by taking bacteriology swabs) to see if someone else is carrying the staphylococcus on their skin, up their nose or around the anus. If they are all negative, it may (rarely) be necessary to continue the patient on long-term low-dose antibiotics in the form of flucloxacillin 250 mg twice a day for about 6 months.

For patients who are allergic to penicillin, erythromycin 250 mg four times daily for one week is an alternative to flucloxacillin.

BOWEN'S DISEASE

All of the following treatments work.
1 Curettage and cautery.
2 Freezing with liquid nitrogen. On the lower leg freeze for 10 seconds after the skin goes white, allow it to thaw and repeat once. Elsewhere freeze for 20 seconds twice. Always use two freeze-thaw cycles.
3 5% 5-fluorouracil cream, applied topically twice a day for four weeks. At the end of treatment, the area will be red and sore; 1% hydrocortisone cream is then used twice a day until the inflammatory reaction has settled (usually 7–10 days).
4 Local excision.
5 Radiotherapy.
   Which is used depends on which will give the best cosmetic result at the site involved. You will need to be particularly careful on the lower leg because most of these treatments can cause ulceration of the skin in the presence of venous disease or a poor arterial blood supply, and this may take many months to heal. Local excision and suture is best if the wound can be easily closed; if not, curettage and cautery is usually the most satisfactory treatment on the legs. It is wise to provide support bandaging such as tapered Tubigrip afterwards until the wound has healed. On the face, neck, trunk and arms, any of the options can be considered.

CALCINOSIS CUTIS

Calcium deposited in the dermis or subcutaneous fat can occur as an isolated problem or be part of some other disease. The first thing to do is to measure the serum calcium. If it is raised, look for the cause, (eg hyperparathyroidism, sarcoid, metastatic carcinoma, myeloma, Paget's disease of bone, the milk-alkali syndrome, etc) and treat that. If it is normal, note where the calcification is.
1 If it is only on the lower legs it will almost certainly be due to long-standing venous disease. It may then interfere with the healing of a venous ulcer and may need to be removed surgically. If it is too extensive to be excised, there is no other way of getting rid of it and the patient may have to live with persistent ulceration.
2 If it is mainly on the finger tips, particularly the palmar surface (and possibly the elbows, knees and buttocks), check whether the patient has scleroderma, dermatomyositis or SLE. Sometimes the calcinosis in these conditions gets better spontaneously. Chelating agents, on the whole, are not helpful. Aluminium oxide decreases the intestinal absorption of phosphate and may be useful. The usual dose is 600 mg four times a day. Small deposits can be excised and sometimes intralesional steroids are helpful.

3 Calcification elsewhere can be left alone, surgically removed or treated with aluminium oxide as above.

Mostly the treatments available are not very effective.

CALCINOSIS—IDIOPATHIC OF THE SCROTUM

Reassurance that it is nothing serious (contagious or cancer) is the main thing that is needed. Very large cysts which are uncomfortable or ulcerated can be excised under local or general anaesthetic.

CANDIDA

Candida albicans occurs in two forms. Throughout the gastrointestinal tract, and in the female genital tract it is present as a harmless commensal organism, characterized by budding yeasts on direct microscopy. The pathogenic form develops from it under certain conditions and shows both spores and hyphae under the microscope. There is always a reason for the presence of the pathogenic form of *Candida* and this should be looked for and treated. The commonest causes are:

- diabetes
- pregnancy
- contraceptive pill
- broad spectrum antibiotics
- immunosuppression
  - AIDS
  - systemic steroids

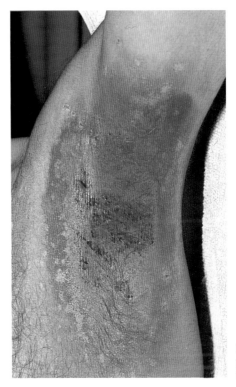

Figure 17 Gentian violet paint applied to the axilla to treat *Candida* infection.

  - cytotoxic drugs
  - cancer
- iron deficiency.

Direct microscopy or mycology culture is recommended before starting treatment because treatment failure may be due to incorrect diagnosis. Nystatin, the imidazoles, clioquinol and gentian violet all work well for *Candida* infections. Nystatin

Table 2   Summary of treatment of Candida infections

Site of infection	Treatment	Comments, side effects and precautions
Vulva	1. Nystatin cream or ointment applied twice daily. If vaginal infection too, use nystatin or clotrimazole pessaries as well (*see* below). 2. An imidazole cream. They all work equally well, so whichever is the cheapest should be used. The choice is between clotrimazole, econazole, ketaconazole, miconazole and sulconazole.	1. Nystatin is yellow and makes a mess of the underwear. Patients prefer an imidazole for this reason. 2. There are no problems with these, but they are more expensive than nystatin.

Vagina	1. Nystatin pessaries (100,000 units) — one inserted high into the vagina at night for 14 nights.
	2. An imidazole pessary placed high in the vagina at night:
	    Clotrimazole (500 mg) — single dose
	    Miconazole (1200 mg) — single dose
	    Econazole nitrate (150 mg) — 3 nights
	The patient's sexual partner should be treated at the same time with nystatin cream or an imidazole cream to prevent reinfection.
		1. They dissolve overnight and make a mess of the patient's underwear the next day.
		2. These make less mess but do also come out onto the underwear. They are more expensive, but more user-friendly!

Recurrent vaginal infection (frequent recurrences)	1. Clotrimazole (500 mg) pessary at night, on the last day of the period, every month for 6–9 months. 2. Clotrimazole (100 mg) pessary every 2 weeks for 6–9 months. 3. Oral itraconazole 200 mg twice daily for 1 day only. 4. Single oral dose of fluconazole 150 mg.	1 and 2. Much cheaper than the oral preparations which are the alternatives. 3. Must be taken after a meal for maximum absorption. Do not use in pregnancy or lactation because embryo toxic. Do not use concurrently with rifampicin. Side effects: nausea, abdominal pain, headache, dizziness and heartburn. 4. Avoid in pregnancy and lactation. May cause phenytoin toxicity.

(Table continues opposite)

Table 2 Summary of treatment of Candida infections (continued)

Site of infection	Treatment	Comments, side effects and precautions
Perianal skin	Nystatin ointment or cream twice a day, together with nystatin tablets 100,000 units 4 times a day until it clears up.	The tablets will not be absorbed but will clear the gut reservoir of *Candida*
Intertrigo (groins, axillae, toewebs, fingerwebs, sub-mammary area and abdominal body folds)	1. Nystatin cream or ointment twice daily. 2. An imidazole cream twice daily. 3. If the skin is very wet, 0.5% gentian violet solution twice daily is preferable.	1. Messy because it stains yellow. 2. More expensive than nystatin. 3. Very messy—stains the skin and clothes purple (*see* Figure 17).
Mouth (white plaques)	1. In infancy, miconazole gel applied directly to the plaques by an adult's finger 4 times daily. 2. In adults, nystatin oral suspension (1 ml) swirled around the mouth several times before swallowing 4 times a day. Continue for 48 hours after clinical cure. 3. Alternatives are nystatin pastilles or amphotericin B lozenges sucked until they dissolve 4 times a day. If the patient is on antibiotics, treatment will need to be continued until they are finished. If the patient has cancer or is immunosuppressed, treatment may need to be prolonged.	1. This is easier than trying to use a suspension of nystatin in a young child. 3. The pastilles and lozenges are more expensive than nystatin suspension, but may be easier for some patients to use.
Mouth (angular cheilitis)	Take the dentures out after every meal and clean them with a hard toothbrush and soap.	This is better for the dentures than soaking in Sterodent overnight as well as getting rid of the angular cheilitis.
Chronic paronychia	Keep the hands dry until a new cuticle has grown (3–4 months). Cotton-lined rubber gloves should be worn for all wet work. A greasy film applied around the nail fold several times a day in the form of Vaseline or nystatin ointment will keep further infection at bay. Do not allow the patient to poke ointments under the nail fold with an orange stick or nail file as this will only damage the cuticle further.	Patients have great difficulty keeping their hands dry, but this is essential at all times apart from washing themselves if the problem is to be resolved.

is the cheapest, but tends to be rather messy. Gentian violet is even more messy (Figure 17). Oral nystatin is not absorbed from the gastrointestinal tract, so is only of use in clearing the gut reservoir of *Candida*. Griseofulvin does not work for *Candida* infections at any site. For treatment of *Candida* infections at the most common sites see Table 2, pages 32 and 33.

CAPILLARITIS

No treatment is necessary as this condition gets better spontaneously. The haemosiderin pigment may take several months to disappear.

CELLULITIS

The cause of this infection is a group A, C or G beta haemolytic streptococcus which gets into the dermis through an obvious portal of entry, eg a leg ulcer, eczema, tinea, etc. *Both the infection and the underlying cause should be treated to prevent recurrent infections.*

Beta haemolytic streptococci are always sensitive to penicillin so intramuscular or intravenous benzyl penicillin, 600 mg every 6 hours, is the treatment of choice. If this is not possible, oral phenoxymethylpenicillin 250–500 mg every 6 hours is an alternative. Treatment must be continued for at least 2 weeks; otherwise relapse is likely. If necessary, oral treatment may be continued after initial parenteral therapy. For patients who are allergic to penicillin, oral erythromycin 250–500 mg 6 hourly can be used. Synthetic penicillins in the form of flucloxacillin or ampicillin are not suitable.

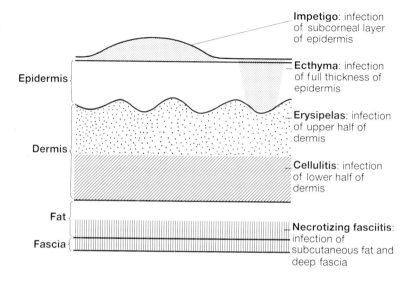

Figure 18 Sites of infections of group A beta haemolytic streptococcus.

If the infection is slow to settle, check that the patient is not diabetic. Cellulitis is always slower to resolve than erysipelas, which usually responds dramatically to penicillin.

CHANCROID

Oral trimethoprim 200 mg twice daily is given for 1–3 weeks. The patient is reviewed weekly and treatment is continued until the ulcer is healed.

CHEILITIS—GRANULOMATOUS

This needs to be distinguished from Crohn's disease of the lips; a biopsy is not necessarily the best way of doing this since they may look remarkably similar histologically. Ask about abdominal symptoms and look inside the mouth for the characteristic cobblestone appearance of Crohn's disease of the buccal mucosa, and if necessary do a barium follow through. If the diagnosis is granulomatous cheilitis, it is worth referring the patient to a dermatologist for patch testing because some patients with this are allergic to mercury in their dental fillings. If the patch tests are negative, injection of triamcinolone 5 mg/ml into the swollen lip is often very helpful.

CHILBLAINS

Prevention is better than cure! Chilblains occur when the skin gets very cold and is then rewarmed too quickly. For those at risk, particularly individuals who work out of doors and the elderly who live in unheated accommodation, wearing warm gloves and boots in the winter and not putting the hands and feet into hot water or in front of the fire when coming indoors should prevent chilblains from occurring. If the ears, nose or thighs are affected rather than the digits, precautions to keep those areas warm are needed.

Nifedipine retard 20 mg three times a day can reduce the pain, soreness and irritation of chilblains. For patients who get severe recurrent chilblains it is worth considering continuing the drug for several weeks if the weather is particularly cold.

CHONDRODERMATITIS NODULARIS HELICIS CHRONICUS

Excision biopsy of the painful papule together with the underlying cartilage is usually curative. Removing the cartilage is more important than removing the skin, and more rather than less should be taken. At awkward sites like the antihelix, it is possible to cut back a flap of skin, remove the cartilage from underneath and sew the skin back over the top (Figure 19).

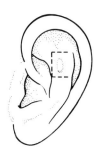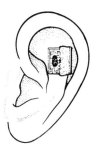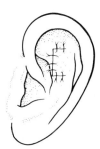

Figure 19

COMEDONES

Open and closed comedones associated with acne should be treated as described on page 18.

Single open comedones can be removed with a comedone extractor—*see* page 19.

Extensive comedones associated with solar elastosis (Figure 20), are not very common and are almost impossible to treat. Topical keratolytic agents can be tried but are rarely helpful. If only a few are present they can be removed with a comedone extractor.

A single giant comedone can usually be left alone once you have explained to the patient that it is harmless. If it is very unsightly it can be curetted out or excised under a local anaesthetic with a circular punch biopsy.

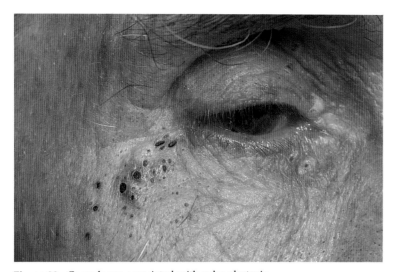

Figure 20 Comedones associated with solar elastosis.

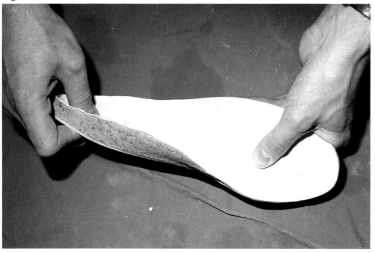

Figure 21 Orthotic appliance for a shoe; made of flexible cork. Courtesy of John Sanders.

CORNS (CALLOSITIES)

Callosities are areas of hyperkeratosis due to continual rubbing or pressure on the skin. Common sites are the sides of the fingers from holding a pen, the palms from manual labour, the backs of the knuckles from chewing, the anterolateral aspect of the ankle due to sitting cross-legged (causing pressure over the talus), and at sites of contact with trusses, callipers and shoes. Explanation of what is happening is all that is required. Some individuals will be able to prevent further friction and the problem will then be resolved. If this is not possible, the thickened area of skin will remain and if troublesome will need paring down with a scalpel.

Corns are localized callosities over bony prominences, usually on the feet. If a bony exostosis is present or there is an obvious anatomical abnormality of the foot, the help of an orthopaedic surgeon may be needed.

The patient should be advised about wearing shoes that fit properly.

The area of hyperkeratosis can be pared down regularly with a scalpel by the patient or a chiropodist and the central core of keratin removed. Alternatively, 5–10% salicylic acid ointment can be applied every night to soften the keratin and make it easier to remove, or salicylic acid plasters can be left on for a week at a time to do the same thing.

Wearing a corn pad or circle of orthopaedic felt around the corn will take the pressure off it and make walking more comfortable. Alternatively, a proper orthotic appliance can be made to fit into the shoe (Figure 21).

Soft corn. Pare away the abnormal keratin with a sharp scalpel (or ask the patient to go to a chiropodist to get this done). Then make the patient stand up straight on a piece of plain paper while you draw a line round each foot in turn. Put her shoes onto the drawing so that she can see that there is a difference between

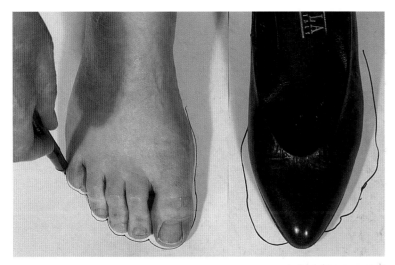

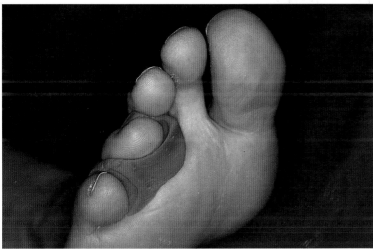

Figure 22 (*above*).
Figure 23 (*below*) Silicone wedge to keep toes apart. Courtesy of John Sanders.

the size of her feet and the size of her shoes (Figure 22). Explain that the corn has developed because she has been wearing shoes that are too narrow for her feet and advise her to get a pair of shoes that fit properly (if necessary give her the drawing that you have just done to take with her to the shoe shop). For the present, keep the affected toes apart with a piece of foam or a silicone wedge (Figure 23).

CUTANEOUS CALCULUS

These disappear on their own in children, so the parents can be reassured that no treatment is needed. They can be excised or curetted off if required.

CUTANEOUS HORN

Provided there is no induration at the base, suggesting an underlying squamous cell carcinoma, they are best curetted off under a local anaesthetic to prevent them being a nuisance. If there is induration present, excision and histological examination is needed.

CYSTS

Dermoid cyst

These should be excised because they frequently become secondarily infected through the punctum on the surface. On the nose they are best removed under a general anaesthetic, since they may extend down between the nasal bones and ordinary elliptical excision will be impossible. Elsewhere, simple excision under a local anaesthetic is effective.

Epidermoid cyst

These can be excised under local anaesthetic if they are a nuisance but do not try to remove them while they are actively inflamed. First excise an ellipse of skin over the surface; the amount you need to remove depends on how big the cyst is and how much redundant skin has been pushed up (Figure 24a). The cyst is then dissected out using a pair of blunt curved scissors (Figure 24b and c). If it has been infected in the past, it may be difficult to remove because it will be stuck down to the surrounding dermis by scar tissue. Cut the surrounding connective tissue carefully away from the cyst while at the same time pulling upwards from the top of the cyst (Figure 24d). It is important to remove *all* of the cyst wall during the procedure; if any of it is left behind, the cyst will recur. If the resultant hole is large, close off the dead space with deep sutures before inserting ordinary interrupted sutures into the skin.

If an epidermoid cyst is seen in a child before puberty, he should be examined for the possibility of polyposis coli by sigmoidoscopy once he reaches his teens. Cysts occurring in childhood are very suggestive of Gardner's syndrome.

Myxoid cyst (mucous cyst)

These can quite safely be left alone. If the patient requests treatment because it is hurting, discharging a clear sticky fluid or causing a groove in the finger nail, the possible options are:

1 Apply a very potent topical steroid ointment such as 0.05% clobetasol propionate (Dermovate) over it twice a day for several weeks.

2 Inject triamcinolone 5 mg/ml into the lesion.
3 Freeze with liquid nitrogen (30 seconds × 2).
4 Excision under local anaesthetic. This is best done by an orthopaedic hand surgeon because they can communicate with the distal interphalangeal joint and unless the communication is removed as well, the cyst tends to recur. A dye is injected into the cyst so that the communication with the joint can be traced and dissected out.
5 Removal by curettage and cautery. Even if the whole thing is not completely removed, there may be enough scar tissue at the base to prevent it refilling from the joint.

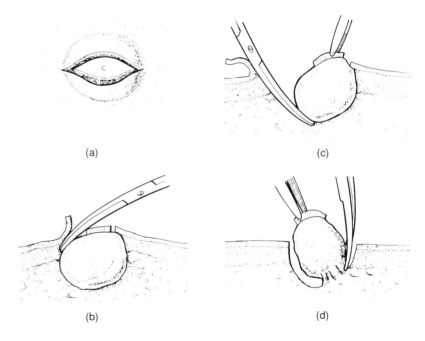

(a)   (c)

(b)   (d)

Figure 24 How to remove an epidermoid cyst.

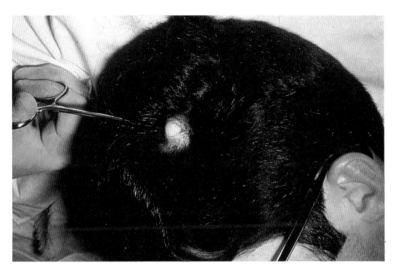

Figure 25 Removal of trichilemmal cyst. The skin is cut open with a scalpel and as soon as you are in the right plane, the cyst will pop out.

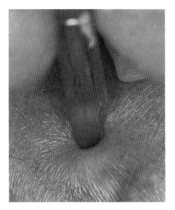
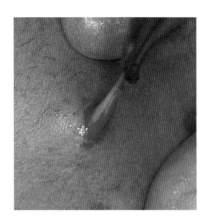

Figure 26 Removal of numerous cysts of steatocystoma multiplex. **(a)** (*above left*) Cut through the skin with a no. 15 scalpel blade held at 90° to the skin. Squeeze out the contents and then **(b)** (*above right*) pull out the cyst lining with a pair of artery forceps.

Pilar or trichilemmal cyst

These cysts shell out very easily under local anaesthetic once you are in the right plane (Figure 25), since they have a connective tissue sheath around them. An alternative method of removal is to cut straight into them with a scalpel, squeeze out the contents and then remove the cyst lining with a pair of artery forceps. It should come out intact and very easily.

Steatocystoma multiplex

Most patients with these do not require any treatment because the cysts do not show. If there is a problem with recurrent infections, long-term, low-dose, broad spectrum antibiotics, as for acne, are used (ie oxytetracycline 250 mg twice daily on an empty stomach, *see* page 19).

Cysts that are cosmetically unacceptable can be excised under local anaesthetic, provided there are not too many.

If huge numbers are present, they can be incised with a no. 15 scalpel blade, the contents squeezed out and the cyst lining removed by pulling out with a pair of artery forceps (Figure 26). You have to pull quite hard to remove the sacs; they do not come out easily like pilar cysts. This will normally need to be done under a general anaesthetic.

DARIER'S DISEASE

For small localized areas of abnormal skin, eg on the forehead or behind the ears, the patient can apply 0.025% retinoic acid cream or gel to the skin twice a day. It works quite well but as soon as the patient stops using it, the disease will recur.

For more extensive disease which is sore or smells, oral etretinate or acetretin will be needed. The dose is the same as for psoriasis (*see* page 168). These patients are best referred to a dermatologist because they will need genetic counselling (the disease is inherited as an autosomal dominant trait) as well as advice on treatment (retinoids are *hospital only* drugs). Retinoids need to be avoided in women of child bearing age if possible because they are teratogenic.

Rarely, retinoids do not help, in which case radiotherapy to the affected areas is another option. It is best not to consider this in teenagers and young adults because of the long-term risks of skin cancer.

DERMATITIS ARTEFACTA

In practice, this is very difficult to treat. The patient (usually female) may not be willing to admit to producing the lesion(s), or to the idea that treatment involves facing up to the problem or conflict in her life which is causing her to damage her own skin. Many patients play a sort of game, pretending that they are fooling the doctor, while all the time knowing that the doctor knows full well that the skin lesions are self-induced. Direct confrontation usually leads the patient to seek help elsewhere. Psychiatrists on the whole are not interested in helping with these patients. Covering the affected area with plaster of Paris or Calaband and Lestreflex (Figures 189 and 190, page 223) will result in rapid healing, confirming the diagnosis, but this is no good as a long-term solution. Unless the underlying problem is dealt with the patient is likely to go on damaging her skin.

DERMATITIS HERPETIFORMIS

A gluten-free diet will eradicate the IgA from the dermal papillae in 9–12 months and the itching will then stop. Although not pleasant, patients should be encouraged to stick to a gluten-free diet to prevent small bowel lymphoma from developing (the risks are the same as in coeliac disease). Most patients with dermatitis herpetiformis have no symptoms of steatorrhoea, so they may eat gluten without realizing it. Many of them, however, will feel a lot better on a gluten-free diet, and only realize after they have started it that they previously felt unwell.

Patients cannot tolerate the itching of dermatitis herpetiformis for 9–12 months until the gluten-free diet works, so initial treatment with dapsone, 50–150 mg daily is required. This will stop the itching within a few hours and is usually dramatic.

Check a full blood count before starting dapsone, because it causes haemolysis of red blood cells. This normally occurs within a few days of starting treatment, so the blood count should be repeated after one week. Most patients will show some haemolysis and will end up with a haemoglobin of around 100–110 g/l. If the fall in haemoglobin is greater than this, the dose of dapsone may need to be reduced. It also causes methaemoglobinaemia so the patient needs to be warned that the lips will look a bit blue. Start with 50 mg dapsone three times a day. Once the itching has stopped and the rash gone, the dose can gradually be reduced down to a maintenance dose of 50 mg daily or on alternate days. Once the haemoglobin has stabilized, it should be checked every 6 months.

Once the gluten-free diet has worked, the dose of dapsone can be reduced and eventually may be stopped.

DERMATOMYOSITIS

In a patient over the age of 40 years, the first priority is to exclude an underlying malignancy. If a tumour is found it should be removed. If this is done the dermatomyositis will get better. If it is not curable, the dermatomyositis will often be extremely difficult to manage; high-dose systemic steroids, 60–120 mg daily, being required.

In a patient in whom there is no underlying malignancy, treatment should be started as soon as possible (once the diagnosis has been confirmed) with prednisolone 60 mg daily. If the creatine kinase (CK) level is high before treatment is begun, serial measurement of this is a good indicator of disease activity, and the dose of steroids can be adjusted accordingly. If there is no fall in CK after a few days, the prednisolone should be doubled to 120 mg daily. Once the CK has fallen back down into the normal range, the dose of steroids can be slowly reduced, aiming to get the patient onto a maintenance dose of between 5 and 10 mg daily until the disease has burnt itself out. Systemic steroids alone may sometimes not control dermatomyositis, and one of the cytotoxic drugs will need to be added, in the form of azathioprine or methotrexate.

During the acute phase of the illness the patient will need to be on bed rest to prevent further damage to the muscles. Once the CK level begins to fall, passive exercises can be introduced. As well as proximal muscle weakness, there may be difficulty with swallowing and breathing and occasionally involvement of heart muscle. Calcification in the skin may be a nuisance particularly if it ulcerates.

This is a very debilitating illness and the patient will take at least a year to feel well even after the initial muscle weakness has recovered. Once better, the disease may relapse on one or more occasions, and the whole process start over again.

DERMOGRAPHISM

This is a self-limiting condition which occurs for a while and then stops spontaneously. It may last for quite a long time (weeks, months or years), but will eventually get better on its own. A long-acting antihistamine, in the form of terfenadine 60–120 mg twice daily, will usually stop it happening. Alternatives are any of the other non-sedative antihistamines taken on a regular basis until it stops (see page 245).

DISCOID LUPUS ERYTHEMATOSUS

This is the only condition for which it is permitted to use a very potent topical steroid on the face. Clobetasol propionate 0.05% (Dermovate) cream or ointment should be applied to the affected areas twice a day until the red plaques disappear. If there are only a few lesions present, this treatment will work well. If it does not work or if the patient has extensive disease, anti-malarials by mouth are more appropriate. Mepacrine 100 mg twice daily is usually effective but has the disadvantage of making the patient's skin (not sclera) go yellow. In some patients this looks like a sun tan, but in others it is a bright fluorescent yellow which is unacceptable (see Figure 32, page 47). It may also cause diarrhoea and vomiting. Most patients tolerate it well. If they do not, hydroxychloroquine or chloroquine can be used instead. These modes of treatment should be initiated by a dermatologist rather than a general practitioner.

The rash is often made worse by sunlight, so a high protective factor sun screen should also be prescribed (Factor 15 or above, see page 140), and the patient encouraged to wear a large hat and long sleeves in the summer.

DRUG RASH

Some drug rashes are life-threatening and it is essential that the offending drug is stopped. Others are no problem at all; they are asymptomatic and get better whether or not the drug is stopped. Unfortunately there are no simple tests for a drug rash and if patients are taking numerous drugs it is often not possible to be sure of the exact cause or even whether a drug is responsible (a viral exanthem may look identical). This leaves the doctor with a problem, not only during the current episode, but also in the future because he needs to know whether it is safe to prescribe the drug again.

If you think the patient has a drug rash, find out:
- what drug(s) he is on
- the exact date each one was started and stopped. It is more likely that a rash is from a recently started drug than one he has been taking for years. He is unlikely to develop a rash in less than 4 days if he has not had the drug before. Most drug rashes take 7–10 days to occur, but they sometimes do not appear for 28 days
- has he ever had the suspected drug before, or any chemically related drug
- has he ever had an adverse reaction to a drug before and if so to which one.

To avoid drug rashes
Only prescribe drugs that are actually necessary.
Always ask the patient if he is allergic to any drug before prescribing.
Make sure you know what is in a tablet or injection when you prescribe it.
Do not give ampicillin for sore throats.

Drug rashes can mimic almost all known skin conditions. The following are the most important reactions.

Exanthematous drug rash

This is the most common kind of drug rash. In the UK, antibiotics, sleeping tablets and tranquillizers are the most frequent causative agents. The rash mimics the common viral exanthems and is made up of symmetrical red or pink macules or papules mainly on the trunk; on the legs it may be purpuric. Almost any drug can cause this kind of reaction but the commonest are:
- ampicillin*
- other penicillins
- sulphonamides
- non-steroidal anti-inflammatory drugs (NSAIDs)
- benzodiazepines
- carbamazepine
- captopril
- phenothiazines
- thiazides
- thiouracils.

If the drug is essential, it is usually safe to continue with it, controlling any itching with calamine lotion or 1% hydrocortisone cream. If the rash becomes extensive or erythrodermic it must be stopped. It will usually clear in about a week.

Erythrodermic drug rash

This is a much more serious problem. The patient is red and scaly all over and may lose both heat and fluids through the skin. The

---

*Invariably causes a rash in patients with glandular fever, cytomegalovirus infection and chronic lymphatic leukaemia.

drug must be stopped and the patient will probably need to be in hospital.*

Drugs which cause erythrodermic drug reactions

allopurinol	cimetidine
barbiturates	gold**
captopril	isoniazid
carbamazepine	nalidixic acid
chlorpromazine	phenytoin
chloroquine	sulphonamides

Eczematous drug reactions

Drugs applied topically are much more likely to cause problems than drugs taken by mouth or by injection. Drugs like penicillin so often cause a contact allergic eczema that they are no longer used topically. Once an allergic reaction has occurred with something applied to the skin, a widespread eczematous rash will occur if the same drug is taken by mouth or parenterally. Those most commonly at fault are topical antibiotics and antihistamines. Some drugs cross-react with others which have a similar chemical make-up, eg sulphonamides, thiazides and chlorpropamide cross-react with benzocaine (in topical local anaesthetics) and paraphenylene diamine (in hair dyes). Aminophylline cross-reacts with ethylene diamine in Tri-Adcortyl cream. The offending drug should be

stopped and the rash treated with 1% hydrocortisone ointment or if it is very bad, 0.025% betamethasone valerate (Betnovate RD) ointment.

Fixed drug eruption

This is a curious reaction whereby, each time a drug is given, a round or oval red plaque occurs at the same site, usually within 2 hours and certainly within 24 hours. The only differential diagnosis is a recurrent herpes simplex infection. Any drug can cause it but in Britain the common ones are:
- sulphonamides
- phenolphthalein (in *over-the-counter* laxatives)
- non-steroidal anti-inflammatory drugs
- barbiturates
- tranquillizers
- quinine (tablets and in tonic water or bitter lemon drinks).

Lichenoid drug reaction

A rash which looks like lichen planus (although usually atypical) can rarely be due to a drug, eg:
- beta blockers
- chloroquine
- chlorpropamide
- gold
- mepacrine
- methyldopa
- penicillamine
- quinine
- thiazides.

---

*This is a particular problem in the elderly.
**The patient will often have a sore tongue, angular cheilitis and proteinuria before the rash occurs.

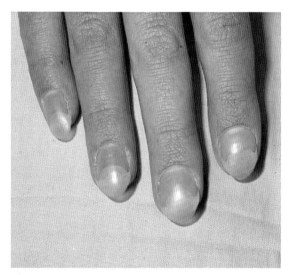

Figure 27 Photo-onycholysis due to demethylchlortetracycline.

Photosensitive drug rashes

There are two types of reaction which involve a drug and the sun. The first is a **phototoxic reaction**, where the skin becomes red and sore like sunburn. Drugs that do this include:

- amiodarone (30–50% of patients on this drug)
- frusemide
- nalidixic acid
- psoralens
- phenothiazines
- sulphonamides
- tetracyclines—especially demethylchlortetracycline.

(Tetracyclines may also cause a photo-onycholysis, with painful separation of the nail from the nail bed, *see* Figure 27).

The second is a **photoallergic reaction** where the rash is identical to a contact allergic eczema but it needs long-wave ultraviolet light (UVA) as well as the drug to cause it. The commonest drugs to cause this are:

- chlorpromazine (Figure 28)
- promethazine
- sulphonamides
- trimeprazine.

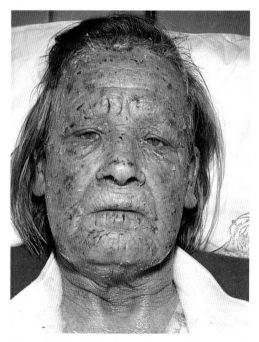

Figure 28 Photoallergic reaction to chlorpromazine.

Urticarial drug rashes

Most urticaria is not due to drugs, nor is it an allergic reaction. Some urticaria is due to a drug, however, and there are three different mechanisms involved:

1 A type 1 allergic response ± anaphylaxis. This is an emergency since, as well as the urticaria, there may be laryngeal oedema and bronchospasm which may cause the patient's death. Penicillin is the most well known drug to do this. Treatment with intramuscular adrenaline (0.5 ml of 1:1000 solution) should be given as soon as possible together with 10 mg of chlorpheniramine (Piriton) intramuscularly.

2 Serum sickness. Urticaria, arthralgia, fever and lymphadenopathy are the hallmarks of this immune complex reaction. It may be caused by:

- penicillin
- nitrofurantoin
- phenothiazines
- thiazide diuretics
- thiouracils.

It may be severe and need treatment with systemic steroids. This is the only reason to give systemic steroids for urticaria.

3 Direct liberation of histamine from mast cells by aspirin, codeine and the opiates. IgE is not involved. This is the commonest cause of infrequent acute episodes of urticaria, when patients take aspirin etc when they have a cold or a headache.

Less common problems with drugs and their causes

Acne—*see* page 22
Erythema multiforme—*see* page 72
Erythema nodosum—*see* page 73

Blisters

Bullous pemphigoid	clonidine
	diclofenac
	frusemide
	ibuprofen
Pemphigus	captopril
	penicillamine
	rifampicin

Coumarin necrosis

2–14 days after starting warfarin or another coumarin anticoagulant there may be massive haemorrhagic necrosis of the skin and subcutaneous tissues. Less often the same thing can occur with heparin. The drug must be stopped and surgical debridement of the affected areas carried out.

Hair loss

Cytotoxic drugs act on all rapidly dividing cells including those of the hair matrix; they therefore cause all the growing hairs to fall out. When treatment stops, the hair will regrow. Meanwhile the patient will need a wig to disguise the hair loss.

The anticoagulants (heparin and warfarin), the anti-thyroid drugs (carbimazole and the thioureas), and the retinoids (etretinate, acetretin and isotretinoin) all cause a shift in the hair cycle towards telogen and therefore an increase in the proportion of resting hairs (a kind of chronic telogen effluvium). This is much less dramatic than the hair loss from cytotoxic drugs but nevertheless real.

Hypertrichosis

An increase in vellus hair all over the body can be due to:

cyclosporin A	minoxidil
diazoxide	penicillamine
diphenylhydantoin	psoralens

Hyperpigmentation

Many different drugs cause a change in the colour of the patient's skin. In some cases this is a post-inflammatory hyperpigmentation following eczema or some other rash. In others it is due to deposition of the drug or its metabolites in the skin. Some drugs stain the skin colours other than brown (*see* below).

Drugs causing increase in melanin in the skin
- amiodarone (Figure 29)
- arsenic (raindrop pigmentation, *see* Figure 133, page 171)
- busulphan
- chloroquine (as well as causing hyperpigmentation of the skin it may cause bleaching of the hair and eyebrows, particularly in red headed individuals)
- contraceptive pill (face only)
- phenytoin.

Drugs causing non-melanin colour change in the skin
Red-pink   clofazimine
Orange   β-carotene
Yellow   mepacrine (Figure 32)
Blue-grey:
- dapsone (due to methaemoglobinaemia)
- gold (mainly sun-exposed sites, due to gold deposition in the dermis—occurs when patient has had more than 150 mg/kg body weight of gold—*see* Figure 30)
- minocycline (mainly legs, but can be on arms and in scars due to deposition of iron in the skin—*see* Figure 31)
- phenothiazines.

Lupus erythematosus

An illness identical to systemic lupus erythematosus can be caused by procainamide and hydralazine.

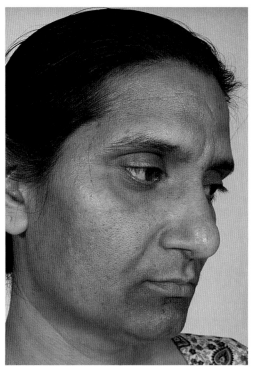

Figure 29
Hyperpigmentation due to amiodarone.

Purpura

Some drugs cause thrombocytopenia with purpura and larger ecchymoses. All such patients should be referred urgently to hospital for investigation. Drugs which can cause a fall in platelet count include:
- all the cytotoxic drugs
- chlorpromazine
- co-trimoxazole
- frusemide
- gold
- indomethacin
- rifampicin.

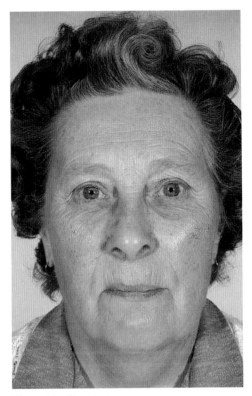

Figure 30 Chrysiasis.

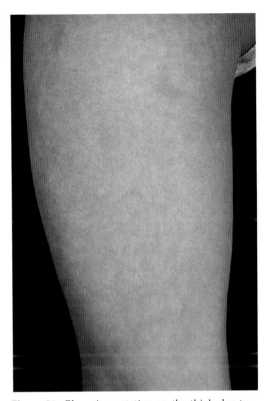

Figure 31 Blue pigmentation on the thigh due to minocycline.

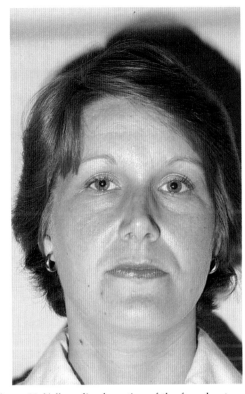

Figure 32 Yellow discolouration of the face due to mepacrine.

Other drugs cause a non-thrombocytopenic purpura, which is likely to be mainly on the lower legs. Drugs which do this include:

- allopurinol
- barbiturates
- carbimazole
- thiazide diuretics.

Toxic epidermal necrolysis

When this is due to a drug rather than a staphylococcal infection it is a medical emergency and such patients should be admitted urgently to hospital. The drugs which most commonly cause it are:

- allopurinol
- barbiturates
- carbamazepine
- NSAIDs
- phenytoin
- sulphonamides.

Vasculitis

A rash due to immune complexes deposited in the blood vessels in the skin is not in itself harmful, but if a similar process occurs in the kidneys it may cause permanent renal damage. It is diagnosed by seeing a polymorphic rash on the lower legs made up of red or purpuric macules and papules, vesicles, pustules and necrotic lesions. The drugs which most commonly cause it are:

- allopurinol
- ampicillin
- gold
- heparin
- hydralazine
- NSAIDs
- thiazide diuretics
- thioureas.

ECTHYMA

A bacteriology swab should be taken before treatment is begun because it can be due to *Staphylococcus aureus* or a group A beta haemolytic streptococcus. Assuming that it is due to *Staphylococcus aureus* (until the swab result comes back), start treatment with flucloxacillin 250 mg four times a day for at least 2 weeks. You may have to continue with systemic antibiotics for 4 weeks or more before it is healed. Topical antibiotics do not work. If the patient is allergic to penicillin use erythromycin 250 mg four times a day instead.

ECZEMA

Eczema is a pattern of disease rather than a definitive diagnosis. Before embarking on treatment, the type of eczema and the cause need to be identified if possible. Where you can find the treatment of the common patterns is outlined below:

Asteototic eczema

The patient should either bath less often or use one of the dispersible bath oils in the bath water each day (*see* page 50). A topical emollient, eg aqueous cream or Boots E45 cream, can then be applied to the dry scaly skin twice a day. Only very occasionally will a topical steroid be needed.

Atopic eczema in infants and young children

Atopic means an inherited predisposition to eczema, asthma and hay fever. 50% of children with this variety of eczema also have ichthyosis (dry, scaly skin). Treatment is usually straightforward, but there are infinite varieties in the patterns of eczema and individual children do not all respond in the same way, so the aim is to find the best treatment for this particular child. In any patient there are three modalities of treatment to be considered.

1 Topical steroids.
2 Emollients.
3 Antihistamines.

1 Topical steroids. Topical steroids are the mainstay of treatment for atopic eczema, even in infancy. If the eczema is active (the skin is red and itchy), they will need to be used. Parents are often afraid of using topical steroids because of the widespread publicity about side effects. You will need to explain that there are different strengths of steroids and that the weaker ones will not harm the skin (even if used over a long period of time — *see* page 8). Start with 1% hydrocortisone ointment applied twice a day. Do not use anything stronger than this on the face however

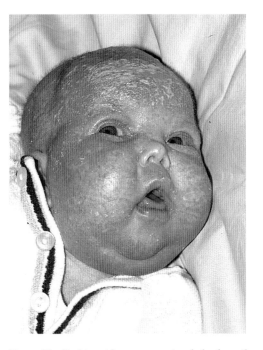

Figure 33 Cushingoid appearance in a baby from the application of very potent topical steroids.

bad the eczema is. On the trunk and limbs, if 1% hydrocortisone ointment is not working, either add 10% urea to the hydrocortisone which makes it much more effective (but do not use it on open skin because it stings) or increase the strength of the hydrocortisone to 2.5%, or use one of the moderately potent steroids (0.05% clobetasone butyrate [Eumovate], or the equivalent — *see* page 8) for short periods until it comes under control.

Ointments work much better than creams since the grease forms an occlusive barrier preventing evaporation of water and delivering the steroid more effectively to the skin.

The aim is to use the weakest possible steroid to control the disease. They are best applied immediately after a bath (*see* emollients, below). It is important to give the parents enough ointment so that it can be used regularly. Infants will need approximately 10 g a day (70 g/week) and a 7-year-old 20 g a day (140 g/week). It is quite safe to use topical steroids in young children if only 1% hydrocortisone is used. If more potent steroids are used, the amounts used will need careful monitoring to make sure that side effects are kept to a minimum (Figure 33). As a general rule do not prescribe more than 30–60 g of a potent steroid each month. This can be used sparingly on any difficult areas and the 1% hydrocortisone used routinely elsewhere (as much as required). Prolonged use of topical steroids can lead to tachyphylaxis (it becomes progressively less effective). One way round this is to rest the skin for 2 days each week, ie use a topical steroid for 5 days followed by a moisturizer only for 2 days.

2 Emollients. If the child has ichthyosis (dry skin) as well as eczema, emollients are an important part of the treatment.

(i) Bath oils. Soaking in a lukewarm bath for 10–15 minutes every day is very helpful, provided one of the dispersible bath oils has been added. There are a number of these on the market all of which work well, although some will suit some patients better than others, eg:

- Oilatum
- Balneum
- Balneum Plus
- Alpha Keri
- Balmandol
- Emulsiderm
- Hydromol.

2–3 capfuls of oil are added to the bath water for an adult-sized bath, half a capful to an infant's bath. If the eczema is very bad, 2 baths a day can be taken. Alternatives are an Aveeno Oilated sachet emptied into the bath or emulsifying ointment (2 tablespoons

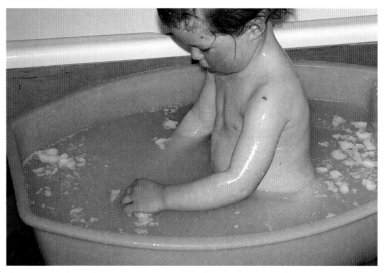

Figure 34 This is how not to use emulsifying ointment. If it is not dissolved in boiling water before being put into the bath water, it will simply float on the surface in lumps.

mixed in boiling water, whisked up until it is dissolved, and poured into the bath water). The latter is cheaper than the bath oils, but most people find it a lot more trouble to use (Figure 34) and it can block the drains! For preparations which can be used in the shower *see* page 59.

Emulsifying ointment or aqueous cream should be used instead of soap for washing, since soaps degrease the skin. Some parents do not like these soap substitutes, preferring something that lathers like real soap which they think gets the dirt off better! Oilatum, Aveeno and Sebamed bars are suitable as alternatives but are much more expensive and are not available on prescription.

(ii) Topical emollients. Emollients can also be applied to the skin during the day between steroid applications. There are a large number available ranging from white soft paraffin (Vaseline) which is very greasy, to Boots E45 cream which is moderately greasy, to aqueous cream which is not greasy at all (*see* page 92). The important thing is to find one that makes the skin more comfortable and which parents will use. It is best to start with something cheap, and only go on to the more expensive preparations if they do not work. Table 3 shows a selection of those that are currently available, including the possible sensitizers which they contain.

Table 3 Emollients available for topical use (*see* also page 92)

Emollient	Contains parabens	Contains lanolin
Alcoderm cream and lotion	Yes	No
Aquadrate cream*	No	No
Aveeno cream	No	No
Aqueous cream	No	No
Calmurid cream*	No	No
Diprobase cream and ointment	No	No
E45 cream	No	Yes
Emulsifying ointment	No	No
Humiderm cream	Yes	No
Hydrous ointment	No	Yes
Lacticare lotion	No	No
Lipobase cream	Yes	No
Locobase ointment	No	No
Natuderm cream	Yes	No
Nutraplus cream*	Yes	No
Oilatum cream	No	Yes
Sential E cream*	Yes	No
Ultrabase cream	Yes	No
Unguentum Merck cream	No	No
White soft paraffin	No	No
White soft paraffin/liquid paraffin mixed in equal parts	No	No

*These preparations contain urea which is very helpful for dry skin but will sting if the skin is open.

3 Antihistamines. If the child is keeping the parents awake at night, it is important to use a sedative antihistamine about an hour before the child's bedtime so that the whole family can get some rest. Parents find it difficult to cope with a constantly scratching child when they have had no sleep for days on end. Antihistamines do not stop the itching, but the sedative variety, if given in adequate dosage, will ensure that the child sleeps through the night. Young children need much larger doses than adults to sedate them; we suggest that you start with trimeprazine (Vallergan) 7.5 mg (5 ml) at night and double it each night until the child sleeps until morning without waking up. You may have to give 45–60 mg to have this effect. Trimeprazine is not addictive and is quite safe in children. Very occasionally children become hyperactive with trimeprazine, in which case promethazine (Phenergan) or one of the other sedative antihistamines can be tried.

R$_x$	
Oilatum	**500 ml**
Put half a capful in the bath each day	
Soak in bath for 10–15 minutes/day	
Emulsifying ointment	**500 g**
Use instead of soap for washing	
1% hydrocortisone ointment	**100 g**
Apply to all affected areas of skin twice a day	
Aqueous cream	**500 g**
Use as a moisturizer as often as required	
Trimeprazine elixir (7.5 mg/5 ml)	**200 ml**
5 ml at night, 1 hour before bedtime	
If the child does not sleep all night, double	
the dose each successive night until he does	
up to a maximum of 30 ml.	

Typical prescription for a young child with extensive atopic eczema

Other measures

Support and encouragement of the parents

Almost all parents who have a child with eczema will need more than repeat prescriptions from their doctor. They will need someone who understands their distress when they see their child scratching himself to bits and they feel impotent to help him. They need someone to talk to about it and someone who is available to see the child if the skin gets worse.

Most children grow out of eczema by puberty but a small percentage will go on getting it all their lives. On the whole these are the individuals who will be the most difficult to manage from the beginning. Early referral to hospital is probably wise.

If there are problems in the home, between the parents or with other members of the family, the child's eczema may get worse. Putting stronger steroids onto the child's skin is not the answer to this and the parents may need help for themselves. Occasionally it is necessary to admit the child to hospital to take the pressure off the family and allow the parents to get some sleep. The change of environment often results in remarkable improvement in the child's eczema.

Parents may want to be put in touch with the National Eczema Society, which has local self-help groups as well as lots of practical information.

There are a number of books available which parents may find helpful, eg:
Your child with eczema—a guide for parents
David Atherton, Heinemann.
Eczema and dermatitis: how to cope with inflamed skin
Rona MacKie, Martin Dunitz.
Learning to live with skin disorders
Christine Orton, Human Horizons Series, Souvenir Press (E&A) Ltd.

There are also some booklets for children, eg:
Edward in toy town by Jenny Creevy and available from E. Merck Ltd.
I have eczema by Althea Braithwaite and available from Dermal Laboratories.

Clothing

Cotton clothes worn next to the skin are much more comfortable to wear than man-made fibres. Wool is particularly irritating, not because of an allergic reaction to the wool, but because the wool fibres themselves tickle. The National Eczema Society provides a leaflet with the names and addresses of mail order companies and department stores which supply cotton clothes for children. Cotton On is perhaps the best known, but there are lots of others.

THE NATIONAL ECZEMA SOCIETY
4 Tavistock Place
London, WC1H 9RA
Tel: 071 388 4097

COTTON ON
29 Clifton Street
Lytham
Lancashire, FY8 5HW
Tel: 0253 736611

Cotton gloves worn at night will prevent some of the damage done by fingernails during sleep. Covering the skin with two layers of Tubegauz (over the topical steroid) at bedtime will also avert some of the damage done by scratching (Figures 35–37).

Treatment of infection

Because of scratching, secondary infection is very common, usually with *Staphylococcus aureus*, but occasionally with a group A beta haemolytic streptococcus. Obvious impetigo, pustules, or splits in the skin, particularly under the ears and over joints, are signs of bacterial infection and this may make the eczema itself worse.

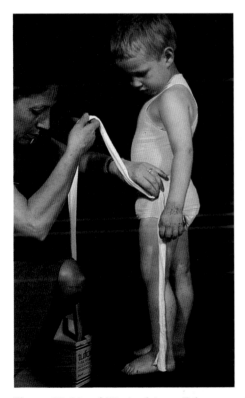 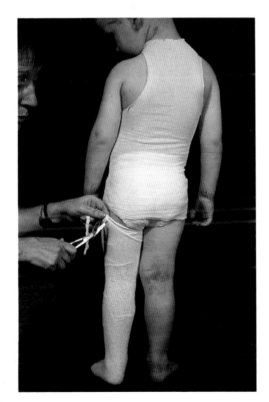 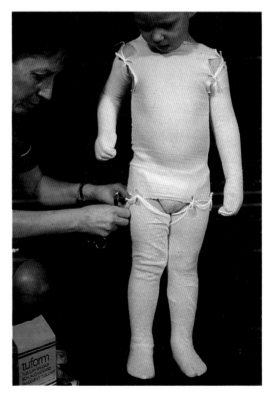

Figures 35, 36 and **37** Applying a Tubegauz suit.

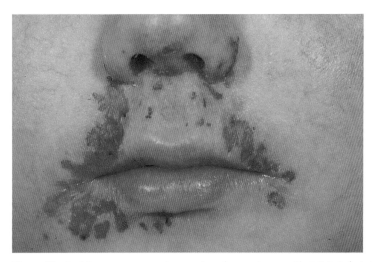

Figure 38 Just because eczema is weeping does not mean that it is infected. This 3-year-old boy has impetigo due to *Staphylococcus aureus* on top of his eczema which needs treating with flucloxacillin.

Early intervention with a systemic antibiotic will prevent a flare-up of the eczema. Erythromycin elixir 125 mg three times a day will cover both staphylococci and streptococci; alternatively, assuming *Staphylococcus aureus* to be the more likely pathogen, flucloxacillin elixir 125 mg three times a day can be given instead. Treatment of open areas of skin with hydrocortisone-tyrothricin lotion may prevent overt infection:

Tyrothricin powder	100 mg
Hydrocortisone powder	500 mg
Cetomacrogol emulsifying wax	2 g
Liquid paraffin	5 g
Glycerine	5 g
Nipagin M	170 mg
Distilled water	to 100 ml

Formula of hydrocortisone-tyrothricin lotion

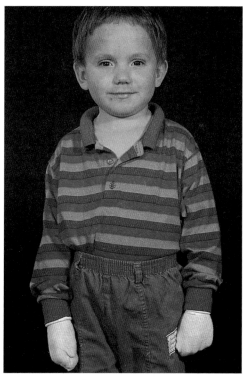

Figure 39 Tubegauz mittens to prevent scratching during the day.

Keeping the fingernails cut short will minimize the damage done by scratching as will wearing Tubegauz mittens (Figure 39).

It is important to exclude **scabies** in a child with infected eczema on the hands, or in any child who has what appears to be infected eczema which is not responding to treatment. Infestation with the scabies mite can easily be missed if it is not thought of, and the telltale burrows on the soles of the feet in infants, and along the sides of the fingers or on the front of the wrists in older children, should be looked for. Sometimes indurated nodules around the axillae or groins are another clue to the diagnosis of scabies.

Viral infections are also more common in children with atopic eczema because they have a defect in cell mediated immunity. Putting topical steroids on the skin can also help them to spread. Widespread warts or molluscum contagiosum occur and are extremely difficult to treat although they eventually get better spontaneously. Herpes simplex can look very similar to a bacterial infection and may be missed; like scabies it should be thought of if an apparent infection does not respond promptly to a systemic antibiotic. Eczema herpeticum, (widespread herpes simplex infection in eczema) is much more serious and is recognized by the fact that the child is ill or that the eczema is painful. It needs prompt treatment with oral or intravenous acyclovir. This is an emergency (*see* Figure 41) and the local dermatologist or paediatrician should be contacted urgently.

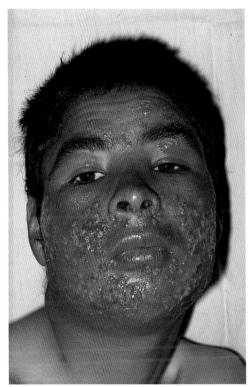

Figure 41 Eczema herpeticum in a 15-year-old boy. This can be a life threatening illness. Note the umbilicated vesicles which are characteristic of this condition.

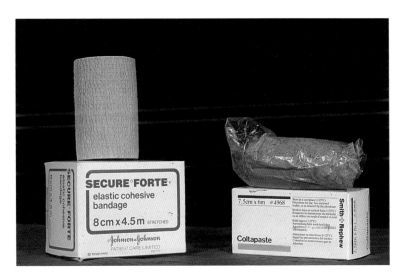

Figure 40 Coltapaste bandage ready to apply. See Figure 42 for how it is done.

Coal tar preparations

Coal tar and ichthammol are very soothing for eczema and particularly help the itching (Figure 42). They are not used much in practice because they are so messy. Tar bandages are helpful when the eczema is mainly on the limbs. Coltapaste or Ichthopaste bandages can be wrapped loosely around the limbs and covered with a sticky elasticated bandage such as Secure Forte to keep them in place (Figure 42). They can be left on overnight, for 24 hours,

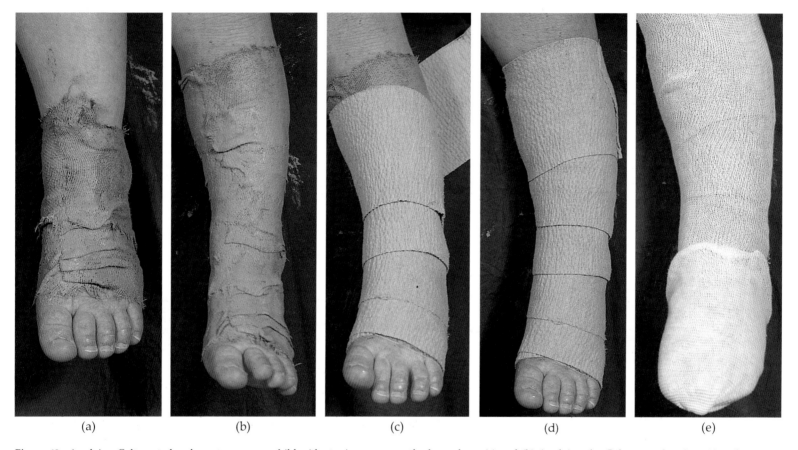

(a) (b) (c) (d) (e)

Figure 42 Applying Coltapaste bandages to a young child with atopic eczema on the lower legs. **(a)** and **(b)** Applying the Coltapaste dressing. **(c)** and **(d)** Covering the Coltapaste with Secure Forte (an elasticated adhesive bandage) to keep the tar off the child's clothes and to provide another layer of bandage which will help keep the child's fingers off the skin. **(e)** These 2 bandages are then covered with Tubegauz.

or for a week at a time depending on how bad the eczema is. The limiting factor is how long it will be before the child scratches them off. If they are allowed to dry out they become very irritating. This can be helped by soaking a flannel in tepid water, and applying it to the bandage every day to keep it moist. Although they are soothing, most children do not like being encased in tar bandages so they are used at times when the eczema is very bad just for short periods, eg in hospital or before a holiday.

Dietary measures

Some children with eczema develop urticaria after eating certain foods. This is a type 1 allergic reaction and is very obvious because the rash develops within a few minutes of eating that particular food. The rash is urticaria rather than eczema and may be accompanied by swelling of the lips. Such foods should be avoided in the future.

Whether foods cause eczema (as opposed to urticaria) is a controversial subject. Most parents are keen to try dietary manipulation to help their child or in fact anything else that might be beneficial. A few children are undoubtedly helped, but the majority are not. Exclusion of milk, dairy products, and eggs is not usually helpful. Going on a *few foods diet* (consisting of lamb, potato, rice, carrot, brassicas and pears) for a trial period of 4–6 weeks can be tried. This should be supervised by a dietitian to ensure that adequate calcium and protein are provided. If the eczema seems better, individual foods can then be re-introduced one at a time to see which one has caused the problem. If such a diet is helpful it should be continued for 6–12 months and then the offending food restarted again to see what happens. It is not likely that the child will need an exclusion diet permanently (50% of children will be back on a normal diet after 9 months, all by 3 years). Often a change in diet seems to help at the beginning, as does almost any change in treatment, but the benefit is not sustained. In that case a normal diet should be resumed.

Most people believe that breast feeding is beneficial in preventing the development of eczema in a child in an atopic family, but the evidence for this is not entirely convincing. The theory behind it is that children who develop atopic eczema have a relative deficiency of IgA. Intestinal IgA mops up allergens in the gastrointestinal tract and if there is not enough of it, food allergens are absorbed and antibodies against them produced. If the child is breast-fed, the child gets IgA from the mother in adequate amounts, and no food allergens are absorbed. Since breast feeding has many other benefits, it seems wise to recommend mothers to do this if there is a family history of eczema at least until there is evidence to the contrary.

Elimination of non-food allergens

House dust mites can be reduced by daily hoovering of carpets, mattresses and bedding, but this is not very practical for most families. An acaricidal spray, Actomite, made by Searle, can be sprayed onto carpets, beds, and soft furnishings; it is said to kill at least 90% of mites within 36 hours and only needs doing every 3 months because it also kills the eggs and larvae. Some children get urticaria from animal fur or saliva and there is no solution to this other than avoiding contact with cats, dogs, horses or whatever animal it is. In a few children the eczema will also flare after contact with animals. There is some evidence that contact with cats (not dogs) in the first year of life is associated with a higher incidence of eczema.

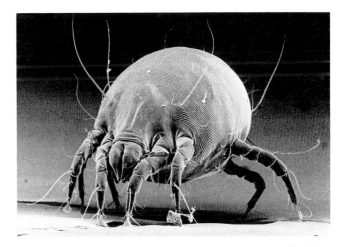

Figure 43 House dust mite (scanning EM picture). Courtesy of Dr Peter Howarth.

Whether or not the eczema flares with these non-food allergens, their elimination is likely to help any associated asthma.

Traditional Chinese herbal remedy (Zemaphyte or PSE101)

Daily boiling up of a decoction of dried traditional Chinese medicinal plants, and then drinking them, has recently been shown to be helpful in some children with atopic eczema (those with widespread non-exudative eczema; not those with weepy eczema or widespread lichenified eczema). The Chinese think that the various plants (*Radix ledebouriella, Herba potentilla, Caulis akebia, Radix rehmannia, Radix paeonia, Herba lopatheri, Cortex dictamni radicis, Fructus tribuli, Radix glycyrrhiza* and *Spica schizonepeta*) act synergistically but what the active ingredient(s) is has not yet been discovered (it is not a steroid). Rather than boil up a selection of dried plants, the remedy is now available in sachets (like large tea bags) from Phytopharm Ltd* and it is available on prescription as Zemaphyte or PSE101. It comes in pairs of sachets, one large and one small, the dose depending on the age of the child:

Age 1–7 years—2 pairs of sachets/day.

Age 8–13 years—3 pairs of sachets/day.

Parents are instructed to put the large sachets in a saucepan containing half a pint of water; it is brought to the boil and then allowed to simmer gently for an hour and a half so that the liquid is reduced to a quarter of a pint. The small sachets, which contain volatile oil are then added for a final 3 minutes. The liquid is then strained off from the sachets and the child drinks it while it is still warm.

Although it works well, both parents and children need to be very highly motivated to use it; the parents because it takes so long to prepare and the children because it tastes really foul. Treatment

*Phytopharm Ltd, Wortley House, 16 Eastbourne Road, Hornsea, East Yorkshire, HU18 1QS.

is continued until the skin is more than 90% clear. The frequency of taking the decoction is then reduced to every second or third day. In this way, the dose is gradually reduced until it can be stopped without a recurrence of the eczema.

So far there have been no serious side effects with it, the main limitations being its exorbitant cost and bitter taste. Nevertheless it is currently recommended that children taking it should have their liver function tests measured before starting treatment and every month while they are on it.

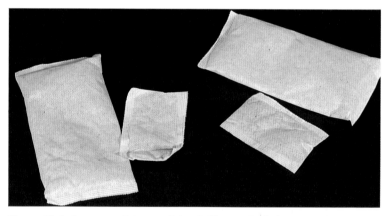

Figure 44 Sachets containing traditional Chinese herbal remedy for eczema.

Evening primrose oil

Deficiency of essential fatty acids causes a rash very like atopic eczema. For this reason and the fact that prostaglandins, thromboxanes and leukotrienes, which are all derived from fatty acids, play a role in inflammation of the skin, it seemed possible that supplementation of the diet with linoleic acid or its metabolites might be helpful in the treatment of eczema. Evening primrose oil contains gamma-linoleic acid. Numerous clinical trials have been carried out to see whether it works, and the evidence is conflicting. Since it is very expensive it should be used as a last resort rather than a standard treatment. If it is used, it should be given in adequate dosage, 6 capsules a day for a young child (12 capsules a day for an adult) for 3 months. Not all patients are able to swallow this number of capsules each day. If there is a problem, they can be snipped open and the oil inside can be swallowed, mixed with milk and drunk, or spread on bread and eaten. If there is no improvement in the eczema after 3 months it should be discontinued.

Atopic eczema in school-age children

The management of eczema in school-age children is basically the same as in young children with topical steroids, emollients and antihistamines (*see* page 49). Use the weakest steroid possible to control the disease because long-term use can lead to skin atrophy (Figure 46), striae (Figure 45), and a number of other problems (*see* page 8). Start with 1% hydrocortisone ointment and only use something stronger than this if it does not work. You should never need to use anything stronger than 0.025% betamethasone valerate (Betnovate RD) ointment or the equivalent (*see* Table 1, page 8). If you must use steroids stronger than hydrocortisone, try to use them for short periods of time just to bring the eczema under control.

The child should soak in a bath containing 2–3 capfuls of one of the dispersible bath oils (*see* page 50) for 10–15 minutes each day. If the family has a shower rather than a bath, there are a number of emollients which can be used there rather than in the bath:
- emulsifying ointment
- aqueous cream
- Oilatum gel
- Unguentum Merck
- Emulsiderm.

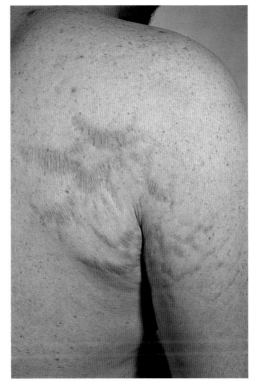

Figure 45 Striae due to application of potent topical steroids for years.

The patient goes in the shower and gets the skin thoroughly wet. The shower is then turned off and one of the shower preparations is rubbed all over the skin. The shower is then turned on again to rinse it off.

Antihistamines at night are slightly more problematic than in younger children, because the child needs to be alert in the morning to go to school. It may be that they can only practically be used at weekends (*see* page 51).

Systemic antibiotics should be used promptly if infection occurs to prevent the eczema getting worse (*see* page 53).

Treatment should be used regularly to keep the eczema under control. This is more difficult to do as children get older and they apply their own ointments. Whereas the parent would apply the ointment every day, children often prefer to do other things! Older children also will often choose not to bath regularly and not use their bath oils as a way of rebelling. All of this makes eczema difficult to control in teenagers. Fortunately the eczema often gets better spontaneously at around puberty, but it may recur later (age 17–18) at the time of exams, a new job or other stress.

Parents should speak to the child's teacher at school so that he or she knows that the child has eczema and that it is not infectious. This should also help to minimize unkind remarks by other children. Emollients and topical steroids may need to be applied during the day at school, particularly in winter, and after hand washing. Swimming can be allowed provided that emulsifying ointment or aqueous cream are used in the shower afterwards. The child must then also apply his topical steroid ointment as he would after a bath at home.

Often the eczema will improve when the family is on holiday in the summer. This is partly due to the sunshine and sea water, but also because the whole family is more relaxed. Sunshine is helpful as long as the weather is not too humid. Swimming in the sea is also beneficial as long as the skin is not infected. Children with eczema should be encouraged to do all the things that their friends are doing; usually with a little care this is possible.

There is a group of children between the ages of 7 and 10 who develop atopic eczema only on their feet. This tends to weep and make a mess as well as being itchy. The feet should be soaked in potassium permanganate, 1:10,000 solution for 10 minutes twice a day (*see* page 61). This coagulates protein and dries up the blisters. After soaking, the skin is patted dry with a towel and a dilute topical steroid ointment applied.

R$_x$

Oilatum	**500 ml**
2–3 capfuls in bath daily	
Aqueous cream	**500 g**
Use instead of soap for washing and as a moisturizer at any time of the day. Use as often as you like	
1% hydrocortisone ointment	**60 g**
Apply to face twice a day	
Betnovate RD ointment	**200 g**
Apply to trunk and limbs twice a day	
Flucloxacillin	**125 mg × 20**
Take one tablet 4 times a day	

Typical prescription for a school-age child with infected atopic eczema

Atopic eczema in adults

Some children grow out of their eczema only for it to return in adult life, either at times of stress or due to unsuitable work. Occupational advice is best given at an early stage, before any training is started. Hairdressing, nursing and other jobs which involve having the hands wet a lot are not suitable, nor is an engineering job where the hands will be covered in oil.

A small proportion of children do not grow out of their eczema and will have it all their lives. Some of these will have it very badly and will need systemic treatment in the form of PUVA, systemic steroids, azathioprine or cyclosporin A. These modalities of treatment should only be initiated by a specialist. For the precautions that will need to be taken with any of these treatments *see* pages 132, 164 and 170.

Figure 46 Steroid atrophy on forearm—note the venules which are visible through the skin.

If the patient has ichthyosis as well as eczema, bath oils and emollients are needed just as they are in children (*see* page 50). If he has had eczema all his life, the patient will be an expert on its management by the time he has grown up and will often know better than the doctor the things that are likely to help. The strength of topical steroids must be kept to the lowest possible to control the disease and minimize skin atrophy etc (Figure 46).

If the eczema begins for the first time in adult life, a dilute topical steroid ointment (1% hydrocortisone ointment) applied twice a day is needed. Ointments may not be very practical if the eczema is widespread because of the mess they make of the clothes. A compromise between what is the best treatment and what is practical may have to be reached. Creams are a lot less messy to use but are absorbed more quickly and so do not have such a lasting effect.

Adding 10% urea to 1% hydrocortisone cream or to 0.025% beta-methasone valerate (Betnovate RD) cream (it will not mix into an ointment) will often be a good solution to the problem if there are not too many open areas. Trial and error is likely to be needed to find the best option for any individual patient.

Holidays in the sun, unless the patient is very fair, often help a lot and many patients will choose to holiday abroad in order to keep their skin comfortable. Artificial sunlight in the form of UVB two or three times a week at the local hospital may help other patients or keep them clear between holidays.

Acute eczema

Acute eczema is characterized by small vesicles in the epidermis which easily break causing exudation of serum (exudate and crust [dried exudate] are not necessarily signs of infection). It is no good trying to apply an ointment or cream to an exuding rash because they will not stay on the skin. The first thing is to dry up the exudate with potassium permanganate. If the rash is on the hands or feet, soak them in a bowl of lukewarm water containing potassium permanganate diluted to a concentration of 1:10,000 for 10 minutes twice a day. This should make the water go a pale pink colour and not a deep purple (Figure 47), or the nails and sometimes the skin will be stained dark brown (Figure 48). Potassium permanganate coagulates protein and dries up the exudate; diluted to a pale pink colour does this just as well as when it is darker.

If the rash is all over the body, use the potassium permanganate in the bath twice a day, again diluted to a pale pink colour. If it is on the face or some other part of the body which cannot easily be put into water, use wet dressings. Soak the dressing in diluted potassium permanganate and apply it to the affected part four or five times a day. If it is weeping a great deal, wet dressings can be

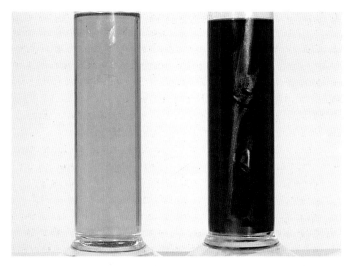

Figure 47 Potassium permanganate solutions. On the left, the pale pink colour is the correct dilution. On the right, the solution is too strong and if used like this will cause brown staining of the skin and nails.

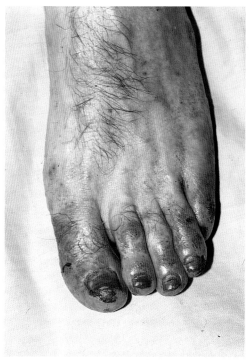

Figure 48 Brown staining due to potassium permanganate. If it is used as a pale pink colour this does not happen.

left in place and kept wet by applying more of the potassium permanganate solution to them every hour.

Once the eczema is dry a dilute steroid ointment can be used. Only use a cream if you are absolutely sure that the rash is not a contact allergic eczema which might be due to a medicament. It is important to find out why the patient has an acute eczema. The common causes are:

- contact allergic eczema (*see* right)
- acute flare of chronic atopic eczema (*see* page 60)
- unclassifiable endogenous eczema (no cause can be found, *see* page 68).

Contact allergic eczema

The first priority here is to remove the patient from the allergen which is causing the rash. This may be easy, eg nickel earrings which can be taken off, or it may be more difficult, eg an acute eczema on the face when nothing new has been applied and the cause is not apparent. Unless the allergen is removed the rash will not get better. Patch testing will be required to find the cause, but this can not be done in the acute phase when there are blisters and weeping.

Management is divided into 4 stages

1 Acute blistering or weeping eczema. Remove the allergen if it is known or can be guessed at and dry up the blisters with potassium permanganate (*see* page 61).

2 Once the eczema is dry, apply a dilute topical steroid ointment two or three times a day. Unless you can be absolutely certain that the rash is not due to a medicament, use a steroid ointment rather than a cream, and one which has white soft paraffin as its base eg 0.025% betamethasone valerate ointment (Betnovate RD ointment) or 0.025% beclomethasone dipropionate diluted 1 in 4 with white soft paraffin (Propaderm ointment 1:4). Avoid ointments which contain lanolin. The reason for this is that all creams contain preservatives which may be allergens, as too may lanolin, and you want to be sure that the treatment does not make things worse or keep the rash going.

3 Once the eczema has settled, patch testing will be needed to find the cause.

4 Once the cause has been identified it should be avoided. This may be easier said than done and may involve the patient in considerable expense, eg buying new shoes and carpets if he is allergic to mercaptobenzothiazole (in the rubber soles of his shoes and in the rubber backing to his carpets), or the need to change his job.

Contact irritant eczema

Almost all contact irritant eczema is on the hands, the dorsum more than the palmar surfaces. Skin irritants are usually weak acids or alkalis. The most common are detergents, shampoos, polishes, cement dust, oils, greases, engineering slurry and some foods (eg citrus fruits, tomatoes, potatoes, flour). Water may even be an irritant. Housewives with young children at home, hairdressers, nurses, cooks, building labourers and those working in the engineering industry are most at risk. Those who have had atopic eczema in childhood or who still have it, also seem to have a higher risk. The problem with contact irritant eczema is that once it has occurred and the skin barrier has been broken, only a minor degree of re-exposure to the irritant will keep it active.

Treatment is aimed at protecting the hands from all skin irritants, which may or may not be possible:

- if it is due to detergents, wearing rubber gloves will prevent it. Some patients find that wearing rubber gloves makes the hands more itchy. If that is the case, cotton-lined, PVC gloves, eg Glovelies, can be worn instead (these are much thicker than ordinary rubber gloves and take some getting used to). It is important that the gloves are worn all the time that the hands are in water, for however short a time. It will be almost impossible for mothers with small children at home, and for nurses, to keep their hands dry all the time or to wear rubber gloves for every piece of wet work

- if it is due to cement dust there is no easy way to avoid it if the patient works on a building site

- if it is due to soluble oil used to cool moving bits of machinery, it is not easy to avoid getting it on the hands. Many engineering jobs are difficult to do wearing rubber gloves, and barrier creams sound like a good idea but in practice do not work. Sometimes it is better to see if there is a different way of doing the job so that the oil does not get onto the skin.

Initially the patient may well have to have some time off work in order to allow the eczema to settle down. Whether, ultimately, he will have to change the nature of his job or give it up altogether is up to him to decide. It may be that he is forced to do so by the persistence and severity of his rash. Some patients are prepared to put up with the eczema to keep working. If he does have to stop work, he may be eligible for industrial benefit, since contact irritant eczema (dermatitis) is an industrial disease (*see* below). Much more time is lost from work due to contact irritant eczema than from contact allergic eczema.

While the eczema is present it can be treated with a moderately potent topical steroid, such as 0.05% clobetasone butyrate (Eumovate) ointment or 0.025% betamethasone valerate (Betnovate RD). Topical steroids alone will never cure this kind of eczema unless the contact with the irritant(s) is removed. Emulsifying ointment or aqueous cream should be used instead of soap for washing the hands and aqueous cream used as a moisturizer afterwards.

Nappy rash in babies, and an identical rash due to incontinence in the elderly, is a form of contact irritant eczema. For treatment of this, *see* page 123.

Occupational eczema (dermatitis)

The terms eczema and dermatitis are used interchangeably but lay people use the word dermatitis to mean a rash due to a job for which compensation can be sought. For this reason we have avoided the term dermatitis except in this instance. Occupational eczema is defined as eczema for which occupational exposure can be shown to be a major causal or contributory factor. In effect, would this patient have developed eczema if he had not done this particular job? The use of this diagnosis implies that an occupational factor has at some time been proved beyond reasonable doubt. The things that point towards such a diagnosis include:

- The patient works in contact with a substance known to cause allergic or irritant contact eczema.
- Other people doing the same job have similar skin problems.
- The pattern of eczema fits with a diagnosis of an allergic or irritant contact eczema, and is similar in all the people doing the same job who have skin problems.

- The eczema occurs after exposure at work and clears when the patient is off work—at weekends, on holiday, and during time off sick.
- Positive patch tests.

Advice about occupational eczema is best given by a dermatologist or doctor experienced in industrial medicine because:

1 Litigation tends to be a long and drawn out process and the patient does not want to start going down that track unless he is likely to be successful. Very often the eczema itself does not clear up while the patient is waiting for the course of the law to take place which often results in more ill health than there would have been otherwise. It may in the end be better to claim dermatitis benefit through the DHSS rather than taking things through the courts.

2 Most manufacturing processes only cause eczema in some workers. Others doing exactly the same job do not get any skin trouble. There must therefore be something wrong with the skin of the individual who gets the eczema. Possibly he may have had atopic eczema as a child.

3 Some jobs are safer than others, eg a young woman with a past history of atopic eczema may have no skin problems whilst working as a secretary, but gets hand eczema if she becomes a hairdresser.

4 Compensation may have to take into account a decrease in income for someone who has to give up a highly skilled job or profession.

Discoid eczema

Start with tar, in the form of 2% crude coal tar in white soft paraffin or Unguentum Merck, applied once or twice a day. The concentration of the tar can then be increased as necessary until the rash is controlled (2%–5%–10%). Patients prefer treatment with a topical steroid but on the whole they do not work very well for this type of eczema.

Hand and foot eczema

Eczema can occur just on the hands and feet or it can be part of a more generalized rash. In either case it may be endogenous or exogenous.

With eczema on the hands it is always worth doing patch tests, because the hands touch a lot of things during the course of a day. If the cause can be found and contact with it stopped, the eczema may be cured. Otherwise the patient will be condemned to using ointments or creams indefinitely.

On the feet an allergic contact eczema is usually more obvious, being confined to the areas in contact with the shoes. Whatever the cause, the treatment will be divided into whether the eczema is acute, chronic or hyperkeratotic.

1 Acute weeping eczema (Figure 49). Initially rest will be required to get the eczema better. Not using the hands or going to bed to rest the feet may be needed. The actual treatment involves soaking the hands or feet in a bowl containing 1:10,000 potassium permanganate for 10 minutes twice a day, patting them dry with a clean towel and then applying a dilute topical steroid ointment which does not contain lanolin (0.025% betamethasone valerate [Betnovate RD] or 0.025% beclomethasone dipropionate diluted with three parts of white soft paraffin [Propaderm ointment 1:4]). Once the very acute phase has passed, the patient can be up and about again. When the eczema has settled properly the patient should be sent for patch testing to see if a cause can be found.

2 Subacute eczema can be settled quickly with occlusive tar bandages. These are very soothing for the patient, will help the eczema to heal and will prevent the patient from damaging the skin further by scratching. On the hands, the bandages are applied around each finger separately (Figure 50) so that they can still be used, and the tar bandages covered with Tubegauz to keep the tar off the clothes, furniture etc.

3 Chronic eczema. The patient will require a topical steroid ointment or cream applied once or twice a day. It will often be a question of trial and error to find the one which will suit this particular patient best. If the skin is very dry or there are a lot of fissures, start with an ointment, probably from the moderately potent group (see page 8). Hydrocortisone is unlikely to be much use. If it is not too scaly the patient may prefer to use a cream.

If the eczema is on the hands and the patient is female, ask her to wear cotton gloves for doing the housework, and rubber gloves or cotton-lined PVC gloves for all wet work, to prevent further damage. A man will also need to protect his hands from irritants as much as possible, and this may involve having time off work if they will not settle down.

If the eczema is on the feet, white cotton socks and leather shoes are likely to be more comfortable than man-made fibres, unless of course the eczema is an allergic contact eczema due to leather.

4 Hyperkeratotic eczema (Figure 52). Here both the eczema and the hyperkeratosis need treating. If the latter is not treated, there is likely to be a problem with painful fissuring.

For the hyperkeratosis the options include:

(i) 5% salicylic acid ointment, either applied alone or mixed with a topical steroid, eg Diprosalic ointment or 5% salicylic acid in quarter strength Betnovate ointment. If the salicylic acid is used alone, it can be applied either in the morning or at night, and a topical steroid used alone the other time. One of the moderate strength steroid ointments, rather than 1% hydrocortisone is normally required (see page 8).

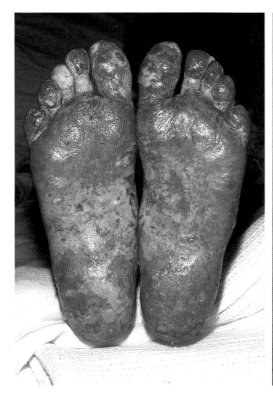

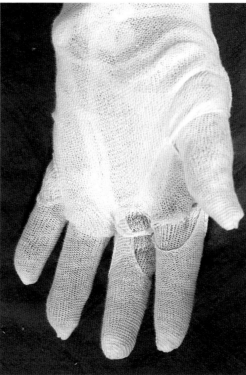

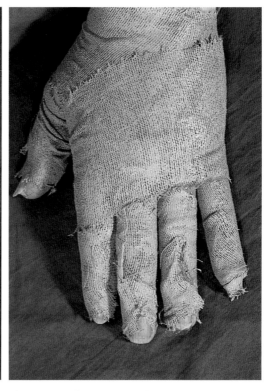

Figure 49 Weeping eczema on the feet. Acute contact allergic eczema due to PTBP formaldehyde resin (glue) in shoes.

Figure 50 Coltapaste bandages applied to a hand. The fingers are each bandaged separately.

Figure 51 Tubegauz applied over tar bandages to keep the tar off the clothes and furniture.

(ii) 50% propylene glycol in water applied under polythene occlusion at night (use plastic bags on the feet and either plastic bags or plastic gloves on the hands). In the morning a moderately potent topical steroid ointment can be applied.

(iii) Soak the hands or feet in 40% urea solution for 10 minutes once or twice a day. This is more expensive than the other two methods, so the liquid should be poured back into the bottle after use and reused.

Haelan tape may also be useful for hyperkeratotic or fissured eczema on the hands and feet. Patients like it because it is not messy. It is however very expensive and is only available in hospitals or on a private prescription.

2 weeks will clear it and it can then be kept clear by using it once every 2 weeks indefinitely. If there is a lot of redness as well as scaling, the patient can apply a topical steroid lotion each night until it is clear. It is best to begin with the weakest possible steroid, eg 0.1% hydrocortisone 17-butyrate (Locoid) lotion, and only use something stronger if that does not work.

If thick scaling is present, you can try either:

- Capasal shampoo, which contains 0.5% salicylic acid, 1% distilled coal tar and 0.5% coconut oil, or
- ung. cocois. co (formula page 176). This is rubbed all over the scalp at night, covered with a scarf or shower cap to keep it off the pillows, and washed off the next morning (Figures 105 and 106, pages 143 and 144).

On the face and trunk

Seborrhoeic eczema tends to come and go, often flaring at times of stress. Treatment should be used when the rash is there and left off when it is not. There are four possible treatments when seborrhoeic eczema occurs on non-scalp skin:

1 2% ketaconazole cream applied twice daily to all affected areas until it is clear. The rationale for this is that seborrhoeic eczema is due to an overgrowth of *Pityrosporum* yeasts.

2 1% hydrocortisone cream applied twice daily until it is clear.

3 1% hydrocortisone ointment mixed in equal parts with sulphur and salicylic acid ointment. This is a lot more messy than hydrocortisone cream, but is very effective. It is worth considering if the other options do not work. It is particularly helpful for the seborrhoeic eczema that occurs in AIDS.

4 2% lithium succinate (Efalith) cream. This is a useful alternative if you do not want to use a topical steroid. It may initially make the skin slightly red, but this tends to wear off after about a week. Use it twice a day until the eczema is clear.

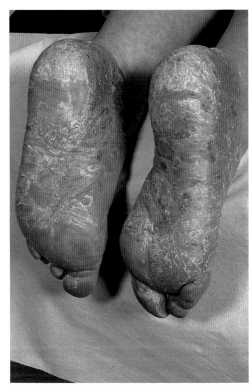

Figure 52 Hyperkeratotic eczema on the feet.

Seborrhoeic eczema

On the scalp

Dandruff is mild seborrhoeic eczema. If it is not very bad, washing the hair more frequently is all that is required. If that is not sufficient, ketaconazole shampoo (Nizoral) used twice a week for

Unclassifiable endogenous eczema

Begin with 1% hydrocortisone ointment or cream applied twice a day. If necessary gradually increase the strength of the steroid (*see* page 8) until the eczema comes under control. Because there is no obvious cause for this type of eczema treatment may have to be continued indefinitely.

Varicose eczema

More important than what is put onto the eczema itself is treatment of the underlying problem (chronic venous stasis due to incompetent valves in the deep veins of the calf) with proper elastic support. Well fitted elastic stockings or two-way stretch elasticated bandages (Blue line, Red line or Molastic bandages) should be worn all the time that the patient is out of bed (*see* also page 221). It is probably best to use elasticated bandages until the eczema is better and then change to elastic stockings because the treatment for the eczema may otherwise ruin the stockings.

For the eczema itself, 1% hydrocortisone ointment can be applied twice a day. The patient may prefer a cream to an ointment, particularly since that will make less of a mess of their bandages. This should be resisted though, because many such patients are allergic to parabens (a preservative in many creams). They become allergic to parabens either by using creams over the years or by using paste bandages which nearly all contain it.

EPIDERMAL NAEVUS

Excision is the only treatment that will get rid of this. Topical keratolytics and dermabrasion have been tried but without much success. Shave and cautery of the prominent warty lesions is easy and quick to do without causing a lot of scarring; it may, however, recur after some years. Often they are quite small and do not need anything doing to them.

EPIDERMOLYSIS BULLOSA

This term encompasses a number of different genetically determined diseases in which blisters appear on the skin in response to trauma. There are three main types depending on where the split in the skin is.
1 Simplex.
2 Junctional (usually lethal in the first 2 years of life).
3 Dystrophic (autosomal dominant and recessive varieties).

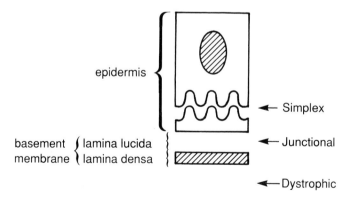

Figure 53 Classification of epidermolysis bullosa according to the site of the blisters on electron microscopy.

In the mildest form of epidermolysis bullosa simplex (Figure 54), blisters only occur when the patient wears a new pair of shoes or if he does a lot more walking than usual. He will quickly learn for himself that new shoes have to be gradually worn in and must fit properly. Cotton socks are more comfortable than nylon ones and will rub the skin less. If the skin is uncomfortable, simple emollients like aqueous cream can be applied morning and night. Generally speaking these patients can lead a normal life and will not need a lot of assistance from doctors.

At the other extreme are patients who are covered with blisters and erosions at birth (Figure 55), who may not survive, and if they do, will be severely disabled because of their skin. A skin biopsy will be needed as early as possible so that the correct diagnosis can be made and genetic counselling given.

Management of the skin

1 Healing of blisters and erosions. There are all kinds of tricks which will help the skin to heal.

- Potassium permanganate in the bath water (so that it is a pale pink colour) to coagulate protein and dry up any erosions. 2–3 capfuls of Oilatum or Balneum can also be added to the bath water to stop the skin drying out.
- Any new blisters can be popped either in the bath or immediately afterwards.
- Open areas of skin can be protected with non-stick dressings such as Jelonet, Melolin, or Kaltostat and covered with lightly elasticated bandages. Sufficient quantities of dressings must be given (Melolin comes in a 7 metre roll as well as in 10 cm squares).
- Jelonet can be applied in strips between the fingers in the recessive dystrophic form of epidermolysis bullosa to try to stop the fingers from sticking together.

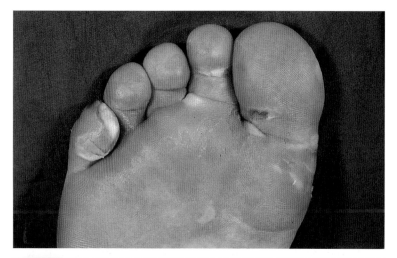

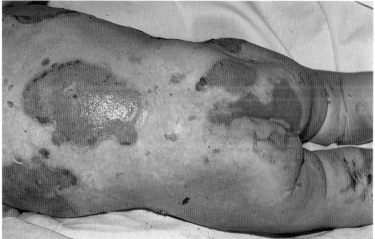

Figure 54 (*above*) Epidermolysis bullosa simplex. Blisters on the right sole of a girl aged 13.

Figure 55 (*below*) Recessive dystrophic epidermolysis bullosa in a new-born infant. Three previous siblings had died of the same condition.

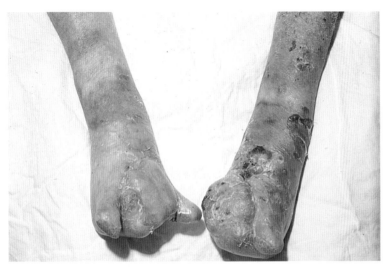

Figure 56 Recessive dystrophic epidermolysis bullosa in a 31-year-old woman. Webbing of the fingers has occurred due to blistering and the open areas of skin sticking together. There is a risk of squamous cell carcinomas developing later in this type of skin.

- Any dressings which are stuck to the skin should be soaked off in the bath rather than pulled off.
- Aqueous cream or some other emollient can be applied to the skin every time the dressings are changed.
  Once the child goes to school, a supply of dressings and emollients will be needed there too.

2 Protection from injury. The skin should be kept covered and the limbs well padded up to prevent injury. If necessary Lyofoam sheeting can replace ordinary cotton sheets, so that the child does not stick to the bedding overnight. Clothes and shoes must not be tight. New shoes are tried with the hands rather than the feet to check that there are no seams that will rub or any rough areas inside. All of this will make a child feel different from other children, which he will not like, but is nevertheless essential to keep injuries to a minimum.

3 Pain relief. The open areas of skin will be painful and adequate analgesia will need to be given, particularly at times of dressing changes. Start with paracetamol an hour before dressings are changed (you may need to use co-proxamol rather than paracetamol).

4 Treatment of secondary infection. If there is secondary infection of blisters and erosions, a systemic antibiotic will need to be given. Topical antibiotics should be avoided because of the risk of sensitization after a period of time.

5 Systemic treatment. There is no cure for this condition. Systemic steroids, phenytoin, retinoids and vitamin E have all been tried in the past but none have stood the test of time.

6 Genetic counselling. Once the diagnosis has been established, the mode of inheritance will need to be explained to the parents (and later to the patient) so that they can make an informed decision about further pregnancies. For some varieties of epidermolysis bullosa prenatal diagnosis is now possible. In some cultures the knowledge that a disease is inherited will be grounds for divorce and this may be difficult to handle.

7 Support for parents. The whole family will need a lot of support to cope with a child with anything but the very mildest kind of epidermolysis bullosa. Health visitors and district nurses need to be brought in early and if possible should liaise not just with the family and general practitioner, but also with the hospital. It will be helpful if they can go to the hospital before the child comes home to see how the dressings are done and the kind and amounts that are needed.

It is sensible to put parents in touch with DEBRA, a self-help group for patients and their families (and if possible another family nearby who are coping with the same thing):

DYSTROPHIC EPIDERMOLYSIS BULLOSA
RESEARCH ASSOCIATION (DEBRA)
Suite 4, 1 Kings Road
Crowthorne
Berkshire, RG11 4BG
Tel: 0344 771 961

ERYSIPELAS

Patients with erysipelas are best treated in hospital since they are constitutionally unwell and intravenous benzyl penicillin, 600 mg 6 hourly, is the treatment of choice. The cause is a group A β-haemolytic streptococcus (*see* Figure 18, page 34) which is always sensitive to penicillin. If the patient is allergic to penicillin, erythromycin 500 mg orally every 6 hours is an alternative. With adequate treatment, the patient should be dramatically better within 24 hours. If he is not, the diagnosis is probably wrong. There is no place for the use of ampicillin, flucloxacillin or other broad spectrum antibiotics in the treatment of erysipelas.

ERYTHEMA CHRONICUM MIGRANS (LYME DISEASE)

Outbreaks of Lyme disease tend to occur in late May and early June when the ticks leave the ground vegetation to feed on their animal hosts (deer and sheep) and wander onto humans by mistake. If suspected the diagnosis can be confirmed by finding antibodies to

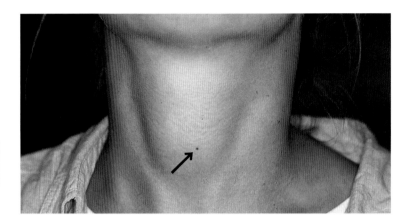

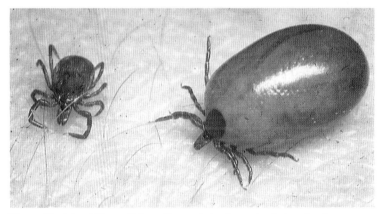

Figure 57 (*above*) Sheep tick on the neck to show size before feeding (approximately 3 mm). The risk of infection with *Borrelia burgdorferi* is low if the tick is removed quickly. To remove ticks—spray with diethyltoluamide (insect repellent) or cover with butter or margarine. Courtesy of Dr Sue O'Connell.

Figure 58 (*below*) Adult female sheep tick *Ixodes ricinus* before (*left*) and after (*right*) feeding. These ticks feed on blood, but only do so once in each stage of their life cycle, ie once as a larva, once as a nymph and once as an adult. The adult enlarges to the size of a coffee bean after feeding. Courtesy of Dr Sue O'Connell.

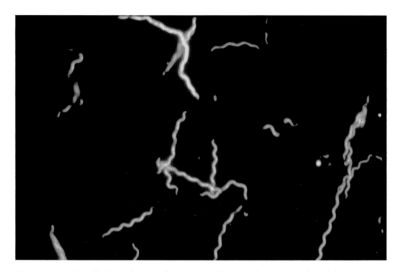

Figure 59 *Borrelia burgdorferi*, the cause of Lyme disease, isolated from an infected tick. Courtesy of Dr Sue O'Connell.

the spirochaete in the patient's serum. There should be a fourfold rise in antibody titre over 2–3 weeks to be significant. The antibody (ELISA) test can be done at your local District General Hospital.

Oral oxytetracycline 250 mg four times a day for 10–14 days is the treatment of choice. In children under the age of 12, who cannot be given oxytetracycline, phenoxymethylpenicillin (penicillin V), 50 mg/kg body weight/day in divided doses is given instead. If children are allergic to penicillin, they can be given erythromycin 50 mg/kg body weight/day in divided doses for 10–14 days.

Providing treatment is given promptly, there should be no long term problems. If there is a delay in treatment, arthritis (initially intermittent swelling of large joints and later a chronic erosive arthritis), meningoencephalitis, facial nerve palsy and heart problems (conduction defects, myocarditis and pericarditis) can occur weeks to months later. These complications need treatment with intravenous cefotaxime or benzyl penicillin so the patient should be referred to hospital.

ERYTHEMA INFECTIOSUM (FIFTH DISEASE)

This is a self-limiting viral infection which gets better on its own in about a week. It needs no treatment.

ERYTHEMA MULTIFORME

The common variety of this disorder disappears in 10–14 days without any treatment. The patient should be reassured that it is harmless and will get better on its own. There may be ulceration of the mouth as well as the rash on the skin, but this is often asymptomatic and will also heal on its own. The cause should be identified if possible so that recurrent episodes can be avoided. The common causes are:

- viral infections, especially herpes simplex
- immunizations
- bacterial infections, especially streptococcal sore throats
- *Mycoplasma pneumoniae* infection
- drugs—sulphonamides, phenylbutazone and other non-steroidal anti-inflammatory drugs.

The commonest cause of **recurrent erythema multiforme** is recurrent herpes simplex infection. Every time the patient gets a cold sore, he gets erythema multiforme 10–14 days later. Treatment of the herpes simplex with topical acyclovir cream, even if begun as soon as the prodromal symptoms occur, will not usually prevent the erythema multiforme from developing. If such episodes are occurring frequently, (several times a year), it is worth putting the patient onto long-term oral acyclovir 400 mg twice daily for at least 6 months. This will often work for frequent recurrences even if there is no history of herpes simplex.

Severe involvement of mucous membranes, **Stevens-Johnson syndrome**, is just one end of the spectrum of this disease. The causes are exactly the same as for the common variety (*see* page 72) although it is more often due to a drug than an infection. The drug should be identified if possible, and not given again; in our experience co-trimoxazole has been the most frequent culprit.

Such patients should probably be admitted to hospital. Ulceration of the mouth is very unpleasant, making eating virtually impossible and even drinking difficult. Frequent mouth washes with glycerine and thymol (made up by dissolving a glycerine and thymol gargle and mouthwash tablet in a tumbler of water), swished around the mouth for several minutes every hour, or applied on a cotton wool swab by a nurse if the patient cannot manage a mouth wash by himself, will keep the buccal mucosa relatively comfortable. If this is not done, the lips can stick together, which initially will make eating and drinking even more difficult, and will at some stage necessitate surgical separation. Benzydamine hydrochloride (Difflam) or chlorhexidine gluconate (Corsodyl) are alternative mouthwashes.

Frequent bathing of the eyes with normal saline and insertion of artificial tears (hypromellose eye drops) will be needed to keep them comfortable.

If there are extensive skin lesions as well as extensive mucosal involvement, the patient may need nursing in a burns unit where there are facilities to prevent ulceration of the skin. There is no evidence that systemic steroids are helpful in this condition. Fortunately it is not common.

ERYTHEMA NODOSUM

Unless the patient rests with the legs up, new crops of nodules will continue to develop until the disease has run its course. It is not usually practical for the patient to go to bed for 3–6 weeks, but putting the feet up whenever possible will help. Alternatively, wearing support stockings or Tubigrip support bandages will often make the legs feel more comfortable. Oral analgesics will probably be needed to alleviate the discomfort (paracetamol or co-proxamol). If an underlying cause has been identified, this also may need treatment (see below).

Common causes of erythema nodosum

Sarcoid
Streptococcal sore throat
Drugs, eg sulphonamides and the pill
Pregnancy
Tuberculosis
Ulcerative colitis and Crohn's disease
Numerous other viral, bacterial and fungal infections

ERYTHRASMA

Erythromycin 250 mg orally four times a day for 14 days will clear erythrasma at any site. Nothing needs to be applied to the skin.

ERYTHRODERMA (EXFOLIATIVE DERMATITIS)

Patients with this should be referred urgently to a dermatologist and may well need admission to hospital. Heat loss through the red skin can cause hypothermia, and malabsorption may cause anaemia. In patients over the age of 50 years, high output cardiac failure and renal failure may also occur.

- If the underlying cause is eczema it can be treated with a 1% hydrocortisone ointment (on the face) and 0.025% betamethasone valerate (Betnovate RD) ointment on the trunk and limbs twice a day.
- If it is due to psoriasis, it must **not** be treated with tar or dithranol or it is likely to get a lot worse, and may be changed to generalized pustular psoriasis. Bed rest and emollients only should be applied (white soft paraffin or aqueous cream). If it does not settle with that, the patient may need systemic treatment with methotrexate (*see* page 161).
- If it is due to a drug rash, the drug must be stopped.
- If it is due to a lymphoma or carcinoma, that will need treating before the skin will get better.

FISH TANK GRANULOMA

Tropical fish infected with *Mycobacterium marinum* die. In their owners it can cause a chronic granuloma in the skin (Figure 60) usually after cleaning out the fish tank when one of the fish has died. In removing the dead fish, the owner can scrape the back of his hand on the gravel at the bottom of the tank and so implant the atypical mycobacterium into his skin. Treatment is with co-trimoxazole 960 mg twice a day, or minocycline 100 mg twice a day until the skin heals (usually 6–12 weeks). He should be advised to remove dead fish wearing rubber gloves in the future.

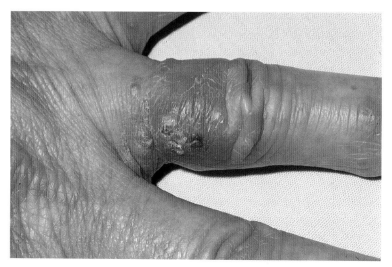

Figure 60 Fish tank granuloma.

FOLLICULITIS

Swabs should be taken from a pustule and from any possible carriage site of *Staphylococcus aureus* (anterior nares, perianal skin, or any rash) for bacteriology culture. Topical mupirocin, fucidic acid or neomycin ointment is then applied, not just where the pustules are, but also to the carriage site(s) four times a day for 14 days.

If these measures do not work, or the patient also has boils or carbuncles, he will need an oral antibiotic too; flucloxacillin or erythromycin, 250 mg four times a day for a week. Sometimes the folliculitis reoccurs when the antibiotics are stopped. A further longer course (4–8 weeks) may be needed.

If the folliculitis has been caused by the application of a greasy ointment to the skin (eg a topical steroid ointment), this should be stopped or changed to a cream. If it has been caused by a tar preparation on the skin, this should be stopped until the folliculitis clears, and an alternative treatment sought for the future.

FOLLICULITIS DECALVANS

This is a chronic infection of the hair follicles with *Staphylococcus aureus*, which leads to a scarring alopecia. Once scarring has occurred the hair will not regrow. It is important therefore to start treatment as soon as possible to minimize the hair loss. Long-term oral antibiotics are required. Flucloxacillin 250 mg four times a day, or Septrin two tablets twice a day can be given for several months. Treatment may have to be continued for 2–3 years, in which case Septrin is more suitable than flucloxacillin.

FORDYCE SPOTS

These are extremely common and completely harmless. They need no treatment. If the patient is anxious he should be reassured.

FRECKLES (EPHELIDES)

Freckles are normal in individuals with type 1 skin (red or fair hair and blue eyes, who burn rather than tan in the sun). Nothing needs doing about the freckles themselves but the patient should be advised about protective sunscreens in the summer, both to prevent sunburn now, and to prevent skin cancer in the future (*see* page 140).

GANGLION

No treatment is usually needed. They can be removed by an orthopaedic surgeon if they are a nuisance.

GENERALIZED PRURITUS

The management of generalized pruritus depends on finding out why the patient is itching when there is no rash to see. Treatment is then of the underlying cause. A full physical examination is essential and if no abnormality is found, a few simple tests are required to try to sort out the cause. We suggest the following:

Investigation	Disease it will pick up
Full blood count Hb WBC and differential ESR	Anaemia, polycythaemia Eosinophilia—worms and reactions to drugs Leucopenia, AIDS Carcinoma, myeloma, infections
Vickers profile Urea and electrolytes Liver function tests	Renal failure Obstructive jaundice
Serum ferritin	Iron deficiency
Serum thyroxine	Hypothyroidism Hyperthyroidism
Auto-immune profile	Thyroid disease Primary biliary cirrhosis
Chest X-ray	Carcinoma of the bronchus Enlarged lymph nodes in a lymphoma
MSU	Diabetes

AIDS

The non-specific itching of AIDS is often helped by ultraviolet light (UVB) two or three times a week (as for psoriasis, *see* page 172 and 173).

Anaemia

If the patient has iron deficiency anaemia, the reason for this must be sought. In a woman it may just be that she is not having sufficient iron in the diet to replace the monthly menstrual loss, but in a man there must always be some other reason, eg bleeding or malabsorption. The cause of the anaemia should be dealt with and the iron deficiency treated with oral iron. Ferrous sulphate, 200 mg three times a day, should be given until the haemoglobin is back to normal and for a further 4 months to replace the body's iron stores. The itching will stop as the haemoglobin rises.

Carcinoma

In the elderly particularly, itching with nothing to see may be due to an underlying carcinoma. Taking a good history is the most important thing to do. If nothing comes to light with this, it is probably worth doing a few non-invasive tests like a chest X-ray and faecal occult bloods.

A more likely cause of itching in this age group is drying out of the skin, which can be alleviated with emollients in the bath and applied topically (*see* page 50).

Diabetes

Occasionally diabetes will present with itching. Usually it is in the flexures and it is due to infection with *Candida albicans*. Always test the urine for sugar in someone who is itching for no apparent reason.

Infestations

(i) Body lice. These will be found along the seams of the clothes. Ordinary washing and ironing of the clothes will eradicate them.
(ii) Onchocerciasis. In patients who have lived or worked overseas, it is important to remember that they may have worms of various kinds. Referral to a doctor with some expertise in tropical medicine is necessary. A high eosinophil count will alert you to the possibility of an infestation.

Jaundice

Itching is a common feature of obstructive jaundice due to deposition of bile salts in the skin (it does not occur with haemolytic anaemia). Itching may occur before the jaundice is obvious clinically. If the obstruction is due to gall stones or a tumour, surgery is required. If it is due to primary biliary cirrhosis, cholestyramine, which binds bile acids in the gut and interferes with their absorption, can be given at a dose of 4–8 g daily. This is usually very helpful in controlling the itching.

Lymphoma

Clinical lymphadenopathy or enlarged lymph nodes on chest X-ray, ± hepatosplenomegaly suggests a diagnosis of lymphoma in an otherwise asymptomatic young adult. Itching may be the first symptom to occur. Referral to an oncologist is essential.

Polycythaemia rubra vera

Characteristically this causes itching when the patient is in the bath. Referral to a haematologist is recommended.

Psychological upset

Many patients itch due to anxiety, depression or an emotional upset. However likely you think that is as the cause, you must also rule out all the physical causes of pruritus or some easily remedial cause can be missed. All types of itching can be made worse by emotional stress.

Renal failure

The itching of end-stage renal failure will make the patient's life a misery. It occurs in 86% of patients on maintenance haemodialysis. Erythropoietin 36 units/kg body weight iv three times a week produces a dramatic improvement after 3–4 weeks. Once better, the dose can be halved but it then needs to be continued indefinitely. Ultraviolet light (UVB) daily or three times a week helps some patients, assuming they are well enough to get to a local hospital for it (*see* pages 172 and 173). Topical steroids and oral antihistamines on the whole are useless.

Thyroid disease

Both hypothyroidism and hyperthyroidism can present with generalized pruritus. As long as you aware of this and do the relevant test, you will not miss it. The itching will stop as the thyroid function returns to normal.

Unknown cause

If no cause is found for the itching, treatment will need to be symptomatic. Start with 10% crotamiton cream twice a day. If it does not help use a topical steroid preparation instead; begin with 1% hydrocortisone and increase the strength to 0.025% betamethasone valerate (Betnovate RD) if necessary. The patient will usually tell you whether he would prefer an ointment or a cream. If the topical steroids do not adequately control the itching and it is interfering with sleep, a sedative antihistamine such as trimeprazine (10–20 mg) or promethazine (25–50 mg) taken about an hour before going to bed may help. The patient will, of course, need to be careful about driving the next day.

GEOGRAPHIC TONGUE

Normally this is asymptomatic. If it is sore, using benzydamine hydrochloride (Difflam) mouthwash several times a day may make it feel more comfortable.

GLOMUS TUMOUR

These are quite safe to leave alone. If they are causing a lot of pain they can be excised under a local anaesthetic.

GOUTY TOPHI

Allopurinol competitively inhibits the enzyme xanthine oxidase, which oxidizes xanthine and hypoxanthine to uric acid. It causes a rapid fall in serum uric acid. Start with 100 mg daily as a single oral dose, and gradually increase to 300–400 mg a day which will need to be continued indefinitely. By gradually increasing the dose you will hope to avoid precipitating acute attacks of gout at the beginning of treatment. If this does occur, give indomethacin 25 mg three times a day for 4–6 weeks. In the long term the tophi will gradually become smaller and disappear.

GRANULOMA ANNULARE

If it is asymptomatic, which it usually is, the patient can be reassured that it is harmless and will eventually go away on its own. It may take quite a long time, months or even years rather than weeks. If it is painful, injection of triamcinolone hexacetonide (Lederspan) 5 mg/ml intralesionally will stop the pain and may make it go away (an alternative is triamcinolone acetonide [Adcortyl] 10 mg/ml).

GRANULOMA FISSURATUM

The patient should take their spectacles back to the optician and get the ear pieces or nasal pads adjusted so that they fit more comfortably.

GRANULOMA INGUINALE

Oxytetracycline 500 mg four times a day is given for 3 weeks. Alternatives are trimethoprim 200 mg twice daily or doxycycline 100 mg twice daily for 21 days.

HABIT TIC NAIL DEFORMITY

Most people with this have no idea that they are damaging their own nails until you point it out to them. Once they realize what they are doing, they can usually stop, although it may be necessary to enlist the help of other members of their family to help them. If they need more help than that, covering the affected nail and cuticle with elastoplast can be helpful.

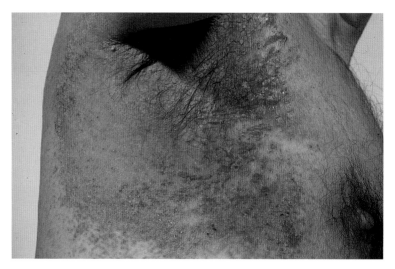

Figure 61 Hailey-Hailey disease and herpes simplex. The blistering is worse than normal, but the severe pain is the thing that should alert you to the possibility of 2° infection with herpes simplex.

HAILEY-HAILEY DISEASE

This disease typically remits and relapses. It is exacerbated by friction, heat, secondary infection with *Staphylococcus aureus*, *Candida albicans*, or herpes simplex and by stress. The patient complains of itching, pain and smell. There may be long periods when the patient is entirely asymptomatic, especially in the winter, but most patients find it a great social handicap. Some patients will need to have time off work when the pain is at its worst.

Wet dressings of potassium permanganate applied to the affected areas once or several times a day, or soaking in a bath containing a pale pink solution of potassium permanganate (Figure 47, page 62) will be all that some patients need. This will dry up the exudate and make them feel more comfortable.

Other patients will need to apply topical steroids. They should use the weakest possible steroid which is effective so as to reduce the risk of skin atrophy in the flexures. This often means using one of the moderately potent group of steroids such as 0.05% clobetasone butyrate (Eumovate), or 0.025% betamethasone valerate (Betnovate RD) cream or ointment twice a day. Once the symptoms are under control, the frequency and strength of steroid application can be reduced.

Secondary infection should be treated early. Infection with *Staphylococcus aureus* is treated with oral flucloxacillin 250 mg four times a day for a week. *Candida* infection is treated with one of the imidazole creams (eg miconazole cream) or nystatin ointment. Severe pain is usually indicative of secondary infection with herpes simplex. This can be confirmed by taking some blister fluid for viral culture, or a Tzanck smear looking for multinucleate giant cells. If herpes simplex is found, oral acyclovir, 200 mg five times a day should be given for 5 days. This will stop the pain almost immediately.

Rarely the above measures will not be helpful and the patient will need systemic steroids, methotrexate, superficial X-ray treatment or even surgical excision of the affected areas.

Since this condition is inherited as an autosomal dominant trait, the rest of the family should be examined, and the patient and his family advised about the genetics (*see* page 90).

HALO NAEVUS

This lesion is usually brought to the doctor's attention because the patient or his parents are worried because of the uneven pigmentation, thinking that it must be a malignant melanoma. It is in fact a perfectly harmless mole and everyone concerned can be reassured that it is not premalignant. When the halo appears around the mole it is often a sign that the mole itself is going to disappear. It will then leave a round white patch which will also go in time.

HAND, FOOT AND MOUTH DISEASE

This condition lasts only a few days, is usually asymptomatic and needs no treatment. It has nothing to do with foot and mouth disease in animals and patients do not need to be isolated.

HEREDITARY HAEMORRHAGIC TELANGIECTASIA

The skin lesions do not need any treatment. Nose bleeds may need cauterizing if they will not stop with ordinary pressure. Anaemia due to recurrent bleeding from the nose or gastrointestinal tract will need treating with oral iron. The familial nature of the disorder should be explained to the patient and his family: it is inherited as an autosomal dominant condition (*see* page 90).

HERPANGINA

Usually no treatment is needed for this viral infection. If the mouth is very sore, glycerine and thymol mouthwash can be used several times a day until the symptoms subside.

HERPES SIMPLEX

Herpes virus hominis types 1 and 2 (HSV-1 and HSV-2) are DNA viruses which, having infected the skin or mucous membranes, remain latent in the posterior root ganglion for the rest of the patient's life. A characteristic feature of such infections is that they tend to be recurrent. Acyclovir is the treatment of choice when treatment is necessary.

Acyclovir (9–[2-hydroxyethoxymethyl] guanine) inhibits virus DNA synthesis without damaging the host cells. It is able to do this because, in order to become active, it must first be phosphorylated by viral thymidine kinase. It also inhibits virus DNA polymerase (the main enzyme responsible for virus DNA replication).

It is available in the following forms:
- 3% acyclovir eye ointment
- 5% acyclovir cream

- acyclovir tablets, 200 mg, 400 mg and 800 mg
- acyclovir suspension, 200 mg/5 ml
- intravenous acyclovir, 250 mg and 500 mg powder in a vial. Made up by reconstituting 250 mg in 10 ml water or 0.9% normal saline and adding it to 90 ml of infusion fluid (normal saline) which is then given intravenously over 1 hour (250 mg/100 ml = 2.5 mg/ml; the dose is 5 mg/kg body weight i.v. every 8 hours).

Which should be used when will be discussed under the different clinical manifestations of herpes simplex infections.

Primary infection with herpes simplex type 1

In the mouth

Most primary infections are asymptomatic, are not recognized and need no treatment. When symptomatic, however, they produce an acute gingivostomatitis which may prevent the patient from eating and drinking. This will get better without treatment, but it is extremely unpleasant for the patient. Oral acyclovir suspension, 200 mg five times a day if the patient can swallow it, will speed up its resolution (provided treatment is started early—within 24 hours of the onset of symptoms). Occasionally it will be bad enough to warrant intravenous acyclovir if the patient cannot swallow or is generally unwell (see under eczema herpeticum, right).

On the skin

In a patient who is not immunocompromised, and who does not have atopic eczema or one of the autoimmune blistering conditions, no treatment is usually needed. If the patient feels unwell or there is severe pain, oral acyclovir tablets 200 mg five times a day can be given for 5 days. This is only of use if it is started early in the course of the infection (within 24 hours). It is particularly useful

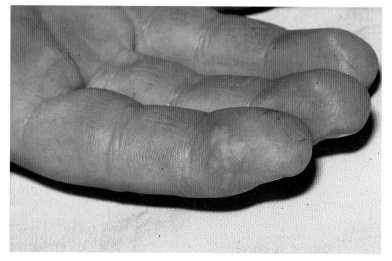

Figure 62 Herpetic whitlow.

for a herpetic whitlow (Figure 62) which characteristically causes exquisite pain.

Eczema herpeticum

Patients with atopic eczema (Figure 41, page 55), pemphigus (Figure 63), pemphigoid or Darier's disease may develop very extensive herpetic lesions with a primary HSV-1 or HSV-2 infection on the skin which occasionally can be life threatening. If the patient is not seriously ill this can be treated with acyclovir orally, 200 mg five times a day for 5 days. If the patient is sick it is better to admit him to hospital so that he can be treated with intravenous acyclovir, 5 mg/kg body weight every 8 hours. This is given slowly over a period of 45–60 minutes to prevent renal damage.

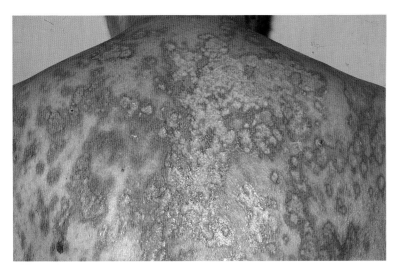

Figure 63 Widespread herpes simplex in a patient with pemphigus; the patient complained of severe pain.

In the eye

3% acyclovir eye ointment is applied five times a day if the patient presents within 24 hours of the onset of symptoms. The associated photophobia is helped by keeping the eye covered between applications of acyclovir.

Recurrent infection with herpes simplex type 1

In the non-immunocompromised host

Most patients with recurrent infections of HSV-1 do not require any treatment. If episodes are extensive or frequent, topical acyclovir can be beneficial. It is most useful in patients who get a prodromal period with itching and/or tingling before the blisters appear. If 5% acyclovir cream is applied at this stage, hourly during the waking hours for 2 days, the attack will usually be cut short, but it will not

prevent further episodes. The patient needs to obtain the cream from the doctor between attacks so that he has it available to use at the start of the prodromal symptoms next time around.

Recurrent erythema multiforme due to recurrent herpes simplex infection

If recurrences are occurring frequently (several times a year) they can be prevented by giving oral acyclovir 400 mg twice daily for at least 6 months; it may have to be continued for a lot longer than this.

In a patient who is immunosuppressed

Recurrent herpes simplex can be a real nuisance in patients with AIDS, leukaemia, lymphoma, carcinoma or those on cytotoxic drugs. Acyclovir should be given topically or systemically at the first sign of infection, depending on the site and extent of the lesions. If episodes are very frequent, oral prophylactic acyclovir can be given, 400 mg twice daily for 6 months or even indefinitely. Very severe infections should be treated promptly with intravenous acyclovir.

Primary infection with herpes simplex type 2

Probably about 50% of primary infections with HSV-2 are asymptomatic. The rest present with localized burning, itching or soreness of the penis, vulva, anus or thighs. Pain may be severe and there may be associated fever, malaise, headache and pain in the back and buttocks. In women there may be dysuria if there are ulcerated lesions on the vulva, and in patients of either sex there can be proctitis with anal infections.

Patients should be seen at a local clinic which specializes in genitourinary medicine. Here the diagnosis can be confirmed virologically, and the presence or absence of other venereal diseases checked for. They are also likely to have some patient information leaflets available which will help to explain to the patient what a herpes infection is and what can be done about it.

In women, oral acyclovir, 200 mg five times a day, should be taken for 5 days because there is almost invariably cervical involvement as well as the superficial lesions. Lignocaine gel can be applied topically to ease the pain.

In men, oral acyclovir is only used if there is a viraemia (the patient feels ill). 5% acyclovir cream can be applied between five and six times a day to the affected area. This will relieve the pain and cut the attack short; it will also decrease the time that the virus will be shed and therefore the time that the patient is infectious. If there is associated lymphadenopathy, there is some evidence that Septrin (trimethoprim 80 mg and sulphamethoxazole 400 mg), two tablets twice a day for 7 days acts synergistically with the topical acyclovir.

The following may be useful to bring symptomatic relief to patients of either sex.

- Soak the area in normal saline (1 tablespoon of salt in a pint of water) for 10 minutes twice a day.
- Put salt or potassium permanganate in the bath water and have a bath twice a day.
- If there is ulceration of the vulva, apply a small strip of Jelonet to prevent the labia minora from sticking together.
- Take aspirin or paracetamol for the pain.
- Apply ice packs to the affected area several times a day (ice cubes wrapped in a clean handkerchief).
- Urinate in a warm bath if there is dysuria.
- Leave the affected area open if at all possible to avoid rubbing from clothes.
- Avoid sexual intercourse until it is better.

Recurrent infection with herpes simplex type 2

Not all patients who have had a primary infection with HSV-2 will get recurrent episodes. For those who do, it is usually a lot less severe than the primary episode. Bathing in normal saline will facilitate healing in 3–4 days in most patients. If healing is delayed for 6–7 days it is worth treating with 5% acyclovir cream as for a primary attack.

In some patients recurrent episodes cause a lot of pain and this may ruin their sex life by causing dyspareunia, frigidity and impotence. If such patients are getting very frequent attacks, long-term prophylaxis with oral acyclovir, 400 mg twice daily can sometimes be justified.

There are two self-help groups for patients with HSV-2 infections:

THE HERPES ASSOCIATION
41 North Road
London, N7 9DP
Tel: 071 609 9061

WOMEN'S HEALTH AND REPRODUCTIVE
RIGHTS INFORMATION CENTRE
52–54 Featherstone Street
London, EC1Y 8RT
Tel: 071 251 6580

Herpes simplex type 2 infections in pregnancy

A primary infection with HSV-2 in the first 3 months of pregnancy can cause infection in the fetus and lead to spontaneous abortion.

If there is active infection with HSV-2 at the time of birth, the child should be delivered by Caesarean section to prevent neonatal herpetic encephalitis.

The use of acyclovir during pregnancy and lactation

Acyclovir is not teratogenic or mutagenic in animals, so it is probably safe to give it during pregnancy. It will normally only be given for serious or life-threatening infections at this time. Given during lactation, acyclovir will be present in the mother's breast milk; since it is not harmful to babies this probably does not matter.

Association of herpes simplex type 2 with carcinoma of the cervix

There is a considerable body of evidence to suggest that genital infection with HSV-2 is one of the causative factors in the development of carcinoma of the cervix. Other factors include early age of first coitus, multiple sexual partners and infection with genital warts. Patients who fit into one or more of these groups should have regular cervical smears taken.

HERPES ZOSTER

Oral acyclovir, 800 mg five times a day for 7 days, works well for herpes zoster causing more rapid healing of the skin lesions and speedy resolution of the pain. In order to work it needs to be given as early as possible in the course of the disease, certainly within 72 hours of the onset of the rash, and preferably earlier than that. Only about 20% of the dose is absorbed when acyclovir is given orally, so high dosage is needed to be effective in herpes zoster.

This makes it a very expensive treatment. It should it be given to:
1 Any patient who is seen while they still have the prodromal symptoms (pain +/or paraesthesia) or who have had blisters for less than 24 hours. The pain of herpes zoster is miserable at any age and the sooner it can be stopped the better.
2 All patients over the age of 70 because they have a very high incidence of post-herpetic neuralgia. There is some evidence that patients with severe pain during the acute phase are more likely to go on getting pain long-term.
3 All patients with ophthalmic herpes zoster. If there is vesiculation along the side of the nose in association with herpes zoster on the forehead (involvement of the nasociliary branch of V^1), there will almost certainly be involvement of the eye. Conjunctivitis, episcleritis, keratitis, corneal ulceration, iritis and glaucoma can all occur in the acute stage. In the long-term there may be scarring of the surrounding skin, ectropion, entropion, scleral atrophy, dendritic ulcers on the cornea (looking very like herpes simplex) and cataract formation. Early treatment will prevent these from occurring. Patients with eye involvement should see an ophthalmologist so that other symptomatic treatment can also be given.
4 Patients who are immunosuppressed for any reason.

Adequate analgesia will be needed for the pain and should be taken regularly. Paracetamol, 1 g every 4 hours or co-proxamol, two tablets every 4 hours will usually be sufficient. The blistered areas should be kept dry by using a few crystals of potassium permanganate in the bath water (enough to make the water go a pale pink colour—see Figure 17, page 62). Topical steroids and topical antibiotics should not be used; if a topical preparation is needed, calamine lotion is as good as anything.

While blisters are present, patients with herpes zoster are infectious to anyone who has not had chickenpox (a patient cannot get herpes zoster from contact with chickenpox, since it is a recrudescence of a previous infection from the patient's own dorsal root ganglion). As a rule it is better to get chickenpox as a child, so patients with herpes zoster do not necessarily need to avoid contact with children unless there are family reasons for the child not getting chickenpox at that particular time (eg holidays).

Treatment of recurrent herpes zoster in patients who are immunosuppressed

Individual episodes can be treated with oral acyclovir, 800 mg five times a day for 7 days. After the first time these patients will know when it is occurring because they will recognize the prodromal symptoms. If they have a supply of acyclovir at home they can start them at the first signs of recurrence. If recurrent attacks are occurring very frequently, they may need to be on long-term oral acyclovir as for herpes simplex (*see* page 81).

If the patient has generalized herpes zoster he will need to be in hospital so that he can be treated with a slow intravenous infusion of acyclovir at a dose of 10 mg/kg body weight every 8 hours for 7 days. This is more likely to be effective than oral treatment.

Treatment of post-herpetic neuralgia

This is a very difficult condition to treat. Straightforward analgesics do not work well although they are often taken for months and years. Carbamazepine, starting at a dose of 100 mg twice a day and gradually increasing until the pain is controlled, is the best of the treatments available. Most patients will need something like 200–300 mg three or four times a day, although a few will need as much as 1600 mg/day. Stellate ganglion block may be helpful for uncontrolled pain following trigeminal zoster.

HIDRADENITIS SUPPURITIVA

Minor degrees of hidradenitis can be controlled by long-term, low-dose antibiotics. Erythromycin, 250 mg twice daily or Septrin, one or two tablets twice a day, given over a period of years will keep some patients free of disease. There will be no effect for at least 3 months so the antibiotic, once started, should be continued for at least this long before considering a change.

If antibiotics do not work, the alternatives are oral etretinate or surgery.

1 Etretinate used at a dose of 0.5–1 mg/kg body weight/day will give an improvement after 8 weeks. It will need to be continued for 6–12 months. This drug is only available on hospital prescriptions and has numerous side effects (*see* page 168). It should not be given to women who might want to get pregnant because it is teratogenic (a woman must be off etretinate for 2 years before it is safe for her to conceive because etretinate has a very long half life).

2 Surgery. All the apocrine glands in the affected area need to be removed. Excision of the abnormal skin together with the underlying sinuses and abscesses is often a major undertaking. In the axillae it is often possible to excise the affected area and close the defect as a primary procedure. In the perineum that is not usually possible, so the patient will be left with a large open wound which is left to granulate up on its own. Although a major undertaking at the time, in the long term, it is often a very worthwhile procedure, leaving the patient pain-free and smell-free.

HIRSUTISM

How much facial hair is cosmetically acceptable in an individual is dependent on many factors, but particularly the patient's country of origin. What is considered normal in many parts of Southern Europe is deemed unacceptable in the UK.

Apart from not liking the look of the excess hair, many women with hirsutism are afraid that they are turning into men. This anxiety will not be helped by the doctor advising them to shave. However much or little hair is present, the patient needs dealing with kindly and sympathetically.

The amount of hair on the face, breasts and lower abdomen in women is under androgen control. Testosterone produced by the ovary is converted to dihydrotestosterone in the skin by the action of 5-alpha reductase and it is this which causes the increase in hair. It is always worth checking the serum testosterone level. If it is more than 5 nmol/l, the patient should be referred to an endocrinologist for a full endocrine work up. If it is less, there is no point in doing any other investigations. On the basis of this one test it is easy to reassure most women that they are not (and will not be in the future) changing sex. Many of them have polycystic ovaries but this does not require any specific treatment.

By the time the patient seeks help from the doctor she will usually have tried all the simple things that do not require medical advice. If she has not, the following are available and may be helpful.

1 Bleaching the hairs with lemon juice or hydrogen peroxide. For patients whose hair is very dark, bleaching will often disguise them enough to be cosmetically acceptable.

2 Depilatory creams. These mainly contain barium sulphide which dissolves keratin. In some patients these creams will make the skin sore by a direct irritant effect; they can also cause a contact allergic eczema and folliculitis. All of these will limit their usefulness.

3 Waxing and sugaring. These are basically methods of mass plucking of hairs. Hot wax or a thick sugar solution is applied to the hairy area of skin; it is allowed to cool, and then peeled off pulling

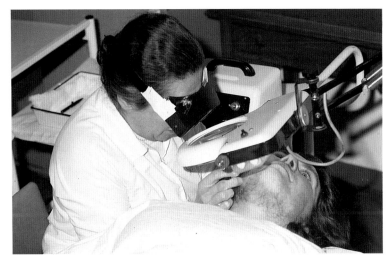

Figure 64 Electrolysis.

the hairs out at the same time. Both methods are available from reputable beauticians. If patients can afford it, this method is suitable for removal of excess hair from the legs and body as well as the face.

4 Plucking and shaving. A surprising number of women still remove unwanted hair by plucking and shaving. Most do not like doing it but they are usually not aware that there are any other remedies available, or they have tried depilatory creams but found that they made their skin too sore.

5 Electrolysis. If the amount of unwanted hair is not too extensive, electrolysis and epilation using a short wave diathermy machine can provide a permanent answer. A fine sterile needle is placed into the hair follicle down to the level of the papilla. A high-frequency alternating current is then passed through the needle for a minuscule period of time. This destroys the papilla permanently and the hair is lifted out without pain. This process works well but is rather time-consuming and expensive. Patients should be careful to be treated by practitioners who are members of the Institute of Electrologists or the Association of Electrologists. Some hospitals provide an electrolysis service under the NHS but many do not.

6 **Anti-androgens.** If there is extensive hirsutism it is worth considering **cyproterone acetate**. This is an anti-androgen which competes with dihydrotestosterone at the hair follicle. Cyproterone acetate 100 mg daily is given on days 5–14 of the menstrual cycle together with ethinyl oestradiol 50 µg on days 5–25 of the cycle. It will be 3–6 months before any noticeable effect is seen. After about 18 months it may be possible to change to a lower dose of cyproterone acetate in the form of the contraceptive pill, Dianette (contains 2 mg cyproterone acetate and 35 µg ethinyl oestradiol), and keep control of the hirsutism. Dianette does not contain enough cyproterone acetate to reverse the excessive hair growth but it may contain enough to keep it under control once the process has been reversed. In patients with extensive hirsutism it may be necessary to keep them on a high dose cyproterone acetate indefinitely. Monitoring of such patients is the same as for women on the contraceptive pill. Do not prescribe this treatment for women who smoke, are hypertensive or have a strong family history of cardiovascular disease or breast cancer. Side effects include weight gain, nausea, depression, headaches and loss of libido.

There is no right answer to this problem which will work for all patients. You will have to discuss the various options with each individual to see which is likely to be the most helpful for her.

HISTIOCYTOMA (DERMATOFIBROMA)

These are completely harmless and the patient can be reassured that they are not malignant and have no malignant potential. They can be excised under a local anaesthetic if they are a nuisance.

HYPERHIDROSIS

Eccrine sweat glands are present in the skin over the whole body surface but they are particularly concentrated on the palms, soles and axillae. Sweating at these sites is often determined by emotion rather than heat. However, in most patients who are complaining of hyperhidrosis, there are no obvious emotional factors involved. Sweat glands are enervated from the sympathetic nervous system but the mediator is acetylcholine. Anti-cholinergic drugs are not often used because in a dose that would be effective in stopping sweating they have too many other side effects (dry mouth, blurred vision etc).

Symptoms usually begin in childhood or at puberty. The sites most commonly involved are the hands, feet, axillae or any combination of these. Treatment is different at the individual sites.

Hyperhidrosis of the axillae

The problem here is of social embarrassment due to staining of the clothes, the need to change the clothes frequently because they are wet, or rotting of the clothes leading to considerable expense. The options available for treatment are:

1 20% aluminium chloride hexahydrate in absolute (or 95%) alcohol. Aluminium ions block sweat ducts; they migrate down sweat ducts and are deposited in the lumen. This effect is only temporary and the ducts become patent again after a few days. The aluminium ions are most available in aluminium chloride hexahydrate. There is, however, an equilibrium between the aluminium ions and the salt and water.

$$AlCl_3.6H_2O + H_2O \rightleftharpoons Al^{+++}.6H_2O + 3Cl^- + H^+ + (OH^-)$$

As you can see from the formula, the dissociation produces both aluminium ions and hydrochloric acid (H^+Cl^-) in association with water. For this reason it is important that the treatment is applied to a dry axilla. If it is wet, the aluminium ions will not be able to migrate down the sweat ducts because sweat is coming out, and the chlorine ions will combine with the water in the sweat to form hydrochloric acid, which will make the skin very sore. It is best used at night just before the patient is going to bed. The axilla is carefully dried before it is applied. The skin can be washed normally the next morning without problem. This treatment is applied every night for about a week, and then only when the sweating returns (usually about every 7–21 days). If there is irritation of the axillary skin, this can be relieved by the application of 1% hydrocortisone cream the next morning.

It takes a long time to dissolve aluminium chloride hexahydrate in alcohol (about 3 weeks), so pharmacists are not too keen on doing it. Fortunately it is now available ready made as:

- Anhydrol Forte (in a roll-on bottle)
- Driclor (in a roll-on bottle).

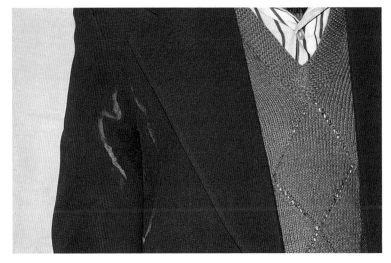

Figure 65 Hyperhidrosis of the axillae can ruin a person's clothes.

A similar preparation, aluminium hydroxychloride, is also available in a roll-on bottle or as a cream (Hyperdrol).

All of these products are flammable and also need to be kept away from jewellery, clothes and polished surfaces.

Commercially available antiperspirants contain aluminium hypochlorite which work well for normal individuals but are ineffective for those with hyperhidrosis. Aluminium hypochlorite is a weak alkali which does not produce hydrochloric acid on dissociation and therefore does not cause soreness of the skin.

2 Surgery. Removal of the axillary vault will remove most of the eccrine sweat glands and so stop sweating. This is normally done under a general anaesthetic.

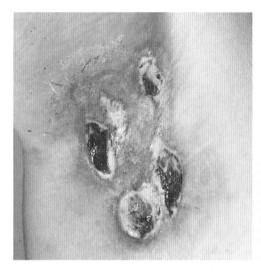

Figure 66 Hyperhidrosis of the axilla treated with cryotherapy. One month later the treated area is still ulcerated. The long-term result was good, but the wounds took about 3 months to heal.

3 Cryotherapy (Figure 66). The eccrine sweat glands can be destroyed by freezing using a cryoprobe. This is an alternative to surgical removal, and what is available locally will depend on the expertise of your surgeons. Both probably work equally well.

4 Sympathectomy. A sympathectomy will completely abolish sweating in the denervated area. Endoscopic transthoracic cervical sympathectomy using an electrocautery to destroy the sympathetic chain will stop sweating of the axilla and palm on that side. Alternatively, excision of the upper thoracic chain (T_{2-4}) will do the same. Both methods can produce a Horner's syndrome.

Hyperhidrosis of the hands and feet

Excessive sweating on the palms can cause problems for a child at school because the ink will run on their school books. The child will often have to put a handkerchief or towel under their hand while writing to mop up the sweat and even so will be hard pressed to keep work neat and tidy. The sweat may also drip from the ends of the fingers at other times and shaking hands is a nightmare. On the feet, shoes and socks can be ruined by the sweat which results in a lot of expense for the patient. Possible methods of treatment include:

1 An alcoholic solution of 20% aluminium chloride hexahydrate (*see* page 87). This is not nearly as useful on the hands and feet as it is in the axillae because it is not usually possible to get them dry enough. It is worth a try however before other measures are tried.

2 5% formaldehyde soaks. For sweaty feet, formalin soaks for 10 minutes once or twice a day are often helpful. It is no good for the hands.

3 Iontophoresis. This involves passing an electric current through tap water or a solution of an anti-cholinergic agent into the skin. Most hospital physiotherapy departments have a direct current apparatus suitable for doing this. It is a useful treatment for both hands and feet. To start with, it is done once a week but once the extremities are dry, the frequency can be reduced to only once every 6–8 weeks.

4 Sympathectomy. For treatment of palmar sweating—*see* left. Lumbar sympathectomy will abolish hyperhidrosis of the feet. It might be worth trying a phenol nerve block of the lumbar sympathetic chain first to see whether a worthwhile effect will be produced.

5 Oral anti-cholinergic drugs. These are not recommended for hyperhidrosis at any site. In order to be effective, doses which cause dryness of the mouth, dilated pupils, blurred vision, constipation and difficulty with micturition have to be given. They are not therefore very practical.

HYPERTRICHOSIS

There is no simple answer to this problem. If it is due to a drug (cyclosporin A, diazoxide, diphenylhydantoin, minocycline, penicillamine or one of the psoralens), and it is possible to stop the drug, the hypertrichosis will be reversible, although it may take up to a year for the hairiness to disappear. Cyclosporin A and diazoxide cause hypertrichosis in everyone; this will always be a problem in females taking them. The other drugs only cause it occasionally.

Bleaching dark hairs with lemon juice or hydrogen peroxide will make them less noticeable. Sugaring can remove the hairs but it will need to be done regularly. A thick syrupy sugar solution is applied to the hairy skin, allowed to dry and then pulled off. In most parts of the country there are beauticians offering this service. It is not available under the NHS.

HYPERTROPHIC SCAR

A hypertrophic scar can be flattened off by:

1 Direct pressure over the scar. A pad of Lyofoam strapped onto the skin with Elastoplast or Micropore will often produce flattening of a scar over several months (if the patient will stay patient for long enough!).

2 Injecting a steroid into it. Triamcinolone hexacetonide, 5 mg/ml (Lederspan) is injected directly into the scar through a 21 gauge needle. It is important to use a fairly large needle or it will be impossible to get the steroid to go into the scar (it will otherwise squirt out between the needle and syringe into your face), at least on the first occasion. The amount of triamcinolone injected will depend on the size of the scar. For a scar which is less than 2 cm long, 0.2–0.3 ml of triamcinolone is sufficient. It is best to err on the side of caution since if too much steroid is injected, dermal atrophy will occur and this is irreversible. If adequate flattening does not occur, it can be repeated once a month until a satisfactory cosmetic result is obtained. Even quite large scars can be treated like this if the patient can cope with the injections. EMLA cream (under polythene occlusion) can be applied to the scar for 90 minutes before the injection to lessen the discomfort in patients with a low pain threshold.

ICHTHYOSIS

The vast majority of patients with ichthyosis will have one of the genetically determined varieties (*see* Table 4, below). A very small minority will have acquired ichthyosis (*see* page 94).

Table 4 Varieties of genetically determined ichthyosis

Autosomal dominant	X-linked recessive	Autosomal recessive
1 Ichthyosis vulgaris	1 Sex-linked ichthyosis	1 Lamellar ichthyosis
2 Bullous ichthyosiform erythroderma		2 Non-bullous ichthyosiform erythroderma
3 Ichthyosis hystrix		

It is important to understand the genetics of these conditions in order to explain the inheritance to the patient and his family.

Autosomal dominant

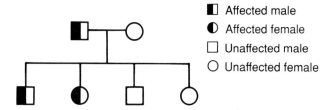

◧ Affected male
◐ Affected female
☐ Unaffected male
○ Unaffected female

Autosomal dominant conditions manifest themselves in the heterozygote individual (◧ ◐). An affected person only needs to receive the abnormal gene from one parent and he (or she) will then pass it on to half of his children irrespective of their sex. The disorder will be seen in each successive generation. An individual who is unaffected cannot pass it on to his children.

Autosomal recessive

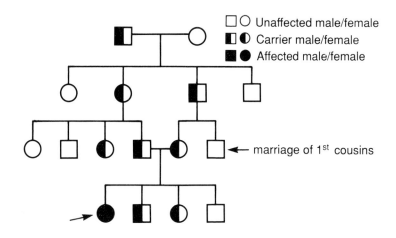

☐○ Unaffected male/female
◧◐ Carrier male/female
■● Affected male/female

◀— marriage of 1ˢᵗ cousins

In the recessive types of ichthyosis the disease is seen only in the homozygous state (■ ●); heterozygous individuals (◧ ◐) are carriers. Affected children need to receive the abnormal gene from both parents; such parents are clinically normal but are usually related to each other. In the pedigree shown above, you can see the marriage of first cousins to produce one affected child (arrowed), two carriers and one normal child, giving what you would expect, one child in four with the disorder. Recessive conditions are seen in siblings but skip generations.

X-linked recessive

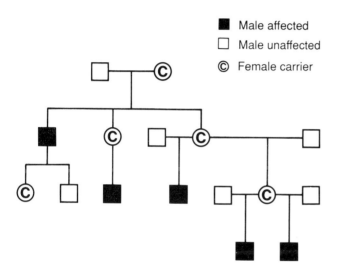

■ Male affected
□ Male unaffected
ⓒ Female carrier

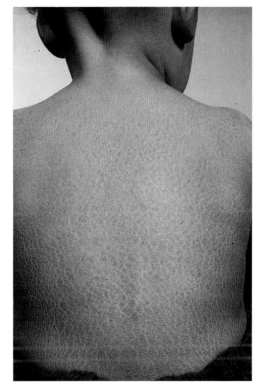

Figure 67 X-linked ichthyosis.

X-linked conditions show themselves only in males and are transmitted by clinically normal females. The parents of boys with X-linked ichthyosis will have a normal skin, but all daughters of such a patient will be carriers. The abnormal gene is carried on the X chromosome. Because the male has only one X chromosome, if it is abnormal he will have the disease. A female has two Xs. If one of these is abnormal she is not affected, but will be a carrier. If both are abnormal she too can have the disease—this could happen if an affected male were to marry a carrier female. A son can never inherit the disease from his father.

95% of patients with ichthyosis will have either ichthyosis vulgaris or X-linked ichthyosis.

Because most patients with ichthyosis will always have it, treatment needs to be simple, cheap, easy to use and cosmetically acceptable. The patient should be discouraged from using soap, which removes the skin's natural grease and makes it even drier. Bathing with one of the dispersible bath oils in the water,* washing with emulsifying ointment or aqueous cream instead of soap, and

*Oilatum, Balneum, Balneum Plus, Alpha Keri, Balmandol, Emulsiderm, or Hydromol (*see* also page 50).

applying some sort of grease with or without a keratolytic agent to the skin after a bath while the skin is still wet will keep the skin comfortable. Many patients find Vaseline or one of the commercially available creams like Nivea as helpful as the ointments prescribed by doctors. It may be worth suggesting that they try

Alcoderm lotion Lacticare lotion
Aveeno cream Calmurid cream** Candermyl cream Diprobase cream Humiderm cream Nutraplus cream** Oilatum cream Sential E cream**
Aquadrate cream **Aqueous cream*** Locobase ointment Natuderm cream Ultrabase cream
E45 cream*
Hydrous ointment*
Unguentum Merck cream
Lipobase cream
Diprobase ointment **Emulsifying ointment*** **White soft paraffin*** **White soft paraffin/liquid paraffin mixed in equal parts***

↑ Decreasing greasiness

*These preparations are cheap.
**These preparations contain urea which is very helpful for dry skin but will sting if the skin is open.

5% salicylic acid ointment, urea or one of the emollients in the list on the left. Which preparation will suit any particular patient will have to be discovered by trial and error.

Patients with ichthyosis vulgaris often improve with increasing age so that the skin is a lot less trouble in adult life than it was in childhood. Some patients improve dramatically in warm weather and may choose to live in the tropics because the disease is then no longer apparent. The heat of an English summer is rarely enough to give more than partial alleviation.

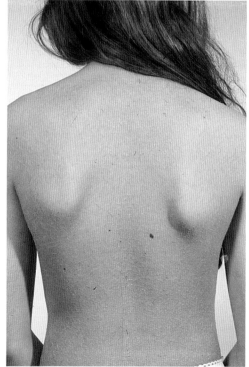

Figure 68 Ichthyosis vulgaris.

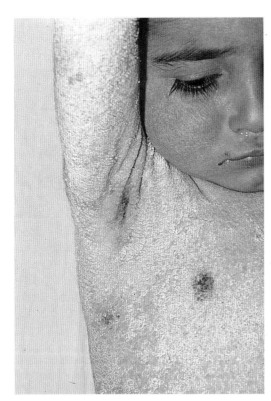

Figure 69 Bullous ichthyosiform erythroderma in a 4-year-old boy.

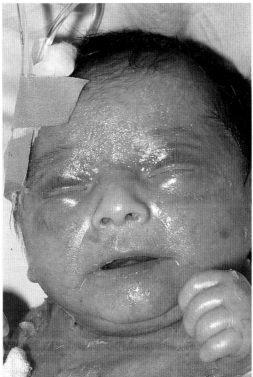

Figure 70 Collodion baby: male aged 6 days. This appearance at birth may be due to non-bullous ichthyosiform erythroderma or lamellar ichthyosis.

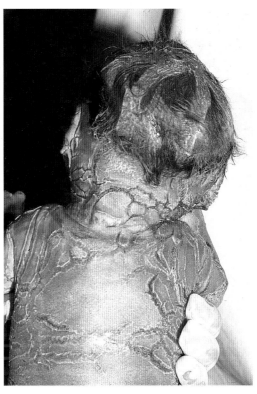

Figure 71 Harlequin fetus: male aged 24 hours.

Patients with X-linked ichthyosis do not improve in the summer or with increasing age, so emollients will be needed all their lives. A few will be bad enough to need one of the retinoids by mouth (*see* page 94).

Patients with the rarer forms of ichthyosis (Figures 69–71) will all be diagnosed at or shortly after birth. They will require emollients just the same as the patients with the commoner varieties, but will probably need the greasier ones, and applied more frequently. If the skin is oozing, they will also need potassium permanganate added to the bath water or used as wet dressings on the skin, and if the skin is infected they will need an oral antibiotic.

Some of these babies will die because of their skin condition, eg harlequin fetus and some with the ichthyosiform erythrodermas. Etretinate (Tigason) by mouth may be life-saving in these situations, but not always. It may also be used in infants who are not *in extremis* but whose skin is not controlled with emollients. The dose is 1–2 mg/kg body weight/day. This is only available in hospitals, but these children will need the help of a dermatologist or paediatrician with some experience in these conditions in any case. Once started, etretinate is likely to be needed for years so the long-term side effects must be borne in mind (*see* page 16), particularly the effects on the bones and joints.

Acquired ichthyosis

The onset of ichthyosis after early childhood is an indication to look for an underlying cause. The ichthyosis can occur before, at the same time as, or after the other signs of the disease. But once it has occurred it then mirrors the state of the underlying disease, disappearing if treatment is successful and returning with a relapse. The most important causes of acquired ichthyosis are:

- Hodgkin's disease
- other lymphomas
- carcinoma
- lepromatous leprosy
- severe malnutrition.

It is possible for the onset of ichthyosis vulgaris to be apparently delayed until adult life, if for example the patient lives in a warm humid environment and later moves to a temperate one. This is seen in England in patients from the Far East, who in their own countries have normal skin, but as soon as they come to England, the ichthyosis becomes apparent.

Treatment while the cause is being investigated is the same as for the common types of genetically determined ichthyoses (*see* page 91).

IDIOPATHIC GUTTATE HYPOMELANOSIS

There is no treatment for this condition. The patient should be reassured that it is as harmless as the freckles that it resembles, albeit in reverse. Because it is due to chronic sun exposure, the patient may be at risk of developing other sun-induced lesions such as solar keratoses and basal cell carcinomas. It would be wise therefore to advise them to use a high protective factor sunscreen (Factor 15 or above, *see* page 140) in the future.

IMPETIGO

This is the one exception to the rule that topical antibiotics should not be used on the skin. Because the infection is so superficial, a topical antibiotic is more effective than one given systemically.

If there are thick crusts on the skin these must be removed before the antibiotic is applied. Arachis oil (or some other oil that the patient has at home such as olive oil or sunflower oil) is applied to the crusts to soften them. After 15–20 minutes the crusts will be soft and can be removed with the fingers. The topical antibiotic ointment (2% fusidic acid [Fucidin], 2% mupirocin ointment [Bactroban], or 0.3% neomycin ointment) is then applied to the area under the crust and up the patient's nose (to deal with the carriage site of the staphylococcus) four times a day until it is better (about 72 hours).

In some parts of the world, where impetigo is more likely to be due to a group of A-beta haemolytic streptococcus than to *Staphylococcus aureus*, phenoxymethylpenicillin (penicillin V)* should be given orally (62.5 mg four times a day to a child under the age of

---

*Erythromycin can be given to individuals who are allergic to penicillin.

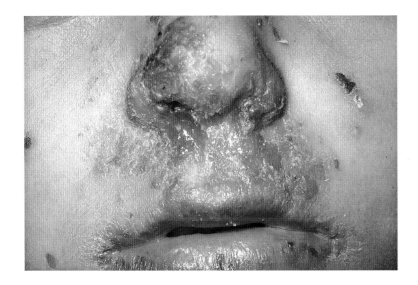

5 years, 125 mg four times a day to an older child, and 250 mg four times a day to an adult) as well as the topical antibiotic to prevent nephritis.

Special forms of impetigo

1 Bullous impetigo in the new-born infant. For some curious reason impetigo in the new-born infant is usually bullous. It is nearly always due to a member of staff in a maternity unit carrying the offending *Staphylococcus aureus* up their nose. As well as treating the infant, the member of staff also needs treatment. Oral flucloxacillin elixir, 62.5 mg four times a day, is the treatment of choice for the child. Topical neomycin ointment up the nose four times a day will be needed for the adult.

2 Impetigo on the scalp is nearly always due to head lice. Unless that is also dealt with, the impetigo will not clear up permanently (*see* page 107).

3 Widespread impetigo. If a child has widespread impetigo there will be some underlying reason for it. Atopic eczema and scabies are the two most common causes. The underlying condition must be treated at the same time as the impetigo or it will simply recur. In both cases it is better to give a systemic antibiotic while treating the eczema or the scabies topically (*see* pages 49 and 191).

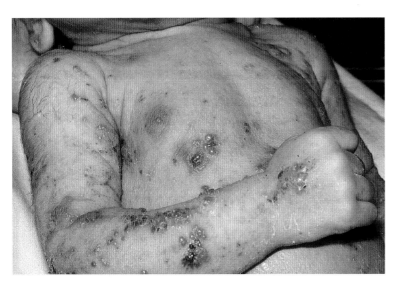

Figure 72 (*above left*) Impetigo in a 5-year-old boy, obviously arising from the anterior nares.

Figure 73 (*below left*) Bullous impetigo in a baby aged 21 days.

INGROWING TOENAILS

The following methods can be tried to resolve this problem.

1 If it is not too bad, the inflammation at the side of the nail will get better spontaneously if the patient wears shoes which are wide enough at the toes so that they are no longer squashed together (*see* Figure 22, page 37). The nail should be allowed to grow up so that its edges are clear of the end of the toe and the nail then cut in a slight curve.

2 The granulation tissue at the lateral nail fold can be destroyed by cauterizing it with a silver nitrate stick, or by freezing it with liquid nitrogen.

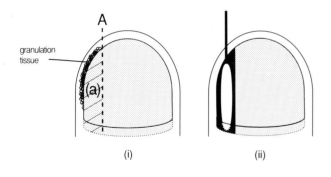

Figure 74 Wedge resection of the lateral nail fold. Anaesthetize the toe with a ring block. (i) Cut down line A and remove the loose nail (a); (ii) Apply phenol on a cotton wool bud to the cavity.

3 Wedge resection of the lateral nail fold and angular phenolization (Figure 74). First anaesthetize the toe with a ring block using 2% lignocaine without adrenaline. Cut down through the nail about 3 mm from the lateral nail fold (line A) with a pair of nail pliers and remove the lateral portion of the nail (a) with a pair of mosquito forceps. Take care to remove all spicules of nail.

Soak a cotton wool bud in liquefied phenol (80%) and apply it to the resulting cavity, (including under the cuticle) with firm pressure for 20 seconds. Do that three times then apply a firm non-adhesive dressing and remove the tourniquet. Cover the dressing with a dry dressing and Tubegauz. Change the dressing after 7 days. The patient then continues with a dry dressing over the area until the wound is fully healed.

4 Removal of the nail together with the nail matrix (Zadek's operation). After this the nail will not regrow and the problem will be resolved permanently. This is not done as the first line of treatment because the nail will then no longer be there to protect the end of the toe.

INSECT BITES

1 Flea bites. Straightforward flea bites are easy to recognize by the fact that they tend to occur in rows or groups—itchy papules with a central punctum at the site of the bites with normal skin in between. Some individuals will get a more generalized rash with lots of excoriations. Although there are 60 varieties of flea in the British Isles, most patients will have acquired cat or dog fleas from their pets. Cats and dogs catch the fleas from other pets and bring them into the home, predominantly during the summer months, and occasionally during spells of warm weather at other times of the year.

Figure 75 Dog flea.

Successful treatment involves treating the animal rather than the human. Regular spraying of the animal's fur, every 7–14 days throughout the summer months, with Novantop (111 trichloro-ethane, fenitrothion and bichlorvos) which is only available from veterinary surgeons will keep them relatively flea-free. If this is not sufficient to prevent the patient from being bitten, the animal's bedding, and any of the armchairs or beds that the pet sleeps on can also be sprayed.

Within a household it is often only one person who gets bitten. No one knows why this is. Many patients are offended when you tell them that they are being bitten by fleas, assuming that you are saying that they are dirty or that they do not take proper care of their pets. It is important to reassure them that all cats and dogs will get fleas in the summer time.

Cats and dogs may have other infestations as well as fleas, eg *Sarcoptes scabei canis* (animal scabies), *Cheyletiella* species and *Forage mites*, all of which can cause undiagnosable rashes in their owners and their families.

To make the diagnosis of an animal infestation, get the patient to stand the pet on a large sheet of newspaper or polythene and brush it fairly vigorously with an animal brush or comb. Wrap the newspaper or polythene sheeting up so that the brushings are safely inside and send these along to the microbiology department of the local hospital. Here the brushings will be spread out onto black paper and examined under a stereoscopic microscope, look-ing for insects, fragments of insects, flea pellets etc. If none are found, the brushings are then put into a pot with 75% lactic acid and left overnight. In lactic acid, mites, fleas, ticks, egg cases etc become detached from the hair sample and float to the top of the liquid. The surface layer is then skimmed off and examined under an ordinary light microscope and the various parasites identified.

The patient is then told what is wrong and they can then go to their vet to get some treatment for the pet. In most cases the human will not need any treatment at all and will quickly become symptom-free when the animal is dealt with. If the itching is intolerable, 10% crotamiton cream (Eurax) can be applied two or three times a day.

2 Bed bug bites. Single large bites occurring on exposed parts of the body each morning when the patient wakes from sleep are suggestive of bed bug bites. It is not possible for the patient to eradicate these from the home and the public health department needs to be called in.

3 Mosquito and midge bites. These insects suck blood for food and can often be seen on the skin having their meal! The diagnosis is not usually in doubt. Mosquitoes are attracted by carbon dioxide in the victim's breath and by some chemicals in body odour. They use these chemicals and other indicators such as temperature to track down their next meal. No one knows for sure why some people are more attractive than others to mosquitoes.

Mosquitoes tend to feed from early evening to daybreak, midges all day long. Once bitten there is not much you can do. Calamine lotion can be applied to the bites. Topical antihistamines should not be used because of the risk of contact sensitization. If there are very numerous bites it may be necessary to give the patient an antihistamine (promethazine 25–50 mg or trimeprazine 10 mg) at night. In this situation the sedative antihistamines work better than the non-sedative ones because you want the patient to be able to get some sleep.

For patients who get bitten frequently, regular use of an insect repellent is advisable. These can be applied directly to the skin or onto clothing adjacent to exposed skin.

Diethyltoluamide* ($C_{12}H_{17}NO$) is the most effective insect repellent available at the moment, but it can cause irritation on the skin and should not be used around the eyes. It is available as a lotion, a stick or a spray.

Other insect repellents contain:

- citronella oil
- dibutyl phthalate*
- dimethyl phthalate*
- ethylaminopropionate
- permethrin.

Lotions are generally cheaper than sticks or sprays. All are equally effective provided they are applied often enough. Aerosols and sprays last 1–2 hours. Liquids, lotions, creams and pump sprays last 2–3 hours. Gels and sticks last 4 hours.

There are a number of insect repellent gadgets on the market too, aimed at keeping flying insects away during outdoor activities in the garden or during the night.

(i) Electric mosquito killers. In these devices a pad containing the insecticides allethrin or bio-allethrin is slowly vaporized by heating. They are very effective in enclosed areas such as a bedroom.

(ii) Insect coils. The coil contains an insecticide. It is lit at one end and should smoulder for 8 hours to give protection through the night. Electric mosquito killers give more reliable protection without the smoke. If an insect coil is going to be used, the patient needs to make sure that it will burn all night; if it burns too fast or goes out, any protection will be lost.

(iii) UV lamps. These are advertised to be used around barbecues: they are supposed to attract insects and electrocute them. They are effective against flies but not against mosquitoes and midges.

(iv) Repellent strips. These contain citronella. They repel insects from the strip but not from humans!

(v) Electric buzzers. These claim to distract biting mosquitoes by imitating the sound of male mosquitoes. Basically they do not work.

4 Tick bites. Ticks also suck blood. They attach themselves to their host and are difficult to pull off. Applying a little butter or margarine will cause them to let go, as will spraying them with an insect repellent such as diethyltoluamide or butopyronoxyl. It is better to tuck the trousers into the socks when walking through the undergrowth during the summer to prevent the ticks from getting onto the skin. Ticks may harbour borrelia which cause Lyme disease (*see* page 71).

INSECT STINGS

There are two distinct families of stinging insects (hymenoptera). The genus Apis contains only the honeybee, whilst the genus Vespidae contains the wasp, yellow jacket and hornet.

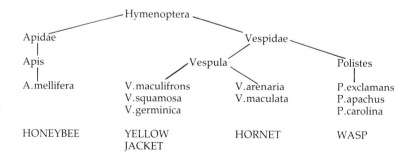

---

*These can also be applied to clothing which is a useful way of protecting children. The insect repellent is applied to clothing near to the exposed skin, rather than on the skin itself so there will be no local irritation and no risk of the child getting it in his eyes.

Bees are entomologically and allergenically distinct from the vespids. Bees sting only in defence, injecting approximately 50 μg of venom into the skin, (the entire contents of the venom sac). The barbed sting is left *in situ*, resulting in evisceration and death of the bee. Wasps can sting several times in succession and it is not clear how much venom is injected per sting.

Most stings cause only a local reaction. A painful swelling, varying in size from 1 cm in diameter to oedema of an entire hand, forearm or leg occurs, which will take several days to subside. Occasional patients, mostly beekeepers who are stung repeatedly, develop an anaphylactic reaction to a bee sting. A patient who has once had an anaphylactic reaction should be taught how to inject himself with 0.5 ml of 1:1000 adrenaline subcutaneously. Unfortunately, a patient who has just been stung and who has had a severe reaction in the past is usually frightened and may find himself unable to open an ampoule, fill a syringe and then inject himself during a time when the symptoms are increasing in severity. Syringes precharged with adrenaline are now available and are available on prescription (Minijet adrenaline 1:1000; they are made by IMS and come in 0.5 ml and 1 ml syringes).

For ordinary stings no treatment is needed, but if the local reaction is severe the symptoms can be improved by taking an oral antihistamine.

INTERTRIGO

In the summer it is impossible to prevent intertrigo from developing in patients who are overweight because the sweaty skin surfaces will rub together. Loss of weight is the only real answer. 1% hydrocortisone cream applied twice a day will alleviate the symptoms and make the skin less red, but this will only help temporarily.

JUVENILE PLANTAR DERMATOSIS

Modern footwear in susceptible individuals is thought to be responsible for this condition. Nylon socks and trainers should be discouraged, and cotton socks and leather shoes worn if possible. Charcoal or cork insoles inside the shoes will also help the sweat to evaporate.

Treatment on the whole is unsatisfactory. Topical steroids are not usually of any help. We suggest you try the following:
1 Vaseline applied two or three times a day. If it does not work, one of the other moisturizers can be tried (*see* list on page 92).
2 2% crude coal tar in Unguentum Merck applied first just at night and later twice a day.
3 2% crude coal tar in white soft paraffin (Vaseline) applied at night only or morning and night.
4 If there are fissures and the feet are painful, they can be wrapped up in Coltapaste occlusive bandages for several days at a time until they settle (*see* Figure 42, page 56).

Although it is no consolation to either the patient or his parents while the condition is there, they can be reassured that it will get better permanently at about the age of 14.

KAPOSI'S SARCOMA

In patients with AIDS the appearance of Kaposi's sarcoma would be a reason to introduce oral zidovudine 250 mg twice daily even with a normal CD_1 count. Once started it should be continued indefinitely.

For the Kaposi's sarcoma itself, no treatment is needed unless the lesions are a problem cosmetically, ie on the face, or they are painful (usually on the soles of the feet). If treatment is needed a course of superficial radiotherapy works well.

In patients without AIDS, the indications for treatment are the same as for patients with AIDS and again radiotherapy is the treatment of choice.

KELOID SCAR

Injection of triamcinolone, 5 mg/ml, into the scar will flatten it off and take away the red colour. Use a 21 gauge needle rather than a smaller one because considerable pressure is needed to get the triamcinolone into the scar tissue. If this does not work, the scar can be re-excised and irradiated with low-dose superficial X-rays (1–3 fractions of 7 Gy) on the same day as the surgery or, at the latest, the next day.

KERATOACANTHOMA

Although this will regress spontaneously, it is usually treated because:
- the patient is alarmed by the rapid growth of the tumour over just a few weeks and is afraid that it is cancer
- it is unsightly
- it will heal with a better scar if removed surgically or treated with radiotherapy
- sometimes it will be misdiagnosed and will in fact be a squamous cell carcinoma.

They are often too large to excise easily, so curettage and cautery is the treatment of choice. If this is going to be done, it is important to do it before spontaneous regression has begun, or the scar tissue which is forming may make it very difficult to curette out. Sometimes they recur after curettage and cautery. This may be because the diagnosis is wrong and it is really a squamous cell carcinoma, or simply because it was not entirely removed the first time. If they recur, they can be curetted out again, excised or treated with radiotherapy.

KERATOSIS PILARIS

This is such a common condition that it can be regarded as one end of the normal spectrum of skin changes. Many patients will not notice it or complain about it. If they do, it is usually a mother anxious about a child with it, not because it is causing any distress to the child but because she is worried about the appearance or afraid that it is something serious. She can be reassured that it is harmless. It often improves spontaneously in the summer. If treatment is required, a topical keratolytic agent can be applied. 10% urea cream (Calmurid), 2% salicylic acid ointment or 0.025% tretinoin cream (Retin-A) put on once or twice a day will not cure it but will remove the rough surface temporarily and make it feel more comfortable.

KOILONYCHIA

Koilonychia classically occurs in patients with hypochromic anaemia, but it is not due to the iron deficiency itself. Most patients with hypochromic anaemia do not in fact have koilonychia, so it is not a reliable physical sign. If the blood picture is normal and the serum ferritin is normal, there is nothing to do about it.

It is extremely common for children under the age of 2 to have koilonychia and this can be regarded as a normal finding. The nails go back to normal without anything being done about them.

KNUCKLE PADS

Although these look like callosities, they are not caused by trauma. Apart from excising them, which is not usually very practical, nothing can be done to get rid of them. The patient can be re-assured that they are not harmful in any way.

LAMELLAR SPLITTING OF NAILS

This change is due to damage to the distal portion of the nail plate by water and detergents. It occurs most commonly in people who have their hands in water all day long. Wearing rubber gloves to protect them and keeping the nails cut short is usually all that is required. A 5–10% aqueous solution of formalin can be painted onto the nails in an attempt to harden them. Some patients will find this useful.

LARVA MIGRANS

The topical application of a 10% thiabendazole suspension to the whole of the track(s) caused by the hookworm larva four times a day for 7 days will usually cure it. An alternative is to freeze just ahead of the track with liquid nitrogen.

LEISHMANIASIS (CUTANEOUS)

In these days of easy world-wide travel, a number of patients will be seen in the UK with tropical diseases like cutaneous leishmaniasis. In its natural habitat, around the Mediterranean, in the Middle

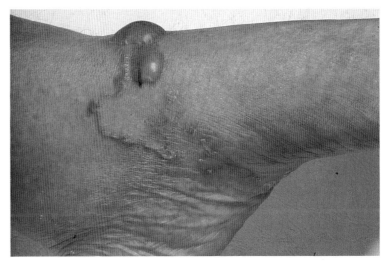

Figure 76 Larva migrans.

East, North Africa, India, Pakistan, Central and South America, the typical boil-like lesion will heal without treatment in about a year. It always leaves an ugly cribriform scar.

Natural history of cutaneous leishmaniasis.

Inoculation of *L.tropica* by sand-fly bite
↓
Boil-like nodule in skin (relatively painless)
↓
Ulcerates ± crusting
↓
Heals
↓
Depressed scar

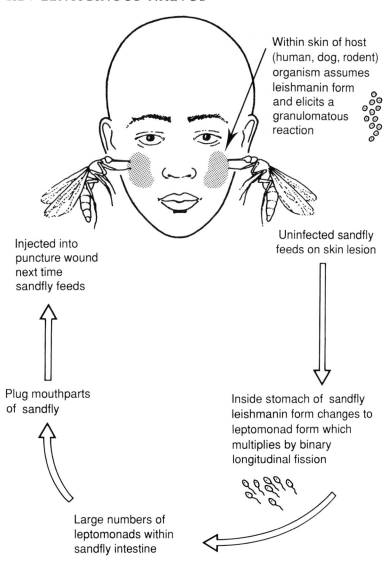

Within skin of host (human, dog, rodent) organism assumes leishmanin form and elicits a granulomatous reaction

Uninfected sandfly feeds on skin lesion

Injected into puncture wound next time sandfly feeds

Plug mouthparts of sandfly

Inside stomach of sandfly leishmanin form changes to leptomonad form which multiplies by binary longitudinal fission

Large numbers of leptomonads within sandfly intestine

Figure 77 Transmission of *L. tropica* and lifecycle of cutaneous leishmaniasis.

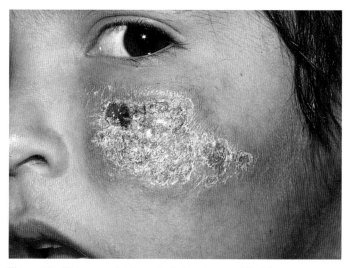

Figure 78 Cutaneous leishmaniasis in a 5-year-old girl.

Pentavalent antimony compounds are the mainstay of treatment but they are largely unsatisfactory. Intralesional injections of sodium stibogluconate (Pentostam) or N-methylglucamin antimoniate (Glucantime) once a week will make the sore heal quicker than it would otherwise. This is unpleasant for the patient and since many of them will be children, it is not very practical. The alternative is to give the antimony by injection (sodium stibogluconate 20 mg/kg body weight im or iv daily until the sore heals [10–30 days]). For most patients it is probably easier to leave well alone.

LENTIGINOUS NAEVUS

These are completely harmless and need no treatment.

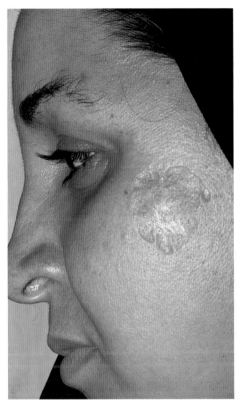

Figure 79 Typical depressed scar of cutaneous leishmaniasis in a 20-year-old Iranian woman.

LENTIGO

These are a normal sign of increasing age. They have no sinister implications. Most individuals will put up with them philosophically once they understand that they are harmless. The various skin-lightening creams that are on the market will not make them go away.

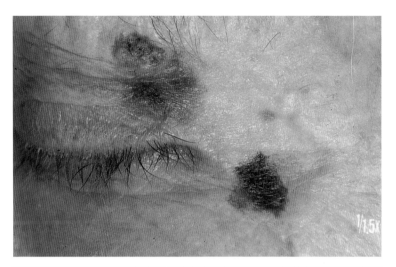

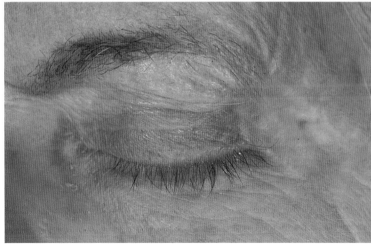

Figure 80 (*above*) Lentigo maligna in a 78-year-old woman.

Figure 81 (*below*) Same patient as Figure 80 after two treatments with liquid nitrogen.

LENTIGO MALIGNA (HUTCHINSON'S FRECKLE)

Ideally these should be fully excised but since they are often large and on the face it may not be practical to do this. Other options can be considered but the diagnosis must first be confirmed by biopsy to exclude a superficial spreading melanoma. Alternatives to surgery are:

1 Radiotherapy. This is a very effective treatment which is likely to give a better cosmetic result than surgery if the lesion is large. It may take up to 2 years for the pigment to disappear after treatment and the patient will need reassuring that it is cured in the meantime.

2 Freezing with liquid nitrogen. Two freeze–thaw cycles:
- freeze for 30 seconds
- allow to thaw which should take at least 90 seconds
- re-freeze for a further 30 seconds.

Freezing works well and can give a very good cosmetic result (Figures 80 and 81). It is important that patients who are treated by this method are followed up regularly to make sure there is no recurrence.

3 Painting with dinitrochlorobenzene (DNCB). 10% DNCB is painted onto the patient's upper arm in order to cause an allergic contact eczema to occur. Everyone with normal cell mediated immunity will become allergic to this chemical if it is applied to their skin. Three weeks later, when they have an acute eczema on the arm, 0.1% DNCB is painted onto the lentigo maligna and this is repeated weekly until the tumour disappears. Again it is important to keep an eye on the patient if they have had this treatment rather than surgery.

LEPROSY

The treatment of leprosy depends on the immune status of the patient, which is what determines the clinical features.

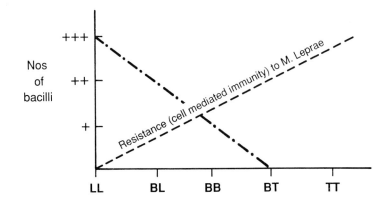

At one end of the spectrum there is tuberculoid leprosy, TT, where the patient has good immunity and the infection remains localized. At the other end there is lepromatous leprosy, LL, where the patient has no resistance to the organism and has widespread disease. In between there are all gradations of immunity and therefore of clinical disease, from borderline tuberculoid, BT, to mid borderline, BB, to borderline lepromatous, BL (*see* diagram above and Figures 82–84).

Patients with leprosy should be under the care of a leprologist or dermatologist with some experience in its management because it is not just a case of giving out pills but careful monitoring of the skin lesions (clinically and by skin smears) and nerve damage (degree of motor loss and anaesthesia, and care of anaesthetic limbs).

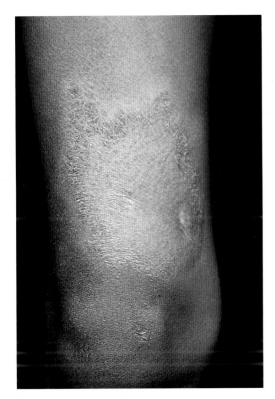

Figure 82 Tuberculoid leprosy: a single anaesthetic plaque.

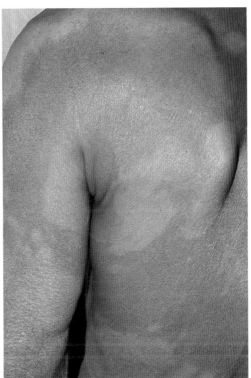

Figure 83 Borderline leprosy: multiple asymmetrical patches and plaques.

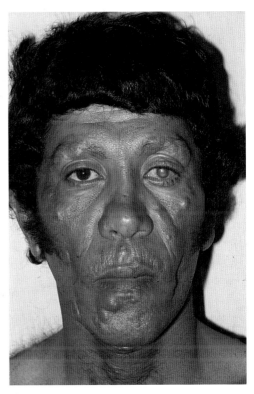

Figure 84 Lepromatous leprosy: multiple symmetrical papules and nodules which are not anaesthetic.

Dapsone has been the mainstay of treatment since its introduction in the 1940s. Because of the risk of drug resistance, the WHO now recommends multidrug therapy.

- For patients with good immunity (TT, BT):
  rifampicin 600 mg orally once a month for 6 months, plus dapsone 100 mg daily for 6 months.

- For patients with not such good immunity (BB, BL, LL):
  rifampicin 600 mg once a month, plus dapsone 100 mg daily, plus clofazimine* 300 mg once a month and 50 mg daily.

*In patients with light-coloured skins where clofazimine may well be unacceptable because of the red colour, ethionamide 250–375 mg daily is an alternative.

Treatment is given for 2 years or until skin smears have been consistently negative for 6 months.

Side effects of anti-leprosy drugs

Dapsone haemolytic anaemia
methaemoglobinaemia
psychiatric problems (psychosis)—rarely

Clofazimine red–brown discoloration of the skin
red–brown discoloration of conjunctivae
red urine, stools, sputum, sweat and tears
dryness of skin

Rifampicin red urine
hepatitis**
thrombocytopenia**
psychosis**
interferes with effectiveness of the pill
decreases effectiveness of systemic steroids

Ethionamide nausea and vomiting
metallic taste in the mouth
rarely, peripheral neuropathy
hepatitis
hypothyroidism
hypoglycaemia
gynaecomastia
optic neuritis (causes ↓ visual acuity and
red/green colour blindness)

**These serious side effects are not usually seen with the once a month dosage.

Care of anaesthetic hands and feet

This is just as important as the drug treatment of leprosy because the care of anaesthetic limbs will need to be continued for the rest of the patient's life. Anaesthetic limbs are continually injured because of the absence of pain so:

1 Patients should be taught to examine their hands and feet every day for minor injuries which would not otherwise be noticed. These must then be treated and protected from further injury.

2 They should be warned against burning their hands. Pots and pans used for cooking (including kettles) must have handles that do not conduct the heat, and patients should be advised to wear thick cotton gloves for cooking or lighting the fire. Smoking should be discouraged.

3 Hot water bottles should not be used in bed because they can cause burns to the arms and legs as well as the hands and feet, and the patient should be warned not to sit too close to the fire.

4 They should wear proper fitting shoes all the time; this means in the house as well as out of doors. The shoes should have Plastazote insoles so that they fit perfectly without slipping or rubbing. Velcro fastenings rather than laces are essential if there is any deformity of the fingers.

5 Callosities on the soles should be soaked in warm water for 10–15 minutes each day and then rubbed down with a pumice stone to keep them flat. Regular chiropody is also essential.

6 If ulceration occurs on the feet it should be taken seriously from the beginning. The area will need to be protected from further injury by padding it up well and keeping the weight off it. A below-knee walking plaster is one of the best ways to get such ulcers to heal (*see* Figure 218, page 244).

The role of surgery in the treatment of leprosy

Corrective surgery can give patients hands and feet that work again (arthrodesis to give a stable foot to walk on; tendon transplants to straighten fingers and toes). Plastic surgery can also be useful for correcting the physical deformities (nasal deformity, facial nerve palsy, excessive folds on the face and gynaecomastia).

LEUKOPLAKIA OF THE MOUTH

Because of the risk of malignant change, leukoplakia should be treated. If the area involved is small, it can be excised; if it is too large for excision, it can be frozen with liquid nitrogen (two freeze–thaw cycles—*see* page 28). Such patients are probably best cared for by an oral surgeon.

LEUKAEMIC INFILTRATE

This will only disappear if the leukaemia is treated.

LICE

Head lice

There are a number of insecticides available which kill both head lice and their eggs (Table 5). All are neurotoxic to the lice. Two treatments should be given, 7 days apart, because young eggs do not possess a nervous system, and may survive a single treatment.

Lotions are better than shampoo formulations because the latter have too short a contact time to be effective. The lotion is applied all over the scalp, left on for 12 hours, and then washed off with a normal shampoo. The permethrin cream rinse is used like a conditioner; after shampooing the cream is put onto the wet hair and left in place for 10 minutes. This leaves the lice and eggs coated with a balsam containing the insecticide, so combining a long contact time with a short treatment time.

Table 5 Treatments currently available

Insecticide	Trade name	Concentration
Malathion	Derbac-M	0.5% lotion*
	Suleo-M	0.5% lotion**
	Prioderm	0.5% lotion**
Carbaryl	Derbac-C	0.5% lotion*
	Clinicide	0.5% lotion*
	Suleo-C	0.5% lotion**
	Carylderm	0.5% lotion**
Pyrethroids		
1 Permethrin	Lyclear	1% cream rinse
2 d-phenothrin	Full Marks	0.2% shampoo

* Water-based   **Alcohol-based

The egg cases can be removed by combing the hair with a nit comb.

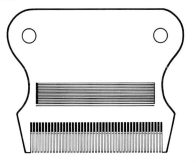

Figure 85 Nit comb.

Problems with treating head lice

1 With time the lice become resistant to the insecticides used in their treatment. It is therefore advisable to change the insecticide you are using every 3 years, using them in rotation (malathion for 3 years; carbaryl for 3 years; permethrin for 3 years).

2 To prevent re-infection the whole family should be treated whether or not they are itching. You may need to involve the health visitor, practice nurse or school nurse to make sure that all the contacts are treated.

3 Many patients with head lice are completely asymptomatic so there are always people in the community who are infested but do not realize it. This is why school nurses check children's heads regularly. There is no one to check on adults in the same way.

4 People are often worried that some of the lice may be missed in children or adults with very long hair. Since the eggs are laid onto the hairs where they leave the scalp, all the viable eggs will be close to the scalp and will be killed as long as the insecticide has been applied all over the scalp itself. In the same way, the adult lice and the immature walking stages have to go to the scalp to feed, so they will be killed by the insecticide then.

5 Only water-based insecticide lotions should be used in patients with eczema because the alcoholic ones will sting the open skin.

Body lice

Body lice live in the clothes rather than on the skin, so treatment has to be directed at them rather than at the patient himself. Malathion powder can be sprinkled along the seams of the clothes but is not usually needed since ordinary washing and ironing will kill the lice. The main thing is to think about the possibility of the diagnosis in anyone who has been sleeping rough and remember to look along the seams of the patient's clothes for the lice and the eggs.

Pubic lice (Crab lice)

0.5% malathion lotion (Derbac-M) or 1% gamma benzene hexachloride lotion or cream (Quellada lotion; Lorexane cream) are applied to the pubic hair and washed off 12 hours later. Treatment is repeated after 7 days. Probably these two treatments should be alternated to prevent resistance (as for head lice). Alcoholic solutions are not suitable for applying to the pubic area. Shaving the pubic hair is another possible solution since the lice need hairs to hold onto while they feed. In individuals who are very hairy the pubic lice can also be found in the axillae, on the body hair and in the eyelashes. These areas should always be checked and, if involved, the whole body treated with gamma benzene hexachloride or malathion lotion (including the eyelashes). Alternatively pick the lice and nits (egg cases) off the eyelashes with the fingers and apply Vaseline three or four times a day so that the lice cannot hold on!

All sexual contacts must also be treated.

LICHEN NITIDUS

This is just a mini form of lichen planus. It gets better on its own over a period of months and no treatment is needed. If lesions are present on the penis the man can be reassured that it is not contagious.

LICHEN PLANUS

Lichen planus on the skin

The rash usually lasts between 9 and 18 months and then gets better spontaneously. No one knows why it occurs and the patient should be reassured that it is not serious or contagious. It is a very itchy condition and the patient cannot be expected to put up with the itching for a year or more. A moderately potent topical steroid cream such as 0.025% betamethasone valerate (Betnovate RD), can be applied twice a day to give relief from the itching (for alternative steroids, *see* page 8). Rarely one of the more potent steroid creams will be needed, but these should be avoided if possible because they will need to be continued until the rash gets better on its own. The steroids will not make the rash go away and you should make this clear to the patient from the beginning. They are very effective in stopping the itching, more so than oral antihistamines, which on the whole are not a lot of help.

Hypertrophic lichen planus

On the legs this may last for years rather than months and is often extremely itchy. A very potent topical steroid cream or ointment, such as 0.05% clobetasol propionate (Dermovate), will frequently be effective when less potent topical steroids have not helped. Occasionally steroids will have to be injected intralesionally in order to be effective (triamcinolone 5 mg/ml).

Lichen planus of the mouth

Most oral lichen planus is asymptomatic and needs no treatment. A few patients get erosive lesions which may go on to frank ulceration and last for years. Once the buccal mucosal surface has been lost, the patient will have a sore mouth and will find eating painful. Treatment of erosive lichen planus is unsatisfactory. The following can be tried.

1 Ordinary mouthwashes, eg glycerine and thymol or benzydamine hydrochloride (Difflam), used several times a day.

2 10% hydrocortisone mixed in equal parts of glycerine and water used as a mouthwash before each meal. It is very bitter and will spoil the taste of the food which follows. It must be spat out after swishing around the mouth rather than swallowed to limit the amount of steroid which will be absorbed.

3 0.1% triamcinolone acetonide in orobase applied to the ulcerated areas several times a day.

4 Prednisone 15–30 mg/day may occasionally be needed for the most severe forms of ulceration. The dose is reduced as soon as the ulceration is healed down to a maintenance dose of 5–10 mg/day. You want to get the patient off steroids as soon as possible because otherwise they will end up taking them for years.

5 Rarely one of the oral retinoids may be needed as an alternative to systemic steroids (etretinate or acetretin, 1 mg/kg body weight/day).

Lichen planus of the scalp

There is no effective treatment for this. High doses of systemic steroids (60 mg prednisolone daily) have been tried but without much success. Since lichen planus causes a scarring alopecia, any hair loss that occurs will be permanent.

Lichen planus of the nails

Longitudinal ridging needs no treatment and most patients who have this change have not noticed it. If pterygium occurs, which will cause permanent scarring of the nails, prednisolone 30 mg/day started as soon as possible will often switch it off. Give this dose for 2 weeks and then gradually tail it off over the next month.

Drug-induced lichen planus

Most lichen planus is not drug-induced. When it is, the rash is likely to be atypical, looking like a mixture of pityriasis rosea and lichen planus. If it is due to a drug, the drug should be stopped. Some of the drugs which cause a lichenoid eruption have a long half life (mepacrine and gold) and stay around in the patient's body for months after it has been stopped. In such cases the rash also will last for many months after the drug has been stopped. Other drugs which can cause lichen planus include the beta blockers, chloroquine, chlorpropamide, methyldopa, penicillamine, quinine and the thiazide diuretics.

A rash that looks like lichen planus but confined to the sun exposed parts of the body can be due to the chemicals involved in colour developing. The diagnosis can be confirmed by patch testing which will give an eczematous response even though the rash is lichen planus.

LICHEN SCLEROSIS ET ATROPHICUS (LSA)

1 Genital lesions in little girls. In little girls the problem is of soreness or itching of the vulva or perianal skin. Both can be helped with topical steroids. 1% hydrocortisone cream or ointment applied twice a day is usually sufficient. Almost all children with LSA grow out of it by the time they reach puberty, so parents can be reassured that it is not serious or permanent.

2 Genital lesions in adult women. Itching is the main problem but soreness and dyspareunia can also occur. It is best to start with a very potent topical steroid such as 0.05% clobetasol propionate (Dermovate) ointment or cream applied twice a day for 2–3 weeks. This dramatically improves the symptoms and makes the patient believe that there is some hope for the future. Once she is

symptomatically better, the strength of the topical steroid can be reduced drastically to 1% hydrocortisone ointment or cream. Some patients will only need to use it once or twice a week, others will need to use it twice a day. A few will find that hydrocortisone is not enough to keep them comfortable and they will need to use a slightly stronger topical steroid. Trial and error may be needed to find which preparation is most suitable for any particular patient. The weakest possible steroid that will control the symptoms should be used to prevent further atrophy from occurring. It is, however, essential to stop the itching, not just for the patient's peace of mind, but also to prevent the development of squamous cell carcinoma in the atrophic skin.

This disease does not remit spontaneously when it occurs in adult women, so treatment will be required for life.

3 Genital lesions in adult men (balanitis xerotica obliterans). Young men with phimosis can be helped by circumcision. Itching and soreness can be controlled with a topical steroid. Start with 1% hydrocortisone cream or ointment applied twice a day. If that is not sufficient, the strength of the steroid can gradually be increased until it works. If there is urethral stenosis with spraying of urine, a more potent topical steroid will be needed (start with 0.05% clobetasone propionate [Dermovate] ointment). This should not be used for more than a few weeks but will be very helpful for alleviating the symptoms. Once the disease is under control it is nearly always possible to keep the patient symptom-free with a less potent steroid. The patient should be reassured that it is not contagious.

4 Non-genital lesions in any patient. The skin lesions of LSA do not respond well to treatment. If the skin feels tight, a moisturizer is as helpful as anything else. Topical steroids are not usually of any benefit.

LICHEN SIMPLEX

What is required here is some way of stopping the patient from scratching (more easily said than done!). A topical steroid ointment of medium potency (0.025% betamethasone valerate [Betnovate RD] or the equivalent, *see* page 8) can be applied two or three times a day. This will often help at first but if it is left off the patient will scratch again. The options then are:

1 Continue with the topical steroids indefinitely.

2 Wrap the leg or arm up in some kind of occlusive bandage so that the patient cannot get at it to scratch (if the lichen simplex is on the arm or leg). Coltapaste covered with Lestreflex (*see* Figure 42, page 56) and left in place for a week at a time will cause the skin to go back to normal in 2 or 3 weeks. It is wise to continue with the bandages for a few weeks after the skin is back to normal so that the patient gets out of the habit of scratching. If nothing else, this treatment will convince the patient that the skin will get better if he can leave it alone. Unfortunately when the bandage comes off he may go back to scratching again.

3 Look for the circumstances in his life that are causing him to subconsciously scratch his skin and help him to come to terms with them or to deal with them.

LIPOMA

Most lipomas are small and asymptomatic and do not require any treatment. Some patients consult the doctor with them because they equate lumps of any kind with cancer. If this is the problem they are easily reassured. If they are large and unsightly or painful they can be excised under a local or general anaesthetic.

LIP SUCKING/LIP LICKING

The first thing is to point out to the patient and his parents (usually the patient is a child) what he is doing; often he will not be aware that the habit exists. Very often he will actually do it while sitting in front of you and you can point that out to him and his parents. Just knowing what is going on will often be enough to stop it. If it is not, something can be applied to the lips and the skin around the lips that will be noticeable when he next does it. This can either be something that tastes horrible or something that cannot be licked off. A thick layer of Lassar's paste is as good as anything; it does not taste nice and is difficult to lick off. Unfortunately some children will wipe it off with their cuffs or even on the furniture! We usually suggest that it is applied as soon as they come home from school and again at bedtime. Vaseline can be used in the morning instead because Lassar's paste is white and will show. It does not take long for a child to get out of the habit.

LUPUS PERNIO

If the patient needs systemic steroids for the rest of his sarcoid there is no problem, the lupus pernio will improve with the rest. If there is no other symptomatic disease and the problem is just in the skin, the treatment is less straightforward. Systemic steroids may still be needed but usually at least 30 mg of prednisolone a day is needed to improve the skin. You have to weigh up the pros and cons of this in the light of the severity of the rash. Injection of triamcinolone (5 mg/ml) intralesionally into the plaques of lupus pernio will sometimes be helpful, as may cosmetic camouflage to disguise the disfigurement.

LYMPHANGIOMA CIRCUMSCRIPTUM

The real problem here is not the vesicles on the surface of the skin, although these do not look very nice and can leak, but a large muscular cistern (or cisterns) lying in the subcutaneous fat just above the deep fascia (*see* Figure 86). To eradicate the lymphangioma circumscriptum this deep cistern must be removed surgically.

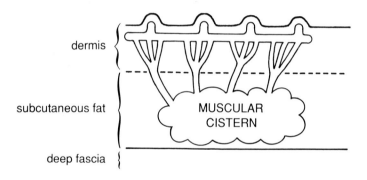

Figure 86.

LYMPHOEDEMA

Although it is not possible to repair damaged lymphatic vessels, the resulting swelling can be improved by compression bandages or a pump, exercise and massage. The physiotherapy department at the local hospital will often be able to advise on all three of these. A Flowtron boot, which is a compression pump that inflates and deflates regularly, can be helpful for some patients and these can either be purchased by the patient or loaned by the local hospital (*see* Figure 88).

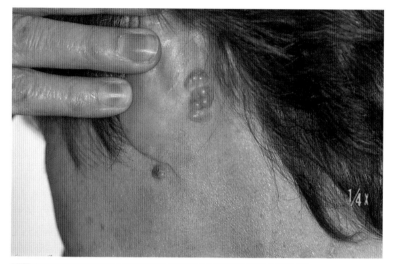

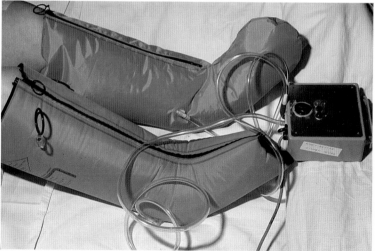

Figure 87 (*above*) Lymphangioma circumscriptum behind the ear.

Figure 88 (*below*) Flowtron boot in use on both legs.

An excellent booklet for patients explaining what to do and when is *Lymphoedema: Advice on Treatment* by Claud Regnard, Caroline Badger and Peter Mortimer (Beaconsfield Publishers Ltd.).

There is also a self-help group for patients:

BRITISH LYMPHOLOGY INTEREST GROUP
PATIENTS' SELF-HELP GROUP

Southern Region	Northern Region
Sister Agnes Williams	9 Melita Street
Sir Michael Sobel House	Darwen
Churchill Hospital	Blackburn
Oxford, OX3 7LJ	Lancashire, BB3 2DA
Tel: 0865 225 864	Tel: 0254 75914

LYMPHOGRANULOMA VENEREUM

Trimethoprim 200 mg twice a day or doxycycline 100 mg twice a day are given for 3 weeks. If the enlarged lymph nodes are fluctuant they should be aspirated.

LYMPHOMA

Patients with lymphomas should be under the care of an oncologist because precise classification is necessary in order to give the best treatment.

MALIGNANT MELANOMA

Prevention is better than cure as far as malignant melanoma is concerned. The most important risk factor is the sun, and 80% of an individual's sun exposure occurs before the age of 18. It is important therefore to get parents to protect their children when they are out in the sun with sun-hats and sunscreens from an early age. For any individual who burns rather than tans in the sun, a high protective sunscreen (Factor 15 or higher) should be used regularly throughout the summer months on all areas of exposed skin. We need to get away from the idea that for people with a white skin, 'brown is beautiful', and discourage sunbathing in the middle of the day (10 am–3 pm). It is sensible for everyone to take care in the sun, but some people are more at risk of developing a malignant melanoma than others, and they should be particularly careful.

- Those with fair or red hair who burn rather than tan in the sun.
- Those who have been badly sunburnt on more than one occasion in the past.
- Those who have large numbers of moles— more than 50.
- Those with atypical moles (irregular shape, variegate colour, some larger than 8 mm in diameter).
- Those with a family history of malignant melanoma.
- Those who have had a malignant melanoma already.
- Children who have had chemotherapy for a previous cancer.

Any patients who fit into one of the above groups should be particularly advised about being careful in the sun, and given a leaflet explaining the signs of malignant melanoma so they know what to look out for. It may be worth running a screening clinic for them once a year, to check their moles.

Treatment of the primary tumour

The prognosis for malignant melanoma depends on the thickness of the primary tumour when it is removed (Breslow thickness—*see* Figure 89).

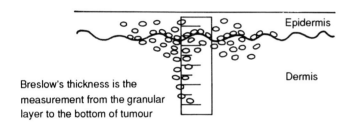

Breslow's thickness is the measurement from the granular layer to the bottom of tumour

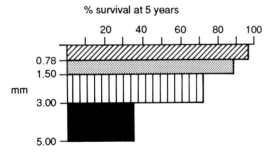

Figure 89 Prognosis of malignant melanoma related to Breslow thickness.

Once a melanoma has occurred, surgical removal is the treatment of choice. There is no scientific basis for the standard practice of removing 5 cm of normal skin around the tumour. Adequate removal is needed but how much that is is open to debate. Probably a 1–2 cm margin is adequate for all tumours. For very thin tumours (less than 0.78 mm thick) it is probably not necessary to remove more than the tumour itself. Regional lymph nodes are not removed unless they are obviously involved (*see* below).

Recurrent disease

Recurrent tumour near to the site of the primary is usually easy to spot. If more widespread disease is suspected, a full clinical examination should be done and if necessary a chest X-ray and liver ultrasound. Other procedures can be done as and when required, *see* Table 6.

Treatment of recurrent disease

1 **Local metastases in the skin.** These can be excised under local or general anaesthetic depending on the site and size of the recurrence. For very large recurrences, radiotherapy can give good palliation, at least for a while.

2 **Metastases in the regional lymph nodes.** Block dissection of the regional lymph nodes is a good treatment when recurrence is limited to the local glands. About 25% of patients with metastases in the local lymph nodes will survive for a further 5 years so the outlook is not necessarily hopeless. The number of involved nodes at surgery plays some part in the likely outcome (if only one gland is involved the outlook is much better than if they all are).

Table 6 Relevant investigations for metastatic malignant melanoma

Site of suspected metastasis	Investigations
Glands	Lymphangiography—gives a very characteristic picture with large round filling defects without involving the edges of the glands Ultrasound CT scan MRI scan—nodes show up as a white colour so quite small glands can be picked up
Lungs	Chest X-ray CT scan—gives a very characteristic pattern MRI scan no good for looking at the lungs themselves; good for evaluating nodes in the mediastinum and heart
Bone lesions	Skeletal survey—will show up lytic lesions, but X-ray changes occur late and by then the patient will almost certainly be symptomatic Bone scan—better for picking up 2°s because it depends on vascularity rather than decalcification
Liver	Ultrasound CT scan—faster and cheaper than MRI scan MRI scan—very accurate
Adrenal	Ultrasound CT scan MRI scan
GI tract	Barium studies—no characteristic pattern for melanoma; need to confirm with endoscopy and biopsy
UG tract	IVP—if 2° in kidney, patient presents with loin pain Urine cytology—if 2° in mucosa, patient has haematuria
Brain	CT scan MRI scan—investigation of choice

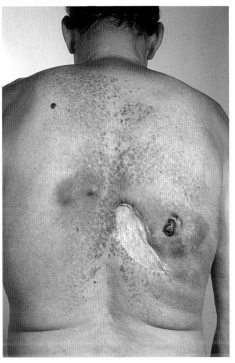

Figure 90 Multiple skin metastases from malignant melanoma. Radiotherapy treatment will give good palliation for a time.

3 Multiple secondaries in the skin, but confined to an arm or a leg. Isolated limb perfusion with cytotoxic drugs (usually melphalan) into the regional arterial blood supply can be effective but is very unpleasant for the patient. Following this treatment the arm or leg will be red and swollen for several weeks.

4 Widespread metastases. A number of cytotoxic drugs, alone and in combination, have been used for patients with widespread secondaries. None of them are particularly good, all giving a partial response in about 25% of patients. Very few patients are alive

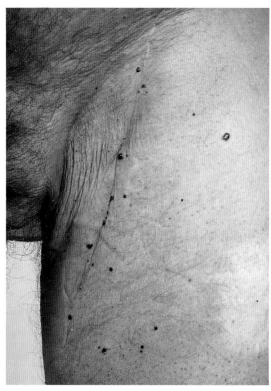

Figure 91 Multiple skin metastases from malignant melanoma. This patient is suitable for treatment with isolated limb perfusion.

Use of radiotherapy in the treatment of malignant melanoma

Malignant melanoma is a radiosensitive tumour but large doses are needed to be effective. It may be used in the following circumstances.

● Primary tumours on the head and neck if it would be difficult to remove the tumour by surgery.
● For treating a primary tumour when the patient is too sick to undergo a surgical procedure (usually because of heart or lung problems).
● For skin or nodal secondaries after failure of surgery. It pays to be aggressive because if the tumour responds to radiotherapy, it is likely to stay away. Generally speaking, small tumours respond much better than large tumours, but radiotherapy is often only used for those that are too big for surgery. In the most advanced tumours, radiotherapy will not alter the prognosis but will give good temporary palliation.
● For bony secondaries.
● For cerebral secondaries.

MEDIAN NAIL DYSTROPHY

The cause of this change in the nails is unknown and it gets better spontaneously after a few months.

MELASMA (CHLOASMA)

1 year after any kind of chemotherapy (this is why it is so important to make the diagnosis of the primary tumour early while it is thin and the prognosis good). Vindesine and dacarbazine (DTIC) are the most commonly used drugs although vinblastine, cisplatin, interferon 2 alpha and interleukin 2 have all been tried.

For patients who develop it during pregnancy or while taking the contraceptive pill, there is a good chance that it will get better spontaneously after delivery or when the pill is stopped. If it occurs during the summer, a high protective factor sunscreen (Factor 15 or above, *see* page 140) will stop it getting darker.

In a few women in whom it develops during pregnancy, it does not get better afterwards, and in others (men and women) it has nothing to do with pregnancy or the pill. In this latter group, a high protective total sun block should be used on the whole of the face whenever the patient is going to be out of doors to prevent the pigment from getting darker in the sun.

There are various skin-lightening creams on the market, none of which are particularly good; they all contain hydroquinone in various strengths. This inhibits the conversion of tyrosine to melanin, it does not bleach pigment that is already there. 2%, 3% or 4% hydroquinone in aqueous cream can be applied to the hyper-pigmented areas twice a day for at least 6 months (it will also lighten normal skin so the patient should only apply it to the abnormal areas). At the same time, the patient should protect herself from further hyperpigmentation by staying out of the sun and using a high protective factor sunscreen. She should apply the hydroquinone cream first and then put the sunscreen on top. If hydroquinone is ineffective 0.05% retinoic acid (Retin-A) cream can be tried instead.

Do not use the monobenzyl ether of hydroquinone by mistake. This will cause complete loss of pigment in a confetti-like pattern which is not confined to the sites of application, and which is permanent (Figure 92).

MILIA

Most patients are not bothered by these small cysts, but a few find them unsightly and want to be rid of them. They are quite easy to remove with a sterile needle. Make a small nick over the centre of the milium as if you were going to remove a splinter. Then put your two thumbnails on either side of the nick and squeeze the cyst until it pops out. The patient can easily learn to do this for himself.

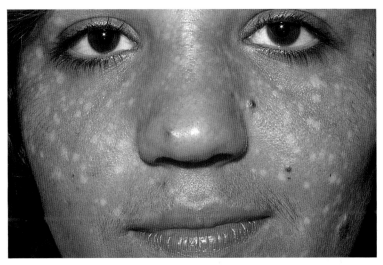

Figure 92 Treatment with the monobenzyl ether of hydroquinone gives this confetti-like hypopigmentation which is permanent.

MILIARIA

This is due to blockage of the sweat ducts in situations of very high humidity and heat. The only way to improve it is for the patient to cool down by taking a cold shower or going into an air-conditioned room.

MILKER'S NODULE

This needs no treatment. It will heal on its own in 4–5 weeks and the patient will then be immune for the future.

MOLES (MELANOCYTIC NAEVI)

Junctional naevi

The only reason for removing these is if they are atypical and cannot be distinguished from a malignant melanoma. Since they are dark brown in colour they may occasionally be mistaken for melanomas, but the round or oval shape and the uniformity of the colour should distinguish them.

Compound and intradermal naevi

These are completely harmless but may be unsightly, particularly on the face, or catch on the patient's clothes. They can be removed by slicing them off flush with the skin (shave biopsy) or by punch biopsy. Both of these will give an excellent cosmetic result (much better than an elliptical excision) and are easy and quick to do.

Congenital melanocytic naevus (giant hairy naevus)

These are always present from birth which ordinary moles are not. They may not be immediately recognizable though because they are often red rather than brown in the first few days of life. In an ideal world they should be removed surgically because they have about a 10% chance of a malignant melanoma developing within them at some later time. Small ones can be excised quite easily but it is often better to delay this until after puberty because it can then be done under a local rather than a general anaesthetic. Also if it is excised early on the scar will grow with the child and may end up a lot bigger than it was at first. If a child has a very large naevus,

he should be seen by a plastic surgeon as soon as possible after birth (within a few days) so that a decision can be taken about whether or not to do anything. It is sometimes possible to expand the skin around the naevus by inserting a balloon underneath the skin and gradually filling it up with water. When the skin has expanded enough, the naevus is excised and the wound closed with primary sutures. For some very large naevi, it is not feasible to excise the whole thing. Dermabrasion immediately after birth, has been tried as an alternative to excision but this has not been very successful; the pigment disappears initially but tends to come back after a few months. It may be better just to keep an eye on the naevus and excise any areas which change or become nodular (some lesions will become papillomatous with time without there being any sinister implications).

Dysplastic naevus

A dysplastic naevus looks like a large junctional naevus but has an irregular edge and different shades of brown within it (Figure 93). It can be very difficult to distinguish from a superficial spreading malignant melanoma and for this reason is best excised under a local anaesthetic.

Dysplastic naevus syndrome (familial atypical mole syndrome)

There are a small number of families where some members have large numbers of moles (more than 100), some of which are more than 8 mm in diameter, and many of which have irregular borders and are variegate in colour (*see* Figure 94). Such individuals have an

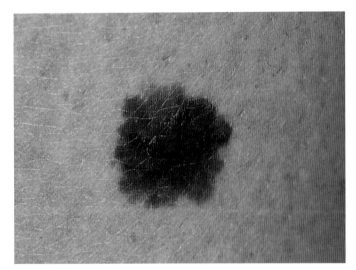

Figure 93 Dysplastic naevus.

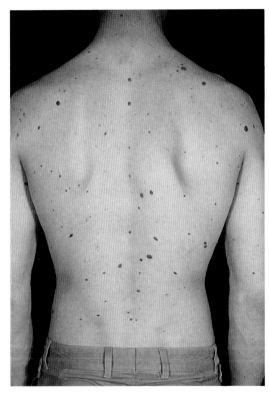

Figure 94 Dysplastic naevus syndrome. The patient has very numerous moles, some of which are large, have an irregular border and a multiplicity of colours.

increased risk not just of developing a malignant melanoma but of developing multiple malignant melanomas. It will be impossible to remove all the suspect moles, but any that are changing should be cut out. It may be helpful to take some colour photographs of the patient (face, chest, back, each arm and leg separately and a close-up of any moles that are very abnormal). If prints rather than slides are taken these can be given to the patient and he can be told to report to the doctor if any of them have changed. A duplicate set can be kept with his medical records so that there is something to compare the patient with if he thinks his moles are changing. It is better to err on the side of caution.

Spitz naevus

These are completely harmless in children and parents can be reassured that they are just a kind of mole. In adults they may be worrying because they can sometimes be confused with a malignant melanoma histologically. At any age they are in fact benign.

MOLLUSCUM CONTAGIOSUM

These are harmless papules due to a virus infection, so they will go away on their own once cell-mediated immunity has developed (usually 9–12 months). In young children it is better to leave well alone and let nature take its course. In adults their resolution can be speeded up by:

1 Sharpening an orange stick to a fine point, dipping it into a saturated solution of phenol and pricking the centre of each spot with it. This usually gets rid of them in a matter of days, but every spot must be treated or they will spread again from any that are left.
2 Freezing each one with liquid nitrogen for 10 seconds.
3 Painting them with 0.5% podophyllotoxin on a cotton wool bud each day until they are gone (2–3 weeks). The patient can do this himself.

Occasionally a molluscum can be confused with a basal cell carcinoma if it is solitary and on the face. If there is any doubt, curettage and cautery, sending the curettings for histological examination, will confirm the diagnosis and get rid of it.

MONGOLIAN SPOT

These usually disappear spontaneously by the end of the first year of life, so need no treatment.

MORPHOEA

Both the plaque form and the linear form of morphoea will resolve spontaneously in time. It may take months or sometimes several years, but eventually the skin will return to normal.

There is a rare and mutilating form of linear morphoea in children in which the underlying muscle and bone are involved as well as the skin, causing problems with growth and permanent deformity. Penicillamine 50 mg orally/day for a month and then gradually increasing up to a dose of 20 mg/kg body weight/day may sometimes improve things. Penicillamine is a potentially dangerous drug with very numerous side effects (anorexia, nausea, blood dyscrasias, proteinuria, systemic lupus erythematosus, pemphigus) so its use should be restricted to hospital use. It must not be given to patients who are allergic to penicillin.

Generalized morphoea, which can cause problems with breathing because of restricting the movements of the chest wall, will also normally resolve on its own in time. If it does not, penicillamine at a dose of 300–600 mg daily may help.

MUCOUS MEMBRANE PEMPHIGOID

Unlike bullous pemphigoid (*see* page 131), mucous membrane pemphigoid does not respond to systemic steroids. Although it is sometimes called *benign* mucous membrane pemphigoid, it can behave in a way which is far from benign, causing blindness due to scarring of the conjunctivae. There is no one treatment that always works and it is a question of finding the right drug for any individual patient. Azathioprine, cyclophosphamide or dapsone can all be used. It is probably best to start with dapsone since this is the safest of the three, although cyclophosphamide is the most effective. The doses and side effects of these treatments are shown in Table 7.

If there is scarring of the conjunctivae, it may sometimes be necessary to inject steroids intralesionally to inactivate the disease. All patients with this rare disorder should be under the care of a dermatologist or ophthalmologist with some experience in its management.

Table 7 Drugs used for treating mucous membrane pemphigoid

Drug and dosage	Side effects	Precautions to take
Dapsone 50 mg three times a day, reducing once the disease is under control	Haemolytic anaemia, methaemo-globinaemia	Check FBC after 1 week and again every 2–3 months. If the Hb falls too much, the dose will need to be reduced
Azathioprine 50 mg three times a day	Nausea, vomiting, diarrhoea and abdominal pain Pancytopenia	Warn the patient about GI upset and tell him to stop immediately if it occurs Check FBC after 1 week and then every 2 months
Cyclophosphamide 50 mg twice a day	Pancytopenia Hair loss Haemorrhagic cystitis	Check FBC after 1 week and again every 1 month Tell the patient to drink plenty of fluids to avoid problems with cystitis

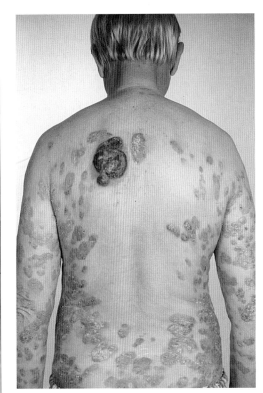

Figure 95 Mycosis fungoides with numerous indurated plaques and a single tumour.

MYCOSIS FUNGOIDES

In the early stages of the disease, which may last for many years, topical steroids are the mainstay of treatment. The patient complains of itching, and topical steroids will help that although they will not make the rash go away. One of the medium potency steroids is needed, 0.025% betamethasone valerate (Betnovate RD) ointment or cream, or its equivalent, applied twice a day as and when required. Most patients will be kept relatively comfortable for years with that.

Once indurated plaques are present, PUVA needs to be considered. Not all patients will need it, some will continue with just their topical steroids quite happily. For those in whom the itching is not controlled at this stage, PUVA twice or three times a week as for psoriasis (see page 164), will not only control the itching, but clear the skin.

When tumours occur, the whole nature of the disease changes. Individual tumours can be successfully treated with radiotherapy (Figure 95). This becomes impracticable if there are lots of tumours. The options then include:

- one of the retinoids, usually isotretinoin, 1–2 mg/kg body weight/day
- gradually increasing doses of interferon by intramuscular injection daily
- quadruple chemotherapy, usually with CHOP
  cyclophosphamide
  hydroxydaunorubicin [adriamycin]
  oncovin [vincristine]
  prednisolone.

NAEVUS OF ITO

A naevus of Ito is a benign flat blue naevus over the deltoid area (it looks just like a Mongolian spot but over the shoulder). It does not need any treatment because it does not show. The patient can be reassured that it is harmless.

NAEVUS OF OTA

A naevus of Ota is a flat blue naevus involving the skin around the eye and of the sclera. It is perfectly harmless but because it shows the patient will often require cosmetic camouflage.

NAEVUS SEBACEOUS

These are perfectly harmless during childhood. Later, any one of the abnormal tissues within the naevus, hair follicle, eccrine or

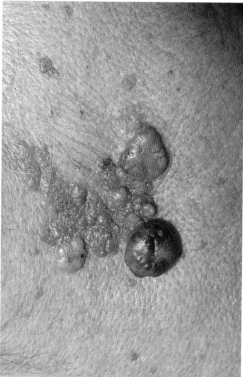

Figure 96 Naevus sebaceous on the right cheek present since birth. A pigmented basal cell carcinoma developed in it when the patient was 60.

apocrine sweat gland or sebaceous gland, can change into a benign or malignant tumour. Basal cell carcinomas are the commonest tumour to develop (Figure 96) although almost any adnexal tumour can occur. When this happens it is usually obvious because there will be a lump within the naevus or a discharge from it. At this stage it is best to excise the tumour, with or without the original naevus, depending on its size. There is no need to remove these naevi prophylactically because none of the tumours that develop are invasive and all will be cured by surgical removal.

NAEVUS SPILUS

These are harmless and need no treatment.

NAPKIN PSORIASIS

Parents are usually very distressed when their child develops napkin psoriasis. This is not because it is itchy or upsets the child in any way, but because it does not look very nice. 1% hydro-cortisone ointment mixed with Vioform (Vioform HC ointment) applied to the affected areas two or three times a day will clear it up fairly speedily. You need to warn the parents that the ointment will stain the nappy, and anything else it gets onto, a yellow colour but they usually do not mind as long as the rash goes away. This rash has nothing to do with atopic eczema or psoriasis but is a type of nappy rash secondarily infected with *Candida*. Once it disappears it does not recur; it is good to reassure the parents on this score from the beginning.

NAPPY RASH

The rash of nappy rash is a mild chemical burn which is caused by ammonia (from the breakdown of urea in the urine by bacteria in the faeces) and detergents (left in non-disposable nappies after washing and inadequate rinsing). It is common in babies with diarrhoea and tends to clear up when the stools return to normal. Ideally the nappy area should be exposed to the air while the skin heals. This is not very practical for most parents, but at the very least the area should be kept as clean and dry as possible. It is impossible to keep a baby completely dry the whole time and all babies will get nappy rash at some time in the first year of life.

Modern disposable nappies are very much better than towelling ones because they contain a material that draws fluid away from the skin keeping it relatively dry. Nappy rash will occur only if the nappy contains more fluid than it can hold, or when loose stools remain in contact with the skin. The nappies should be changed as soon as they are wet or soiled and the skin cleaned and dried. A moisturizer such as zinc and castor oil cream is then applied to the area which is about to be covered by the nappy.

Towelling nappies should not be used in babies with nappy rash unless the parents cannot afford good disposable ones. If they are used, they should be changed frequently and boiled (not just washed on the hottest setting of the washing machine) so that any bacteria in the faeces will be destroyed. They should also be very thoroughly rinsed so there is no detergent left on the nappy. Plastic pants should be left off unless absolutely essential since they will just hold the wet alkaline solution onto the baby's skin.

If the rash is very bad and does not improve after taking the simple measures outlined above, 1% hydrocortisone ointment can be applied twice a day for a few days to speed things up.

NECROBIOSIS LIPOIDICA

Many patients with necrobiosis lipoidica have diabetes so this should always be checked for. Treatment is aimed at stopping the plaques on the front of the shins from enlarging. If they have a raised mauve border, it is likely that they are in the process of getting bigger and treatment should be advised. A topical steroid ointment or cream, eg 0.025% betamethasone valerate (Betnovate RD) or the equivalent (*see* page 8) can be applied twice a day until the edge has flattened off. The patient should be warned that the treatment will not get rid of the marks altogether.

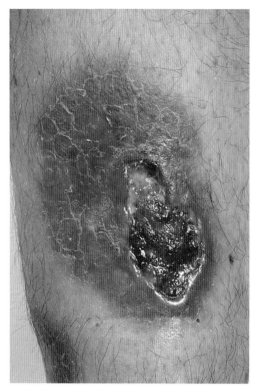

Figure 97 Necrobiosis lipoidica on the leg of a 21-year-old diabetic man. Ulceration has occurred after minor trauma.

If the edge is not raised, and the area of skin merely discoloured, treatment with topical steroids will not help. Patients do not like the look of the marks on the legs and are often not at all happy that you have no means of getting rid of them. Cosmetic camouflage in a woman can help a great deal by disguising the blemishes and enabling her to wear a skirt.

The affected areas of skin are atrophic and occasionally may ulcerate after trauma (usually obvious trauma like being knocked with a supermarket trolley or kicked by a football boot). If this happens it can be very difficult to get the ulcers to heal. They should be carefully protected from further trauma, and a non-stick dressing like Jelonet applied and covered with a dry dressing. The dressings can be changed twice a week until the ulcer(s) heal.

If there are no signs of healing after a few weeks, a skin graft may be required. Pinch grafts seem to work well and this can be done under a local anaesthetic (*see* page 235). If an area of necrobiosis lipoidica has been ulcerated in the past, the patient should take every care to protect the legs from further injury in the future. This may involve wearing shin pads under the trousers for a man (all the time, not just for playing football, and not just for men whose injury occurred whilst playing football) and even getting someone else to do the shopping to avoid injury from shopping baskets and trolleys.

NECROTIZING FASCIITIS

The most important thing here is to think of the diagnosis in any patient who has what looks like erysipelas or cellulitis which does not begin to improve with penicillin or erythromycin after 24–48 hours, or who has dusky purple areas appearing within the larger red swollen area (Figure 98). The diagnosis can be confirmed by finding a high level of anti-DNAase B in the patient's serum, if your local microbiology department can measure it.

It can be an acute fulminant illness with the patient dying almost before you can think of the diagnosis, or it can be a much slower process with the necrotic tissue gradually separating from the surrounding normal skin (Figure 99).

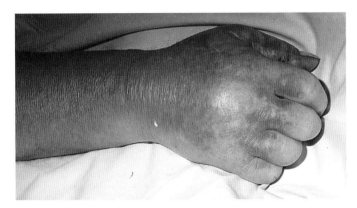

Figure 98 Acute fulminating necrotizing fasciitis.

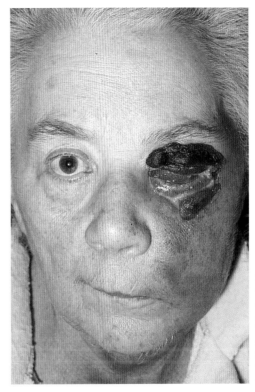

Figure 99 Chronic variety of necrotizing fasciitis 4 weeks after the onset. The black eschar will eventually slough off. This patient later needed plastic surgery to reconstruct her eyelids.

Patients should be admitted urgently to hospital so that wide surgical debridement of the affected skin can be carried out. Although this disease is usually due to a group A beta haemolytic streptococcus, antibiotics alone are not sufficient treatment. This is because the streptococci produce a toxin which causes the blood vessels in the affected area to thrombose. This not only causes the necrosis of the skin, which is the hallmark of the disease, but also prevents the antibiotics from getting to where they are needed. Without surgery some patients with necrotizing fasciitis will die and others will spend many months in hospital.

NEUROFIBROMATOSIS (VON RECKLINGHAUSEN'S DISEASE)

This disease is inherited as an autosomal dominant trait, although 50% of all patients are new mutations. This means that an affected individual will pass on the abnormal gene to half of his children, but the risk to subsequent children in a family who have a child with it 'out of the blue' is very low (*see* page 126). The abnormal gene is on chromosome 17 and prenatal diagnosis is now possible using linked DNA markers.

Inheritance of neurofibromatosis

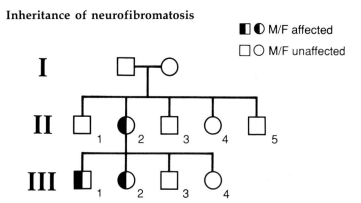

■ ● M/F affected

□ ○ M/F unaffected

Proband II₂ is a new mutation. Parents and subsequent sibs. unaffected.
50% of her children (III₁₊₂) are affected, with equal numbers of males and females.

Café-au-lait patches begin in the first 5 years of life, so if a child in an affected family reaches the age of 5 without having café-au-lait patches he is almost certainly unaffected. Neurofibromas begin at around puberty; the number that a patient has being very variable. If there are only a few and they do not show, no treatment will be needed. Some patients have enormous numbers and it will then be quite impracticable to remove them even if the patient wants it done. Individual neurofibromas which are very unsightly or which get in the way of the patient's clothes can be excised under a local or a general anaesthetic. There is no way of preventing them from occurring.

Patients should be seen by their GP once a year, so that any lumps that need removing can be dealt with, and at the same time the more serious complications of neurofibromatosis can be looked for by checking the blood pressure, examining the back and checking the visual acuity and fields.

Table 8 Major complications of neurofibromatosis

Complication	How to diagnose it
Plexiform neuroma and neurofibrosarcoma	Large multilobular lesion most often on the head and neck. If it becomes painful, or any other lump becomes persistently painful or uncomfortable, consider malignant change.
Scoliosis	Check the spine every year after the age of 6. If the curvature increases, bracing or spinal fusion will be needed.
Phaeochromocytoma	Check the blood pressure regularly. Consider the diagnosis also if there are intermittent episodes of unexplained anxiety, agitation, palpitations or sweating. Confirm by checking 24 hour urinary VMA and then by abdominal CT or MRI scan.
Optic glioma	Suspect if problems with visual acuity. Confirm with CT or MRI scan of the orbit.

Patients may want to be put in touch with others with the same thing. LINK is a self-help group for patients and their families:

LINK
120 London Road
Kingston upon Thames
Surrey, KT2 6QT
Tel: 081 547 1636

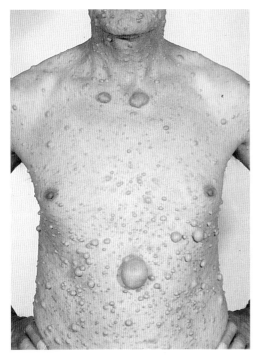

Figure 100 Neuro-fibromatosis. Large neurofibroma on the abdomen gets in the way of the patient's clothes and can be excised. It is quite impractical to think of excising all the lesions.

NODULAR PRURIGO

In order to get this better the patient must somehow stop scratching and picking the skin. If it is confined to the arms and legs, they can be wrapped up in Coltapaste occlusive bandages covered with Lestreflex for a week at a time (*see* Figure 42, page 56). When these bandages are first applied they are very soothing, but as the paste dries out the skin becomes itchy again. Every day a flannel, soaked in lukewarm water and wrung out, should be placed on top of the bandages for 10–15 minutes to keep them moist. This will keep them comfortable and enable the patient to keep them in place for longer. If the patient's fingers can be kept away from the nodules they will heal in 2–3 weeks. Unfortunately, when the bandages are taken off the patient will often begin to scratch again.

If the face and trunk are involved, paste bandages are not an option. Topical steroids can be helpful in alleviating the symptoms, although they will seldom cure the disease. Start with 1% hydro-cortisone ointment or cream, and do not progress to anything stronger than this on the face. On the trunk, if hydrocortisone does not work, one of the moderately potent group of steroids can be used (0.05% clobetasone butyrate [Eumovate], 0.025% betametha-sone valerate [Betnovate RD], or 0.00625% fluocinolone acetonide [Synalar 1 in 4 dilution]) twice a day. It will often be necessary to find the right ointment or cream by trial and error for any individual patient. In some instances, taking the patient into hospital to break the itch-scratch cycle will be helpful. The treat-ment in hospital is the same as at home, but taking the patient out of the normal environment ± some sedation will often do the trick.

Patients will often tell you that they feel unclean with this con-dition and it is important that this is expressed and any feelings of guilt dealt with. Nodular prurigo may begin at a time of stress in the patient's life and it can sometimes be helpful to explore this avenue with him (her) before the skin will improve. Whatever the underlying cause and however slow the improvement, it is im-portant not to leave the patient without hope for the future.

ONYCHOLYSIS

Most doctors assume that onycholysis is due to a fungal (dermato-phyte) infection. This is not the case; dermatophytes primarily affect the toenails and cause thickening rather than detachment. If the nail itself is not thickened (and there are no white streaks), then a fungal infection can be confidently dismissed. If you are not sure, send some nail clippings for mycology culture.

The first thing is to try to determine the cause of the onycholysis.

1 If it is due to trauma, this should be avoided in the future. Cleaning under the fingernails with a nail file is forbidden. The involved nail(s) should be cut back as far as possible to stop it catching on things, which would stop it sticking back down. If it follows a subungual haematoma it will recover as the new nail grows out.

2 If it is due to psoriasis, it will come and go in the same way that the skin lesions do. There is no specific treatment for the nail changes but if the skin disease is bad enough to need a systemic treatment (methotrexate or etretinate—see page 161) the nails will clear as the skin does.

3 If it is due to poor peripheral circulation, the hands and feet should be kept warm in cold weather.

4 If it is due to thyrotoxicosis, the nails will go back to normal when the thyroid disease is under control.

Whatever the cause, the onycholysis can be hidden in women by covering the nails with a coloured nail varnish.

ORF

This needs no treatment. It will heal on its own in 4–5 weeks and the patient will then be immune in the future.

OTITIS EXTERNA

Otitis externa is seborrhoeic eczema of the external auditory meatus. For most patients the treatment is the same as for seborrhoeic eczema elsewhere, with 1% hydrocortisone cream or ketaconazole cream applied twice a day when the rash is there, and left off when it is not (see also seborrhoeic eczema, page 67). However, because of the narrow ear canal there are problems which are unique to this site:

- scale tends to accumulate blocking the ear and causing pain
- secondary infection (with *Staphylococcus aureus*, gram negative organisms, *Candida albicans* and aspergillus) is common especially in wet and humid conditions (eg after swimming)
- the itching encourages the patient to poke things down the ear.

If the eczema is dry and scaly, the treatment is the same as for seborrhoeic eczema elsewhere (1% hydrocortisone cream or ketaconazole cream used twice a day until it is better).

If there is a lot of scale and/or pain, the patient should see an ENT surgeon. A perforated ear drum and a co-existant otitis media must be excluded. Aural toilet with removal of the excess scale can be done in the ENT clinic which will help the pain.

If there is an acute weeping eczema, do not be tempted to use one of the topical steroid/antibiotic (± antifungal) ear drops or sprays. You will only make things worse by exposing the patient to the risk of developing an acute contact allergic eczema on top of what he already has. Take a swab for bacteriology and mycology culture. If there is a bacterial infection present, use a systemic antibiotic depending on the sensitivities (probably flucloxacillin or erythromycin 250 mg four times a day for 7 days). If there is a fungal infection, ketaconazole will be required rather than a topical steroid. First dry up the exudate with an astringent such as 13% aluminium acetate ear drops. When it is dry, use 1% hydrocortisone cream or ointment twice a day until it is better. Some patients with recurrent problems find tar more soothing than topical steroids, and an ichthammol wick inserted into the ear canal will be very soothing.

PACHYONYCHIA CONGENITA

There is no cure for this condition. Regular chiropody will be needed to keep the toenails as flat as possible to stop the toes from hurting when the patient is wearing shoes.

PAGET'S DISEASE OF THE NIPPLE

Because this can look very like eczema, it is essential to confirm the diagnosis by biopsy before embarking on treatment. Once it has been confirmed the patient should have a mammogram done looking for the microcalcification of an intraduct carcinoma. It is essential to check the other breast at the same time.

Treatment involves doing a simple mastectomy. Anything less than that has a high incidence of recurrence 5–10 years later. There is no need to do an axillary clearance because it is extremely rare for there to be involvement of the local lymph nodes.

Extramammary Paget's disease (of the anogenital area or axilla)

The diagnosis needs to be confirmed by biopsy. Treatment then involves surgical excision of the abnormal area of skin and of the underlying carcinoma.

PALISADING ENCAPSULATED NEUROMA (PEN)

These little papules, which look a bit like intradermal naevi (Figure 101) are completely harmless. The diagnosis is usually made when

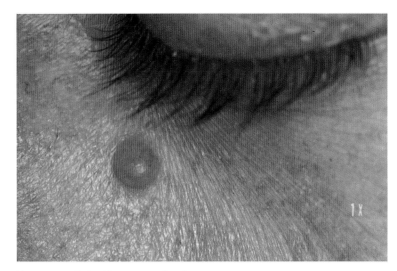

Figure 101 Palisading encapsulated neuroma.

one is excised because the patient did not like the look of it. The histology report often comes back as *neurofibroma* which is wrong. This lesion has a very specific pathology and it is nothing to do with neurofibromatosis. If they are unsightly, they can be removed under a local anaesthetic; otherwise they can be left alone.

PANNICULITIS

Panniculitis needs to be distinguished from other causes of tender red nodules on the lower legs by biopsy if necessary (Table 9). There are some specific causes of panniculitis and these should be asked about and looked for:
- cold, especially in the newborn

- trauma to heavy breasts and buttocks
- associated with pancreatic disease (Ca pancreas)
- associated with discoid lupus erythematosus
- artefact from self-injection of oily liquids (look for the needle mark!).

Table 9 Causes of tender red nodules on the lower leg

Erythema nodosum	Tender red nodules on front of shins Individual lesions only last 7–14 days Associated fever and arthralgia Mainly young women
Panniculitis	Single or multiple red nodules, mainly on lower legs but can be any area of subcutaneous fat Lesions last weeks or months Heal with scarring
Nodular vasculitis	Impossible to distinguish from panniculitis except on biopsy of an early lesion Mainly lower legs Lesions last weeks or months
Polyarteritis nodosa	Benign form associated with livedo reticularis and/or ulceration on lower legs Generalized form. Patient unwell with involvement of lungs and kidneys High ESR
Thrombophlebitis	Lesions over superficial veins

In most patients the cause will not be known. The patient is otherwise fit and well but has painful lumps on the legs which may continue for years. Systemic steroids are the most useful treatment starting with prednisolone 30 mg daily and gradually reducing as soon as the disease comes under control to a maintenance dose of 7.5–10 mg daily. Since treatment may have to be continued for many years, it will be wise to refer the patient to a dermatologist for the diagnosis to be confirmed and the necessary investigations carried out.

PARONYCHIA

Acute paronychia

This is caused by *Staphylococcus aureus* or a group A beta haemolytic streptococcus. If the digit is red and exquisitely painful but there is no pus visible, start the patient on oral flucloxacillin or erythromycin, 250 mg four times a day for 7 days. If there is obvious pus present, it should be lanced to let it out. Once it is better the patient should be advised about keeping the hands dry so that a new cuticle will grow (*see* below).

Chronic paronychia

The commonest pathogen here is *Candida albicans*, but it is not necessary to treat that specifically. The real cause is the loss of the cuticle, which has disappeared totally or partially by being soaked in water for long periods of time and then traumatized. This produces a gap between the posterior nail fold and the nail itself which allows entrance for bacteria and fungi. The paronychia will only get better permanently if a new cuticle can be induced to grow.

The patient must keep the hands dry by wearing rubber gloves or cotton-lined rubber or PVC gloves for all wet work until a new cuticle has grown (3–4 months). A protective film of Vaseline can be applied around the nail several times a day to keep water out.

Some doctors suggest that nystatin ointment is applied around the nail fold during the day and neomycin or gentamycin ointment at night, to get rid of *Candida* and bacteria, but there is no evidence that this is more effective than Vaseline.

PEARLY PENILE PAPULES

No treatment is needed for these. If the patient is anxious he can be reassured that they are perfectly harmless, and not contagious.

PEMPHIGOID (BULLOUS PEMPHIGOID)

The diagnosis should be confirmed by skin biopsy (for histology and immunofluorescence), and by looking for basement membrane antibodies in the serum. For a few patients, in whom the blisters are localized to just a small area of the body, topical steroids in the form of 0.025% betamethasone valerate (Betnovate RD) ointment or cream (or the equivalent) can be applied twice a day. This may control the blistering for many months but eventually the blisters will become more widespread. At this stage systemic therapy will be needed and the two drugs that are most commonly used are prednisolone and azathioprine.

Prednisolone 30–40 mg daily should be started immediately. The blisters will begin to dry up within 48 hours. The steroids are kept at this dose until all blistering has stopped, and then reduced fairly rapidly to a maintenance dose of 5–7.5 mg a day.

We usually reduce it from:
40 mg to 30 mg
30 mg to 25 mg
25 mg to 20 mg
20 mg to 15 mg
15 mg to 12.5 mg
12.5 mg to 10 mg
10 mg to 7.5 mg
7.5 mg to 5 mg;

with a change of dose twice a week. If blisters recur, the dose will need to be increased again by going up 2 points on the above scale. Once a maintenance dose has been reached it is wise to keep the patient on it indefinitely. This is why it is essential to confirm the diagnosis before treatment is started. In a few patients the blisters will not stop with 30–40 mg prednisolone, and the dose will have to be increased to 60 mg a day. This is fairly unusual. Again, once the disease is under control, the dose of steroids should be reduced as soon as possible.

If it is not possible to get the maintenance dose of systemic steroids down to an acceptable level (5–7.5 mg daily), which is very unusual, azathioprine should be added. Azathioprine is not used as the first line of treatment because it takes 6 weeks to work. It does however work very well for pemphigoid and may be safer, in the long term, than prednisolone. Start with 2 mg/kg body weight/day, ie 50 mg two or three times a day. Providing there are no side effects (fall in blood count or diarrhoea and vomiting), this dose can be continued indefinitely. Once the blisters are under control, the dose of prednisolone can gradually be reduced with the aim of either getting down to a very low maintenance dose or getting the patient off steroids altogether.

Table 10 Management of the patient on systemic treatment

Drug	Side effects and precautions to be taken against them
Prednisolone	1 Salt and water retention may put the patient into congestive cardiac failure. Weigh patient before treatment begins and then weekly. Look out for ankle oedema. Add a diuretic if dose cannot yet be reduced. 2 Weight gain. Patient should be warned that this may occur (due to salt and water retention and increase in appetite) and encouraged to eat less. The typical Cushingoid facial appearance does not usually occur until the disease comes under control, so is not seen early on when the patient is on the highest dose of steroid. 3 Increase in blood pressure. Check before treatment is begun and then once a week until the dose is stabilized. After that it can be checked once a month. 4 Glycosuria. Latent diabetes may be brought to light. Test the urine once a week. If the patient is going to have to stay on treatment indefinitely, insulin may be needed. If the dose is coming down it may be possible to await events provided the patient is not unwell. 5 Easy bruising and tearing of the skin. Warn the patient that this may occur and that it is nothing to be alarmed at. If the patient (and his carers) are careful, not too much damage will be done. 6 Tendency to infection. Being aware that this can occur is the most important thing and looking for the site of infection if the patient develops a fever or becomes unwell.

Drug	Side effects and precautions to be taken against them (continued)
Prednisolone	7 Osteoporosis and fractures of the head of the femur and spine. Think about it if there is pain in the back, hips or knees; X-ray to confirm the diagnosis and reduce the dose as soon as possible. 8 Proximal muscle weakness may make it difficult for the patient to get out of bed and walk. Be on the look-out for it, and reduce the dose as soon as possible if it occurs. 9 Peptic ulceration. Prophylactic cimetidine should be given to a patient with a previous history of peptic ulceration.
Azathioprine	1 Diarrhoea and vomiting. This can be very severe and cause rapid dehydration. Warn the patient that it might occur and tell him to stop the tablets and call the doctor immediately if it does. If it is going to happen, it usually does so in the first week of treatment so you will know very quickly whether it is going to be alright or not. 2 Pancytopenia. Check a full blood count before treatment begins and again after 1 week and 1 month. After that, once every 2–3 months is sufficient unless bleeding or infection occur. Warn the patient to get in touch immediately if he gets a sore throat or chest infection. If the haemoglobin, WBC or platelets fall a little, the dose should be reduced; if they fall a lot the drug must be stopped.

In patients in whom there are contraindications for giving systemic steroids, azathioprine should be started from the beginning. Generally speaking, patients cannot put up with widespread blisters for 6 weeks, so prednisolone will have to be given as well for the first 6 weeks. The steroid dosage is then reduced as soon as possible and stopped once the azathioprine has taken effect. For the side effects of prednisolone and azathioprine *see* Table 10.

In all patients the blisters can be dried up by using potassium permanganate in the bath (diluted so that the bath water is a pale pink colour). If secondary infection of the blisters occurs, flucloxacillin or erythromycin 250 mg four times a day should be given for 7 days.

Pemphigoid should be thought of in all patients over the age of 70 who present with a very itchy rash even if there are no obvious blisters. Looking for basement membrane antibodies in the serum is a useful thing to do, but it is only present in 70% of patients, so if it is negative it does not rule out the diagnosis completely. Alternatively, a skin biopsy for immunofluorescence will be positive at that stage and will confirm the diagnosis.

PEMPHIGOID (HERPES) GESTATIONIS

Fortunately this condition is uncommon. It is extremely itchy and will make life intolerable during the day and stop the patient sleeping at night. Ice placed directly onto the itchy plaques and blisters will bring symptomatic relief, but only temporarily. If it occurs near full term, the patient can often be kept going until after delivery with topical steroids (eg 0.025% betamethasone valerate [Betnovate RD] ointment). If it occurs earlier and the itching is intolerable she may need to be given systemic steroids (usually prednisolone, 30 mg daily). Such patients should be under the care of a dermatologist. Systemic steroids do not seem to have any adverse effects on the fetus.

PEMPHIGUS
Pemphigus vulgaris

Pemphigus is a very uncommon disease in spite of the name which refers to the commonest form of pemphigus. It is much more serious than pemphigoid and without treatment most patients will die (of fluid loss or secondary infection). All patients with pemphigus should be admitted to hospital until the blisters are under control because very high doses of systemic steroids are needed to control it. Skin biopsy of a new blister (for histology and immunofluorescence) and serum for circulating intercellular antibodies must be taken before treatment is begun, because once started, systemic steroids will be needed for the rest of the patient's life. If there are no obvious blisters but only erosions, particularly early on when the blisters may be confined to the mouth, the diagnosis can be confirmed by finding acantholytic cells on a Tzanck smear. (A Tzanck smear is taken by scraping the base of a blister or an erosion with a blunt scalpel and putting the fluid you get on a clean glass slide. This is then stained with H & E or any other stain you like).

Treatment is started with prednisolone 120 mg daily until the blisters stop. The dose is then gradually reduced to a maintenance dose of 5–10 mg a day. What often happens is that the blisters dry up initially, but once the dose is down to about 50 mg a day, new blisters appear. If this happens, the dose has to be raised again until the blisters stop, and then reduced again. At this stage it is often a nightmare for patient and doctor alike.

If the blisters cannot be controlled with a reasonable maintenance dose of steroids, azathioprine can be added at a dose of 2 mg/kg body weight/day. This will take 6 weeks to work, so is no good as an initial treatment to control the disease. In any patient in whom there are contraindications to long-term treatment with systemic steroids, azathioprine can be started at the same time as the prednisolone with the idea of stopping the steroids as soon as the azathioprine has worked.

Because such large doses of steroids are needed, all patients will run into problems with side effects (this is a reason for these patients being in hospital initially). The precautions that are needed are the same as in pemphigoid, *see* Table 10, page 132. In the long term, the lowest dose of systemic steroids that will control the disease is given, but it may have to be higher than you would like.

If prednisolone and azathioprine do not work, methotrexate, gold or plasmapheresis are alternatives.

As well as systemic treatment, the patient will need potassium permanganate in his bath water to coagulate protein and help to dry up the blisters. Initially he may need intravenous fluids to counteract fluid loss through the skin and antibiotics if there is any sign of bacterial infection. If he complains of severe pain in the skin, consider the possibility of infection with herpes simplex (*see* Figure 63, page 81); if this occurs, intravenous acyclovir will be required (*see* page 80).

Pemphigus foliaceous

Pemphigus foliaceous is a more superficial variety of pemphigus with the blister just under the granular layer of the epidermis. It is less common than pemphigus vulgaris and less serious. It can often be controlled just with a moderately potent topical steroid such as 0.025% betamethasone valerate (Betnovate RD) cream or ointment (or the equivalent) applied twice a day. Sometimes the blisters are bad enough to require systemic treatment, in which case methotrexate often works better than prednisolone. Patients should be referred to a dermatologist so that the diagnosis can be confirmed and the best treatment sorted out.

PERIORAL DERMATITIS

Since this is usually due to the application of a topical steroid cream or ointment stronger than 1% hydrocortisone to the face, the first thing is to stop it. The rash will then get better, but it often takes several months. Oxytetracycline 250 mg twice a day on an empty stomach (half an hour before food or one hour after) for 6 weeks will get it better quicker. How it works is not known. When the topical steroid is stopped the rash may initially get quite a lot worse. The patient must be actively discouraged from using the topical steroid again at this stage, preferably by removing the tube from him! We usually tell the patient that the rash cannot be cured while the topical steroid is used. If the skin is very dry and some kind of topical preparation is needed, aqueous cream is a very pleasant moisturizer for the face, and it can safely be applied as often as the patient likes.

PERSISTENT SUPERFICIAL DERMATITIS

This is just a type of eczema, although it is often confused with mycosis fungoides. Ultraviolet light works better than any ointments or creams. The patient may find that it improves spontaneously in the summer if he is able to get out into the sunshine. If he lives or works near a hospital with facilities for outpatient UVB therapy this can be given two or three times a week for 6–8 weeks. Alternatively a dilute topical steroid can be tried. Start with 1% hydrocortisone ointment and increase to something stronger only if it does not work. Generally speaking, UVB works better than topical steroids.

PHIMOSIS

If there is no obvious infection present the patient will need to be circumcised; he should be referred to a surgeon. If you suspect that there is an underlying infection present, of which the commonest are chlamydia, gardnerella and *Candida*, the patient should be referred to the local hospital department of genitourinary medicine so that the diagnosis can be confirmed. Sometimes the penis is so tender that it is impossible to take urethral swabs. In that case the patient's sexual partner should be examined and the diagnosis confirmed from her. If no infection is found, ice or 1% hydrocortisone cream applied twice a day can be helpful.

PHOTOSENSITIVITY RASHES

In a patient with a rash due to sunlight it is not just a matter of staying out of the sun or using a sunscreen, but of making a definite diagnosis. To do this, the important questions to ask are:

1 How long does it take after exposure to sunlight for the rash to occur, and if you come in out of the sun, how long will it take before the rash goes away?

2 Do you get the rash through window glass on a sunny day?

1. Timing. Solar urticaria occurs within a few minutes of sun exposure and clears in about an hour. Polymorphic light eruption, which is the commonest rash due to the sun, does not appear for several hours after sun exposure and lasts several days. Patients with porphyria get burning ± blisters within a few minutes of sun exposure but the skin changes last for several days. Patients with Hutchinson's summer prurigo or photosensitive eczema will usually deny any relationship between their rash and sun exposure, although it is obvious from the distribution of the rash that it must be due to the sun.

2. Window glass. Window glass cuts out short-wave ultraviolet light (UVB), so if the patient is getting the rash on a sunny day when they are indoors with the windows shut, it must be due to long-wave ultraviolet light (UVA). This has implications for the treatment because the ordinary absorbent sunscreens only block out UVB. If the rash is due to UVA the patient will need a reflectant sunscreen containing titanium dioxide or zinc oxide which will be much less cosmetically acceptable (*see* page 140).

Solar urticaria

Because this is a type 1 allergic response, an antihistamine should be useful. Begin with one of the non-sedative ones such as terfenadine 60 mg twice a day, and increase it to 120 mg or even 240 mg twice a day until it works (astemizole 10 mg daily and cetirizine dihydrochloride 10 mg at night are alternatives). At the same time it is worth the patient using a high protective factor sunscreen which should be applied at least half an hour before going out (*see* pages 140 and 141).

A few patients will not be helped by these simple measures. They should be referred to the local dermatologist so that light testing can be carried out and the diagnosis confirmed. Some of them will have erythropoietic protoporphyria or systemic lupus erythematosus and not solar urticaria at all. Others will need to be desensitized to ultraviolet light by giving very small doses of UVB each day and gradually increasing it until the patient can tolerate ordinary sunlight. It is an extremely tedious procedure for the patient; if he stops for any reason, he will be back to square one. So once started the daily UVB has to be continued indefinitely and the patient will have to be very well motivated to persevere with it.

Polymorphic light eruption

The cause of this very common rash is unknown. There is no question that it occurs after sun exposure, but often it cannot be verified by light testing. Some patients will only get it if the weather is exceptionally hot or if they go abroad on holiday, others will develop it on the first sunny day in spring in the UK. All patients show some degree of tachyphylaxis, ie if they go on being exposed to the sunlight, the rash will gradually get less and less until it stops. In Britain it is not often possible to rely on continuous sunshine day after day, so it is better to get the patient to use a high protective factor sunscreen (Groups 1, 2 or 3 in Table 13, page 141) before going out into the sun. In countries where sunshine is more reliable it is better to tell the patient to put up with the rash until they have developed tolerance to it (a few weeks).

Some patients do not improve using ordinary non-opaque sunscreens, and find that having the rash severely curtails their activities in the summer months. Some of them will benefit from PUVA therapy given two or three times a week for about 6 weeks in the early spring to prevent the polymorphic light eruption from developing. Others will be helped by PUVA as an actual therapy for the rash. It is again given two or three times a week for 6–8 weeks (for problems with PUVA see page 166). Any patient who does not improve with sun-protective creams and sensible protective clothing should be referred to a dermatologist.

Porphyria

There are many different forms of porphyria, all of which will need specialist help to confirm the diagnosis, offer genetic counselling and to sort out an appropriate treatment. Some patients need treatment other than protection of the skin from the sun—see Table 11.

Table 11 Main types of porphyria

Type of porphyria	Treatment
Erythropoietic protoporphyria (EPP)	Beta carotene 50–200 mg daily (enough to maintain a serum level of 500 µg/100 ml). Cholestyramine may help to reduce the liver damage but some patients may eventually need a liver transplant.
Variegate porphyria	Avoid any drugs that can precipitate acute attacks—barbiturates, chlordiazepoxide, danazol, dapsone, ergot preparations, erythromycin, griseofulvin, halothane, meprobamate, methyldopa, oestrogens, pentazocine, phenytoin, sulphonamides and sulphonylureas.
Porphyria cutanea tarda (PCT)	Stop all alcohol intake. If the symptoms do not go away, consider monthly venesection (500 ml) until the serum ferritin is back to normal or symptoms have abated or chloroquine 200 mg twice a day.

These patients react to long-wave ultraviolet light at 400 nm. Ordinary non-opaque sunscreens will not be of any help and they will burn or blister on a sunny day indoors since light at 400 nm will come through window glass. Indoors, therefore, the curtains will need to be kept closed if the weather is sunny or Uvethon-Y screens should be placed over the windows (see pages 137 and 138).

Babies with EPP should be kept out of the sun; it is not enough to allow them to sit out in a pram with the hood up. Titanium dioxide or zinc oxide must be used as a sunscreen (*see* page 139) whenever they have to be taken out of doors, and the skin covered as much as possible with thick cotton clothes (which are cool but do not allow UVA to penetrate) and the head with a broad-brimmed hat. The same precautions need to be taken for older children and adults.

Adults with variegate porphyria or PCT will also need titanium dioxide or zinc oxide opaque sunscreens and advice on suitable protective clothing.

Hutchinson's summer prurigo

Like patients with polymorphic light eruption, light testing of patients with Hutchinson's summer prurigo is often unhelpful. A high protective factor sunscreen should be used throughout the year (Group 1, Table 13, page 141). If this is not enough to get rid of the rash and the symptoms, the patient should be referred to a dermatologist so that the diagnosis can be confirmed and other treatments tried. PUVA or chloroquine are used and sometimes help.

Photosensitive eczema (Chronic actinic dermatitis; actinic reticuloid)

This is a disease in which there is extreme sensitivity both to ultraviolet light (UVB and UVA) and visible light. It is an extraordinarily distressing condition for the patient, usually a middle-aged or elderly man, because it is very itchy, looks horrible, interferes with his work and/or hobbies, stops him going out of doors and may even necessitate him living in semi-darkness (Figure 102). Added to this is the fact that, although a few patients will get better spontaneously, most do not and the condition persists indefinitely. Most patients have difficulty in accepting that their rash is due to the sun and this too mitigates against them getting better because unless they accept it and take steps to avoid it, there is no chance of it improving.

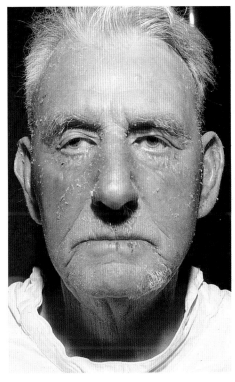

Figure 102 Photosensitive eczema in a 78-year-old man.

It is probably wise to arrange for a patient with this to be admitted to hospital when the rash first begins. At this stage it is likely to be pretty bad and very likely he will be grateful that you are doing your best to help.

In hospital:

1 He can be nursed in a room with Uvethon-Y* screens at the windows so that all the ultraviolet light is screened out. This will cause a dramatic improvement in the rash within 24–48 hours.

*Uvethon-Y available from, May and Baker Plastics Products, Dagenham, Essex, RM10 7XS.

2 He can be helped symptomatically by the application of a dilute topical steroid ointment to the skin twice a day (1% hydrocortisone ointment on the face and 0.025% betamethasone valerate ointment [Betnovate RD] elsewhere).

3 The itching is controlled with chlorpheniramine 4–8 mg four times a day (sometimes as much as 16 mg four times a day is needed). Trimeprazine or promethazine, which are usually used for eczema, should not be used because the phenothiazines can sometimes cause photosensitivity.

Once the skin is better:

4 He can be light tested to find out how much of the UV spectrum he is reacting to, and therefore which sunscreens are going to be most appropriate.

5 He can be patch tested and photopatch tested to see if there are any topical or systemic agents that he should avoid. It is quite common for these patients to have an allergic contact eczema to one or more substances, including sometimes the chemicals in sunscreens.

6 The cause of the rash can then be explained to him, together with the precautions he will have to take in the future.

7 He can be shown how to use the ointments and sunscreens that he will have to use at home, and he can be supervised until both he and the staff are confident that there will not be any problems at home. The topical steroid is applied first and the sunscreen is put on top 10 minutes later. The patient is advised to put both on first thing in the morning and again early–mid afternoon. Unless he is going to use a commercially available sunscreen, he will need to be shown how to mix burnt sugar and ferric oxide with his titanium dioxide sunscreen so that the colour matches his skin (*see* page 140).

8 Ideally he will then be nursed in a room without any specific protection to see how he gets on just with the treatment he is going to be using at home. If the rash recurs when he is nursed in a room

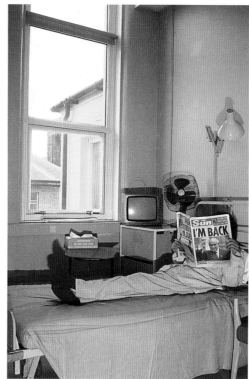

Figure 103 Uvethon-Y screened room.

without Uvethon-Y screens at the windows, he will have to have Uvethon-Y screens or blinds fitted to the windows of his house, or at least to the windows of the room(s) where he spends most of his time. Usually one of the patient's relatives can fit the Uvethon-Y; if not it will have to be arranged through social services. It is not very pleasant being in a Uvethon-Y screened room because the light is yellow and many patients and their families find it depressing to live in a kind of perpetual twilight.

Once the patient goes home, he must avoid the sun. He should not go out, even with his sunscreen on, in the middle of the day (10 am–3 pm) unless it is absolutely essential because the intensity of UVA is about 100 times stronger then. When he goes out he should wear a hat, gloves and a long-sleeved shirt, preferably made of thick and tightly woven cotton. If he holds his shirt up to the light and he can see through it, it will let the light through to damage his skin. He should wear clothes that he cannot see through when he holds them up to the light. A neckerchief worn around the neck will protect his neck from the sun and his collar from the mess made by his sunscreen.

He should not go abroad to the sun for his holidays, and he must understand that sitting in the shade is not safe because of reflected light (from sand, water, a path or grass). Nor is it safe to be out if the weather is cloudy, because clouds do not screen out ultraviolet light. He may have to avoid occupational exposure to ultraviolet light (arc welding and fluorescent light tubes if they are not protected with a plastic diffuser). He may have to fit diffusers to his fluorescent lights at home or just use tungsten lighting.

He will need to use one of the opaque sunscreens, which are a lot less cosmetically acceptable than the ordinary ones which protect against UVB. Commercially available sunscreens which are supposed to protect against UVA are rarely sufficient, although it is obviously worth trying something like SUN E45 SPF 25, Uvistat 20 or 30, or Soltan 20 in the first instance. If they do not work a mixture such as the one shown *right* will be needed. This is very effective but makes a mess of the patient's clothes, particularly his collar and cuffs. It also looks like a foundation cream. Most women will find it perfectly acceptable because they can put their ordinary make-up on top, but most men will find it difficult to use.

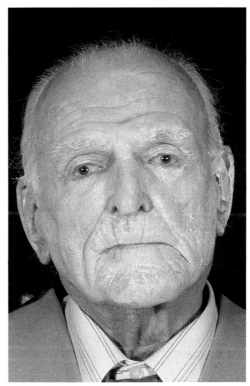

Figure 104 Patient with titanium dioxide sunscreen without any added colouring material. This is too unsightly for the patient to cope with.

Titanium dioxide powder	15 g
Aqueous cream or Uvistat cream	285 g
Burnt sugar and ferric oxide are added to make it match the patient's skin colour.	

Some patients will go on having problems in spite of doing their best to avoid the sun. In that case, azathioprine 2 mg/kg body weight/day, ie 50 mg twice or three times a day, can sometimes transform their lives back to normal. A full blood count should be done before azathioprine is started and again after 1 and 4 weeks because it can cause pancytopenia. Once the patient is stabilized on azathioprine, the blood count needs checking only every 2–3 months (*see* also Table 10, page 132). If the blood count falls or if the patient cannot take azathioprine because of gastrointestinal symptoms (diarrhoea, vomiting and abdominal pain), cyclosporin A is the only alternative (for the side effects associated with cyclosporin A, *see* page 170).

Photosensitive drug rashes

Patients with photosensitivity due to drugs (*see* page 44) will first of all need to stop the offending drug. Sometimes this is not possible, particularly with amiodarone when there is no other drug which will effectively stop the patient's arrhythmia. In that case a sunscreen containing titanium dioxide or zinc oxide must be used. Almost all drug-induced photosensitivity rashes are due to UVA so the patient will need protection with one of the opaque sunscreens (*see* below).

Sunscreens

Sunscreens work either by absorbing ultraviolet light or by reflecting it. Most absorbent sunscreens only protect the skin against UVB. The reflectant ones contain inert mineral pigments, which basically put an opaque barrier between the sun and the skin and protect against both UVB and UVA (Tables 12 and 13).

Patients who are very sensitive to UVA will not find these commercially available sunscreens adequate protection, even those in Group 1. They should use 5% titanium dioxide mixed with

Table 12 Chemical composition of sunscreens

Chemicals in absorbent sunscreens	Chemicals in reflective sunscreens
1 Para-aminobenzoic acid (PABA)* 2 PABA esters*, eg octyldimethyl PABA (padimate) 3 Cinnamates, eg 2-ethylhexyl *p*-methoxycinnamate 4 Benzophenones**, eg oxybenzone and mexenone 5 Dibenzoylmethanes**, eg butyl methoxy dibenzoyl methane	6 Titanium dioxide 7 Zinc oxide

*Only active against UVB; penetrate into the stratum corneum after half–2 hours, so not easily removed by water. PABA preparations often sting the skin and stain the clothes yellow.
**Give a little protection against UVA too.

aqueous cream. This is very white and looks unsightly (Figure 104). Burnt sugar and/or ferric oxide can be added to make it more or less the same colour as the patient's skin. There is no set formula for working out how much of either to use; it is just a question of adding a little of each and trying it out until the colour match is right.

Protection from the sun is needed for everyone with a Caucasian skin if they are going to be exposed to ultraviolet light (especially children). Keeping the skin covered with clothes and the head with a wide-brimmed hat are sensible precautions that anyone can take. On holiday, sunbathing should be avoided in the middle of the day, and exposure to the sun should be increased gradually to avoid getting sunburnt. Sitting in the shade or swimming will not protect against sun damage even though the person feels cool.

Table 13 Available sunscreens

Sunscreen	Main ingredients (numbers = chemicals in Table 12)
1 High protection against UVB and UVA*	
SUN E45 25	6
Soltan 20	6
Uvistat cream 30 and 20	3 + 4 + 5 + 6
2 Medium protection against UVB and UVA**	
Piz Buin total sunblock lotion 24	3 + 5 + 6
RoC Total Sunblock cream Over 15	3 + 4 + 7
SpectraBAN Ultra 17	2 + 4 + 5 + 6
SUN E45 15	6
Uvistat cream 15 and 10	3 + 4 + 5
Uvistat cream 8 (water-resistant)	3 + 4
3 High protection against UVB	
Almay Total Sunblock cream 15	2 + 4
Coppertone Supershade 15	2 + 4
Coppertone Ultrashade 23	2 + 3 + 4
RoC invisible sunscreen 10–15	3 + 4 + 5 + 6
RoC sunscreen stick 10–15	3 + 5
SpectraBAN 15 lotion	1 + 2
4 Medium protection against UVB	
Almay ultra protection lotion 12 (water-resistant)	1 + 4
Piz Buin creme SPF12 lotion	3 + 5 + 6
Piz Buin creme Allergy lotion	3 + 5 + 6
SpectraBAN 10	3 + 4

*The number refers to the SPF against UVB. The SPF for UVA is approximately 10. **The number refers to the SPF against UVB. The SPF for UVA is between 4 and 7.

Which sunscreen to use when

Type of patient	Type of protection
Normal individual with Type 1 (always burns, never tans), or Type 2 skin (always burns, sometimes tans) Vitiligo Albino	Need protection against sunburn in the short term and skin cancer in the long term. Use sunscreen with high SPF, 15–20 (Groups 1 and 3) throughout the summer months. No need for SPF >25 because unlikely to be exposed to that much sun in a day
Normal individual with Type 3 (sometimes burns, always tans), or Type 4 skin (never burns, always tans)	Need protection against skin cancer in the long term. Use sunscreen with medium protection against UVB (Group 4) for holiday times. Do not need protection for ordinary sun exposure
Patients with solar urticaria, polymorphic light eruption and discoid or systemic lupus erythematosus	Use sunscreen from Groups 2 or 3 throughout the summer months to prevent rash from occurring or getting worse
Patients with photosensitive eczema, drug-induced photosensitivity, Hutchinson's summer prurigo or porphyria (and patients in group above who have not improved)	Use sunscreen from Group 1 in Table 12. If it does not help, get the chemist to make up a 5% titanium dioxide mixture (formula on page 139)

PHYTOPHOTODERMATITIS

For phytophotodermatitis to occur the patient needs to have had contact with a plant containing psoralens and exposure to the sun. The commonest plants to cause problems belong to the *Umbellifera* and *Rutacea* families, most being wayside flowers although some are garden shrubs. Wild parsnip, wild chervil, cow parsley, giant hogweed and rue are the main culprits in the UK, although it can also be due to bindweed, carrot, dill, fennel and St John's wort. The diagnosis can be difficult because the patient may not know the names of the plants that he has been in contact with. Ideally the plant responsible should be identified so that it can be avoided in the future. If the rash has occurred after strimming in the garden, the patient should be told to wear his trousers tucked inside his socks or Wellington boots when doing this in future. If the rash is very acute with blistering and weeping, the patient will need to soak in a bath containing potassium permanganate (so that the water is a pale pink colour) for 10 minutes to dry it up, or apply wet dressings of potassium permanganate to the affected area for 10–15 minutes twice a day. Once it is dry, 1% hydrocortisone ointment can be applied twice a day until the rash clears.

PIEBALDISM

The affected areas of skin will have no protection from ultraviolet light and will burn in the sun and have an increased risk of skin cancer. A high protective factor sunscreen (one from Groups 1, 2 or 3 in Table 13, page 141) should be used twice a day (early morning and mid-day) throughout the summer months. A patch of white hair can be dyed to match the rest of the hair if the patient does not like it.

PIGMENTED PURPURIC ERUPTION

If the rash is itchy it should be treated like eczema with a dilute topical steroid ointment or cream. Begin with 1% hydrocortisone cream (or ointment) and increase to 0.025% betamethasone valerate (Betnovate RD) if necessary. If the rash is not itchy, but merely discoloured due to haemosiderin deposition in the dermis, no treatment is needed because macrophages in the skin will gradually remove it. This is likely to take quite a long time, but the patient can be reassured that it will eventually get better. If there is associated venous disease, wearing elastic stockings will be helpful.

PILONIDAL SINUS

The sinus needs to be opened up, laid open and allowed to granulate up from the base. This is best done by a surgeon under a general anaesthetic.

PITTED KERATOLYSIS

This is a bacterial infection of keratin softened by sweat and occurs only in individuals with very sweaty feet. Rapid improvement can be gained by using 3% fusidic acid cream twice a day, or oral erythromycin 250 mg four times a day. In practice, helping the sweaty feet works better than specifically removing the causative organism. The feet should be soaked in a 5% solution of formaldehyde for 10–15 minutes once or twice a day. This usually works well; if it does not, iontophoresis can be tried instead (*see* page 88).

PITYRIASIS ALBA

Pityriasis alba is a very mild variety of eczema, which shows itself in the summer when the surrounding normal skin tans. If the child is very fair, the rash will be invisible, but if the child's skin tans easily, the rash will show as white patches in the summer. The child's parents should be reassured that it is nothing serious and that it will get better spontaneously. Usually no treatment is required but if it is, 0.5% sulphur in aqueous cream works as well as anything. Topical steroids are not needed.

PITYRIASIS AMANTACEA

This can be due to eczema or psoriasis. The treatment is the same whatever the underlying cause. Coconut oil compound ointment (Ung cocois co.) is rubbed into the thick scale at night just before the patient goes to bed, and washed off the following morning with a tar based shampoo (eg Polytar) or whatever other shampoo the patient likes. Because it makes a mess, the head should be covered overnight with a scarf or shower cap to keep the ointment off the pillow (*see* Figure 106). This treatment is repeated each night and washed off each morning until the scalp is clear. This usually takes 7–10 days. Once it is clear the treatment can be done once a week or once a fortnight to keep it clear. Alternatively once it is clear, the scalp can be washed with Capasal shampoo (which contains coal tar, salicylic acid and coconut oil) once a week to keep it clear.

Coconut oil compound ointment can be made up by the chemist, in which case it must be kept in the refrigerator when it is not being used, otherwise it becomes very runny and makes a mess everywhere.

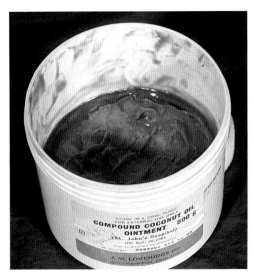

Figure 105 Coconut oil compound ointment ready for use.

Coconut oil compound ointment is made up as follows*:

Emulsifying wax BP	650 g
Yellow soft paraffin BP	450 g
Precipitated sulphur BP	200 g
Salicylic acid	100 g
Coal tar solution BP	600 ml
Coconut oil BP	3000 g

In contrast, Capasal shampoo contains 0.5% salicylic acid, 1% coconut oil and 1% distilled coal tar.

*A commercial form of this is available as Cocois ointment (made by Bioglan Laboratories).

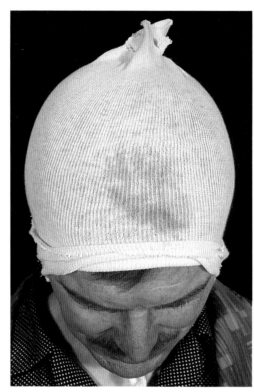

Figure 106 Patient with coconut oil compound ointment and a Tubegauz bonnet, ready for bed. A scarf or a shower cap are alternative head coverings.

PITYRIASIS LICHENOIDES CHRONICA (PLC)

This responds well to ultraviolet light. If it occurs in the summer, the patient can be encouraged to get out into the sunshine as much as possible and expose the affected skin. If the patient does not have access to a garden where he can sunbathe, or if there is no sunshine, a course of ultraviolet light treatment (UVB) at the nearest hospital can be arranged by the local dermatologist. It is

usually given as a sub-erythema dose two or three times a week for 6–8 weeks. Rarely PLC is bad enough to consider treating with PUVA. This works well but is not without its hazards (*see* page 166). It is given twice a week for 6–8 weeks.

PITYRIASIS ROSEA

This is a self-limiting condition which gets better in about 6 weeks. In most patients it is asymptomatic and needs no treatment other than reassurance that it is harmless. If it is very itchy, calamine lotion or 1% hydrocortisone cream will stop the itching until the rash clears on its own.

PITYRIASIS RUBRA PILARIS

Pityriasis rubra pilaris is an uncommon condition which is usually misdiagnosed as psoriasis. It looks very like psoriasis, being bright red in colour, but there are very obvious follicular lesions (*see* Figure 107) and thick hyperkeratosis on the palms and soles. In most instances it gets better spontaneously after 1–3 years but until then the patient will certainly require some treatment. It does not respond to topical steroids, and topically white soft paraffin is as useful as anything. The patient should be referred to a dermatologist so that the diagnosis can be confirmed and treatment with one of the retinoids instituted (etretinate or acetretin). The dose is the same as is used in psoriasis, *see* page 168.

PITYRIASIS VERSICOLOR

The rash is often more extensive than it first appears. Undress the patient so that you can see the full extent of it. If it is not all treated

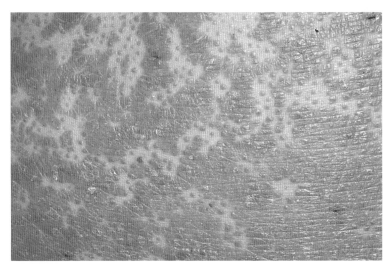

Figure 107 Part of the rash of pityriasis rubra pilaris. If you look carefully there are always follicular lesions present. Note that the colour is very similar to that of psoriasis.

it will recur by spreading from what was left behind. It is due to a yeast infection (*Malassezia furfur*) not a dermatophyte fungus so drugs like griseofulvin and terbinafine do not work. The treatments which do work are:

1 20% sodium thiosulphate solution applied to the whole of the affected skin at night before the patient goes to bed, every night for 6 weeks. It has a very slight smell, which does not seem too bad when it is in the bottle, but which patients do not like when they have to lie covered in it all night. They can wash it off in the morning so they do not have to put up with the smell all day too. It works very well and is cheap.

2 2.5% selenium sulphide shampoo (Selsun) can be applied to the affected skin twice daily for 2 weeks. It is only left on the skin for 20 minutes after it is applied because it can sting the skin and be quite uncomfortable.

3 A topical imidazole cream applied twice a day for 2 weeks. Clotrimazole, econazole, ketaconazole, miconazole and sulconazole cream all work equally well; use whichever one is cheapest. They are all more expensive than sodium thiosulphate and selenium sulphide.

4 Ketaconazole 200 mg daily for 10 days, or fluconazole 200 mg daily for 7 days are useful treatments for patients with recurrent extensive infections with pityriasis versicolor. They are not recommended as a first-line treatment because of the danger of liver disease with ketaconazole (although this is unlikely to occur with just 10 days treatment) and the expense and gastrointestinal side effects of itraconazole.

If the rash is made up of white macules and patches rather than the orangey–brown or dark brown variety, you will need to warn the patient that the rash will look the same after treatment. The scaling will be gone but the white patches will still be there. This is because the fungus produces something which inhibits tyrosinase and prevents melanin from being produced in the affected skin. Once the fungus is gone, the melanocytes will again be able to produce melanin, but will usually only do so when the patient has been out in the sun. With the orangey–brown and dark brown varieties of pityriasis versicolor, the treatment will eradicate the rash.

POLYMORPHIC ERUPTION OF PREGNANCY

Because this rash is very itchy, most women will not be able to put up with it until it clears on its own 2–3 weeks after delivery. 1% hydrocortisone ointment, or if it does not work, 0.025% betamethasone valerate ointment (Betnovate RD), can be applied twice a day to relieve the itching. Occasionally an oral antihistamine will also be needed, such as chlorpheniramine 4–8 mg four times a day.

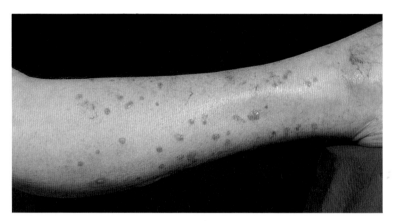

Figure 108 Disseminated superficial actinic porokeratosis on the lower leg treated with liquid nitrogen 24 hours ago. Most lesions have blistered. It is usual to have this number of lesions.

POROKERATOSIS—DISSEMINATED SUPERFICIAL ACTINIC

This is a very common problem on the lower legs and forearms (mainly in women). Small (0.5 cm), round, slightly scaly papules all have a raised edge that looks like a thread of cotton stretched around it if you look carefully. It is completely harmless but patients often complain that they are sore in the sun. If they are causing symptoms they can be frozen with liquid nitrogen for 5–10 seconds each. Warn the patient that she will get blisters where they have been treated (Figure 108), but these heal in 7–10 days. If they are asymptomatic they are best left alone.

PORT WINE STAIN

In a port wine stain the abnormal blood vessels are all in the upper 0.6 mm of the dermis, an area which is readily accessible to the light beam from an argon or tuneable dye laser. These lasers are very successful in improving the look of a port wine stain although they will not get rid of it completely. The aim of treatment is to coagulate the abnormal blood vessels in the dermis without damaging the epidermis, the dermal collagen or the skin appendages. With the flashlamp-pumped tuneable dye laser even very young children can be treated (from 3 months of age); in fact the cosmetic result is better the younger the patient and the lighter the port wine stain. The argon laser is not quite so good and can result in some scarring (*see* Figures 109 and 110); it works best in older patients with purple lesions. There is a list of hospitals where laser treatment is available inside the front cover. Port wine stains can also be disguised with cosmetic camouflage so that the patient looks normal to the outside world.

Sturge-Weber syndrome

Some patients with port wine stains will also have congenital glaucoma (or develop glaucoma later in life) and meningeal angiomas. The glaucoma can be treated just as it is in patients without the Sturge-Weber syndrome with pilocarpine eyedrops and oral acetazolamide if necessary. The diagnosis should be considered in a patient with a facial port wine stain who develops epilepsy and/or a contralateral hemiplegia. The meningeal angiomas can be diagnosed on a skull X-ray (*see* Figure 111), but there is no way of treating them at present. The epilepsy is treated with anticonvulsants.

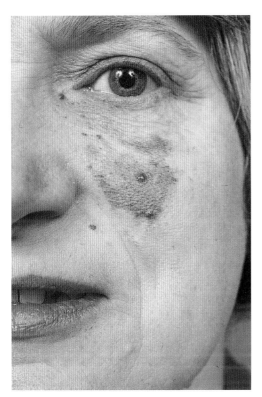

Figure 109 Port wine stain before treatment. Courtesy of Mr J Carruth.

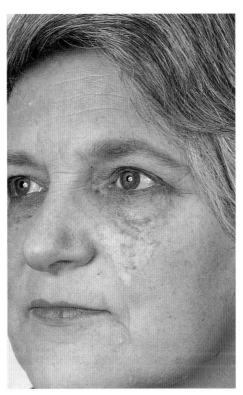

Figure 110 Same patient as Figure 109 after treatment with the argon laser. There is some scarring but the patient was pleased with the result. Courtesy of Mr J Carruth.

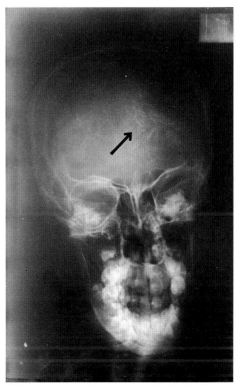

Figure 111 Skull X-ray in a 7-year-old girl with Sturge–Weber syndrome. Note the calcified vessels on the left of the picture.

POST-INFLAMMATORY HYPERPIGMENTATION

In most patients hyperpigmentation occurring after inflammation of the epidermis will get better spontaneously as macrophages remove melanin which has fallen into the dermis. Unfortunately it takes quite a long time for this to happen (months rather than days or weeks), especially in those individuals with pigmented skins who are most concerned by the colour changes. Skin-lightening creams such as 4% hydroquinone cream do not usually work very well and the only thing to do is to be patient until it improves. Cosmetic camouflage may be helpful in the interim.

POST-INFLAMMATORY HYPOPIGMENTATION

Some patients develop hypopigmentation after inflammatory conitions of the epidermis. This usually gets better more quickly than post-inflammatory hyperpigmentation. If the underlying condition clears up, the skin will repigment once the patient goes out into the sun and retans without any help from the doctor. If it is very unsightly, cosmetic camouflage can be offered until it improves spontaneously.

PRURITUS ANI

Check first to see whether your patient has a rash around the anus. Many patients who complain of pruritus ani have a straightforward skin condition to account for it, eg:

- psoriasis
- eczema
- lichen planus
- scabies
- candidiasis
- lichen sclerosis et atrophicus.

It is essential to examine the whole of the patient's skin in order to make a diagnosis. If one of the above conditions is found involving the perianal skin, it is treated as follows.

1 Psoriasis. 0.05% clobetasone butyrate (Eumovate) cream or 0.1% hydrocortisone 17-butyrate (Locoid) cream is applied twice a day until it is clear. Ordinary hydrocortisone cream is ineffective. Flexural psoriasis is the exception to the rule of not using topical steroids to treat psoriasis. Tar and dithranol tend to make the perianal skin very sore.

2 Eczema. 1% hydrocortisone cream or ointment can be applied twice a day when the eczema is there and left off when it is better. Ideally a lotion or a gel should be used on a moist area of skin, but all the topical steroid lotions have an alcoholic base, so they will sting open areas of skin, and the only steroid gel (0.025% fluocinolone acetonide [Synalar]) is in the potent group so is not suitable for this area. In practice most patients will find a cream or ointment satisfactory although they may have to try both to see which they prefer.

3 Lichen planus. 0.025% betamethasone valerate (Betnovate RD) ointment or cream can be applied to the perianal skin twice a day as to the rest of the rash to alleviate the itching until the rash gets better spontaneously (*see* page 108).

4 Scabies. A 25% emulsion of benzyl benzoate or 1% lindane lotion are applied to the whole body surface except the face (*see* page 191).

5 Candidiasis. First test the urine for sugar to exclude diabetes as the cause. If the rash is only around the anus the most likely reason for it is that the patient has been on a course of broad spectrum antibiotics. These should be stopped and the patient given nystatin tablets 100,000 units four times a day to clear the *Candida* from the gut; nystatin cream can also be applied topically twice a day until the rash is better (*see* also Table 2, page 32).

6 Lichen sclerosis et atrophicus. 1% hydrocortisone cream or ointment can be applied to the itchy skin twice a day. Increase the strength of the topical steroid only if the hydrocortisone does not work (*see* page 110).

If the patient has no obvious skin disease, they should be asked about **threadworms** which are easily seen in the faeces (or the ova can be found on a Sellotape sample from the perianal skin). Threadworms are a common cause of pruritis ani in children, but they can also be found in adults.

The female threadworms come out of the anus to lay their eggs (ova) on the surrounding skin at night and when they do so cause itching. Scratching leads to the ova being transferred to the patient's fingers and fingernails and thence to the mouth (directly, or indirectly on food eaten with unwashed hands). Inside the patient's large bowel the ova mature and the cycle starts again. The whole family should be treated with mebendazole 100 mg orally as a single dose (except for pregnant women and children under the age of 2). If re-infection occurs it can be repeated after 2–3 weeks. Children under the age of 2 are treated with piperazine 50 mg/kg body weight daily for 7 days. As well as the drug treatment, the patient should be told to wash the perianal skin first thing in the morning to remove any ova laid during the night, and to wash his hands and scrub under his fingernails with a nail brush after going to the toilet and before meals.

If the patient has no skin disease and no threadworms, a rectal examination should be carried out to exclude anal and rectal pathology. Patients with poor perianal hygiene, particularly if they have diarrhoea or soft stools, may itch because faeces are left on the skin after defaecation. You can check for this by looking; if it is not obvious, try wiping the perianal skin with a gauze swab—any trace of brown or yellow indicates that the hygiene of the area is not ideal. In the same way any kind of discharge from the anus, whether mucus, blood or faeces, will keep the perianal skin wet and itchy. For this reason, haemorrhoids, a fistula in ano or a carcinoma of the rectum can all present with pruritus ani and will need dealing with surgically.

There remain a large number of patients (mainly men) with pruritis ani for whom no physical cause can be found. 1% hydrocortisone cream applied twice a day is often helpful in breaking the itch–scratch cycle. Whatever the original cause of the itching, scratching damages the skin and makes it itch more. In addition he should wear loose fitting cotton underpants to keep the area as cool as possible and he should pay particular attention to keeping the perianal skin clean and dry. He should wash his bottom after defaecation with soap and water. A bidet is very helpful in this respect and if the patient does not have one, he might find it helpful to buy a plastic one (from a boat shop or a surgical appliance department) which can be placed over the toilet. If these simple measures do not work he should be referred to a dermatologist so that the diagnosis can be confirmed and patch testing carried out. Very often such patients are allergic to local anaesthetics which they have used inadvertently in creams advertised for use in pruritis ani and for haemorrhoids which they have bought themselves. If one cream has made the itching worse, the patient may well have changed to another one containing the same local anaesthetic.

There may be some psychosexual problem or some other anxiety as the cause of the itching, and unless that is sorted out the itching will continue. It is a mistake to think that it is just a question of finding the right cream or ointment to use.

PRURITUS VULVAE

Like pruritus ani in men, pruritus vulvae in women can go on relentlessly for years without the cause ever being found. Before assuming that it is due to an emotional problem (guilt about her own or her partner's adultery or impotence, a previous abortion or sexual abuse in childhood), it is important to examine the vulva, pubic area, perianal area and the rest of the patient's skin for evidence of a straightforward cause. Table 14 on page 150 outlines the common causes and what to do about them. In some patients

Table 14 Causes and treatment of pruritus vulvae

Diagnosis	How to make the diagnosis	Treatment
Candida albicans infection	Patient may be sore as well as itchy. Thick white vaginal discharge. Spores and hyphae on direct microscopy of the vaginal discharge. *Candida albicans* grown on culture of vaginal discharge. (Test the patient's urine for sugar to exclude diabetes as the cause.)	1 Nystatin ointment or cream applied to the vulva twice a day, together with: 2 Nystatin pessary (100,000 units) inserted high into the vagina at night for 14 nights, or an imidazole pessary placed high in the vagina at night: Clotrimazole (500 mg), single dose Miconazole (1200 mg), single dose Econazole nitrate (150 mg), 3 nights. 3 The patient's sexual partner should be treated at the same time with nystatin cream or an imidazole cream to prevent re-infection.
Trichomonas vaginalis infection	Frothy greenish–white vaginal discharge. Direct microscopy of the discharge will show the protozoa.	Both the patient and her sexual partner should be given metronidazole 200 mg orally three times a day for 7 days (alcohol must be avoided while taking metronidazole).
Gardnerella vaginalis infection (also called bacterial vaginosis)	Vaginal discharge with a fishy smell. Wet smears of the discharge show clue cells (multiple organisms stuck to the epithelial cells); gram staining shows gram-negative rods.	Both the patient and her sexual partner should be given metronidazole 200 mg orally three times a day for 7 days (alcohol must be avoided while taking metronidazole).
Psoriasis	Bright red, well demarcated rash, probably best seen on the pubic area rather than the vulva. Look on the elbows, knees and sacrum for the more typical bright red plaques with silvery scaling. The patient is very likely to have some ordinary psoriasis too.	0.05% clobetasone butyrate (Eumovate) ointment or cream, or 0.1% hydrocortisone 17-butyrate (Locoid) ointment or cream, or Calcipotriol ointment (Dovonex), applied twice a day.
Eczema	Poorly defined pink scaly rash with lichenification. May be blisters and weeping if it is a contact allergic eczema. Patient may well have eczema elsewhere.	1% hydrocortisone ointment or cream applied twice a day. It will rarely be necessary to use a steroid stronger than 1% hydrocortisone on the vulva.

(Table continues opposite)

Table 14 Causes and treatment of pruritus vulvae (continued)

Diagnosis	How to make the diagnosis	Treatment
Lichen sclerosis et atrophicus	White atrophic plaques confined to the vulva and perianal skin ± follicular plugging and haemorrhagic blisters. Very severe itching with or without dyspareunia in an adult.	In adults, use 0.05% clobetasol propionate (Dermovate) cream or ointment twice a day for 2–3 weeks until the itching has stopped, and then a weaker topical steroid such as 1% hydrocortisone cream or ointment twice a day on a regular basis. In children just use 1% hydrocortisone cream or ointment twice a day.
Lichen planus	Typical flat-topped mauve papules on flexor aspects of wrists as well as on the vulva ± white streaks in the mouth.	0.025% betamethasone valerate (Betnovate RD) cream or ointment applied twice a day will give symptomatic improvement until it gets better on its own (9–18 months).
Scabies	Look for burrows along the sides of the fingers and on the front of the wrists.	25% benzyl benzoate emulsion or 1% lindane solution applied to the whole body surface except the face and scalp on two successive nights.
Pubic lice	Look for nits attached to the pubic hairs; these are easier to see than the lice themselves.	0.5% malathion lotion or 1% lindane lotion or cream is applied to the pubic hair and washed off 12 hours later. This should be repeated after 7 days.
Herpes simplex	Often pain as well as itching. Blister fluid can be examined by electron microscopy or by viral culture for herpes simplex. Patients should be referred to local department of genitourinary medicine so that other sexually acquired diseases can be excluded.	For a primary infection, oral acyclovir 200 mg is taken five times a day for 5 days because there is nearly always involvement of the cervix too. Lignocaine gel is helpful topically to relieve the pain. For a recurrent infection bathing in normal saline is usually sufficient. Topical 5% acyclovir cream can be used five or six times a day if the lesions are on the vulva.
Vulval warts	Obvious viral warts. May cause itching because they stick out and the patient finds that irritating.	10% podophyllin in tinc. benz. co. applied once a week by the surgery nurse. The patient should be instructed to wash it off after 4 hours the first week, 6 hours the second week, 8 hours the third week.
Threadworms	In children you may see the worms on the vulva as well as in the stools. Sellotape stripping from around the anus will show the ova on microscopy.	Mebendazole 100 mg orally as a single dose will cure it. Treat the whole family. In children under the age of 2, use piperazine 50 mg/kg body weight/day for 7 days instead.

no cause for the itching can be found. There is nothing abnormal to be seen on the vulva or on the rest of the skin. It is worth exploring with the patient whether there is some anxiety at the bottom of it. Meanwhile the application of 1% hydrocortisone ointment twice a day is likely to be helpful in stopping the itching.

PSORIASIS

The pathology of psoriasis is well understood, but what causes these changes to occur is not. Traditionally, treatment has been aimed at reducing the rapid cell turnover of the epidermis, but more recently newer treatments have sought to alter the immune response. It is inevitable that in a chronic disease for which the cause is unknown, there will be no single treatment which is satisfactory for every patient. The following is a list of the drugs which are currently used for the treatment of psoriasis, either singly or in combination.

Topical treatment	Systemic treatment
Calcipotriol	Methotrexate
Dithranol	Azathioprine
Tar	Hydroxyurea
Salicylic acid	Etretinate
Emollients	PUVA
Ultraviolet light (UVB)	Cyclosporin A
(Topical steroids—flexures and scalp only)	Arsenic

Treatment of the different patterns of psoriasis can be found on the following pages:

Explain to the patient that the cause is not completely understood and that the course of the disease is very variable. It tends to run in families and can be made worse by infections (guttate psoriasis is usually induced by a streptococcal infection), stress (especially bereavement), trauma (psoriasis occurs at sites of cuts and scratches—Koebner's phenomenon) and hormonal changes (it often begins around puberty, improves during pregnancy and gets worse post partum and at the menopause). Some drugs make psoriasis worse and should be avoided if at all possible.

Drugs which make psoriasis worse

Lithium
Antimalarials (chloroquine)
Beta blockers
Withdrawal of systemic steroids. When systemic steroids are stopped or the dose reduced, psoriasis can get a lot worse (rebound phenomenon) or it can change into generalized pustular psoriasis which can be a life-threatening condition.

Psoriasis is not caused by food and a patient should be discouraged from going onto any special diet as a treatment. On the other hand, sunshine is often helpful (unless the patient is very fair and burns in the sun). Many patients choose to go abroad on holiday once or twice a year simply to keep their psoriasis at bay. Others would be helped by sunshine but are too embarrassed to expose their skin in case other people look at the rash and make adverse comments. The disease has natural remissions and relapses; it may last for life or only be present for a few months.

It is important to understand what it is like to have psoriasis from the patient's point of view. It is very common to find that a patient feels unclean because of his rash; he feels that people are looking

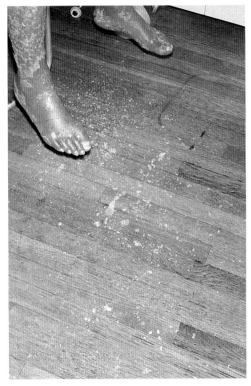

Figure 112 Scales on the floor from a patient with psoriasis who has just got undressed.

at him and that they will be afraid to come close to him or touch him in case it is contagious. The 'leper complex' is still very much alive and well. If the rash is on the face or backs of the hands it may be impossible to hide it and the patient may lose his job or be afraid that he will.

As well as looking awful, it also makes a mess. It is said that a patient with psoriasis has to take his own dustpan and brush with him when he goes on holiday. Certainly it is true that the psoriatic scales make a mess when they are shed, on the collar and over the shoulders from the scalp and on the floor when the patient gets undressed (Figure 112). Obviously the more extensive the rash the more mess it will make; some patients resort to covering their skin with cling film to keep the scales in place. For a woman, wearing tights and/or a body stocking will keep most of the scales on the skin during the day so that the scales do not make a mess on the carpet at home or at work.

Although the various treatments that are available do not cure psoriasis, they are very helpful and it is important to give the patient hope that something can be done. Treatment of an individual patient will depend on the pattern and extent of his psoriasis and what he is able to use. The treatment options for the different patterns of psoriasis are outlined below.

Chronic plaque psoriasis

If there are not too many plaques, the options lie between calcipotriol, dithranol and tar. Topical steroids should not be used because hydrocortisone is ineffective, and the more potent steroids have many side effects when used long term (*see* page 8). There is the added danger that when the steroids are stopped, rapid relapse of the psoriasis (rebound phenomenon) or generalized pustular psoriasis can occur.

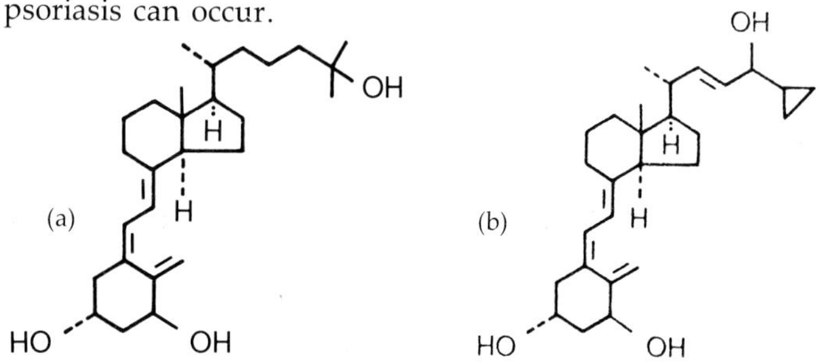

Figure 113 (a) 1,25-dihydroxy vitamin D_3. (b) Calcipotriol.

CALCIPOTRIOL Calcipotriol is a Vitamin D_3 analogue which, like its naturally occurring counterpart, slows down epidermal proliferation (it also has an effect on T lymphocytes and it is a potent inhibitor of interleukin 1). Theoretically it could cause hypercalcaemia and hypercalcuria (and therefore kidney stones and soft tissue calcification), but in practice, at the dose used in the ointment (50 μg/g), these effects are not seen. Less than 1% of the calcipotriol applied to the skin is absorbed systemically, and any that does get absorbed is rapidly transformed to inactive metabolites.

Calcipotriol ointment (Dovonex) is applied to the psoriatic plaques twice a day and an improvement in the rash should begin to be seen in 1–2 weeks. It does not smell or stain the skin (or clothes), but it can cause redness and irritation of the skin, particularly on the face (tell the patient to wash his hands after applying the calcipotriol ointment to avoid getting it on the face). Provided that no more than 100 g/week is used, there is no limit to how long it can be used for; the only limiting factor will be how much psoriasis the patient has. It seems to be very effective in flattening the psoriatic plaques and removing the scale but not quite so good at getting rid of the redness. It is certainly as effective as tar and dithranol. Its great advantage is that it is not messy to use (just greasy), so it is probably the treatment of choice for ordinary plaque psoriasis as long as it is not too extensive.

DITHRANOL Dithranol is a synthetic derivative of anthracene, and is derived from a natural product, chrysarobin, the active constituent of Goa powder, a herbal remedy derived from the bark of the Brazilian tree *Andira ararotea*. It is a yellow powder which can be made up into a cream, ointment, stick or paste.

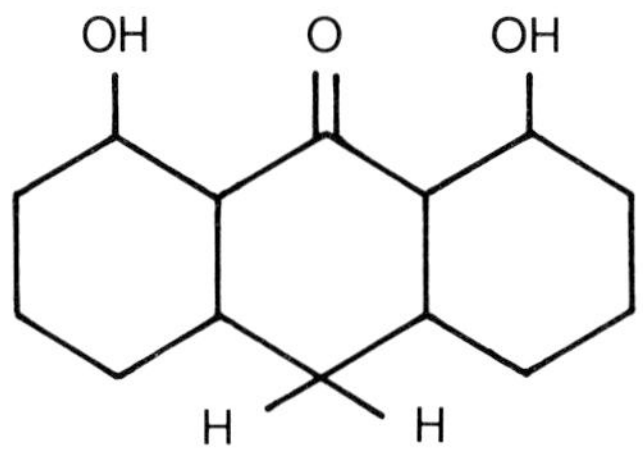

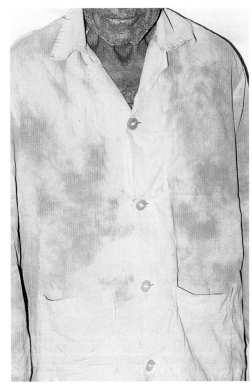

Figure 114 Dithranol.

Its breakdown products are unstable and are easily oxidized causing irritation, burning and brown discolouration of normal skin, and mauve/purple staining of the patient's clothes (Figure 115), which will not wash out. The skin staining is a useful indicator of disease activity (and whether the patient is actually using the treatment).

Some patients tolerate dithranol well, others badly (especially those with very fair skin). Because it causes irritation and burning of normal skin, it must be applied carefully just to the plaques of psoriasis. Always start with a weak concentration of dithranol and gradually increase its strength.

There are numerous preparations containing dithranol (or synthetic derivatives of it) on the market (*see* page 156) but Dithrocream is by far the most widely used. It can be used in one of two ways.

1 At night. Starting with the 0.1% cream, the patient applies the cream at night, by rubbing it in carefully just to the plaques of psoriasis. He then wipes it off with a tissue or flannel so that there is no cream left on the skin to stain the clothes or bedding. This is repeated each night until the psoriasis is gone. The patient will be able to tell when it is clear, not because the skin looks normal but because the patches are brown rather than red. Once the epidermal cell turnover has returned to normal, the breakdown products

Figure 115 Dithranol staining of the clothes.

which stain normal skin will be seen where the psoriasis once was (*see* Figure 122, page 160).

2 Short contact therapy. Again starting with the 0.1% cream, the patient applies the dithranol to the psoriatic plaques. 30 minutes later he washes it off. This is repeated once a day until the skin is clear.

With both methods, if the skin is not clearing, the strength of the Dithrocream can be increased every 2 weeks from 0.1% to 0.25% to 0.5% etc. It is a good idea to know the colour of the tubes of the

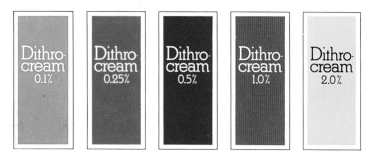

Figure 116 Colours of the tubes of different concentrations of Dithrocream.

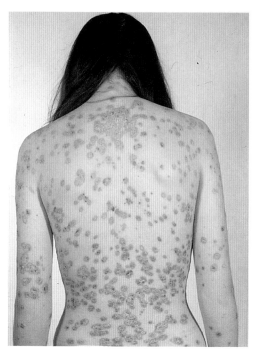

Figure 117 Extensive plaques of psoriasis. Not suitable for treatment with dithranol because it would take too long to apply, or calcipotriol because > 100 g/week would be needed.

various strengths because the patient is more likely to remember the colour of the tube than the concentration of the dithranol (Figure 116).

Dithrocream is fairly easy for the patient to use providing there are not too many plaques to treat and they are accessible. If the plaques are very small, the Dithrocream can be applied with a cotton bud to make sure that it does not get onto the normal skin. If possible the patient should be shown how to apply the cream rather than just given the tubes to take away.

If the patient has very numerous plaques like the girl shown in Figure 117, Dithrocream is not the answer, however willing the patient and family are to co-operate. It would simply take too long to apply the cream for it to be practical. If the patient is single and lives alone and the psoriasis is on his back or buttocks, Dithrocream is not practical because he will not be able to apply it carefully to the plaques without getting it on the normal skin.

Other dithranol preparations which can be used as alternatives to Dithrocream are shown in the table *right*. The ointments and wax sticks can all be used in the same way as the creams, ie apply at night and wipe off immediately or as the short contact method.

Ready-made preparations of dithranol (and its derivatives)

Alphodith ointment (0.4%, 1%, 2%, 3%)
Anthranol ointment (0.4%, 1%, 2%)
Antraderm wax stick (1%, 2%)
Dithrocream (0.1%, 0.25%, 0.5%, 1%, 2%)
Dithrolan ointment (0.5%) [with salicylic acid]
Exolan cream (1%) [dithranol triacetate]
Psoradrate cream (0.1%, 0.2%, 0.4%) [with urea]
Psorin cream (0.11%) [with coal tar and salicylic acid]

Dithranol is most effective when used in a paste which can be applied to the plaques and left in place for 24 hours. This is too time-consuming for most patients to contemplate at home, and makes too much mess of the clothes, but it is the mainstay of in-patient therapy for psoriasis (*see* page 158).

TAR Crude coal tar is the sticky black liquid left behind when coal has been heated to remove the volatile constituents. It is a complex mixture of hundreds of different hydrocarbons; which of these are the active constituent(s) is unknown. It is assumed that it works by decreasing mitotic activity in the epidermis. Coal tar solution (liquor picis carbonis, LPC) is further refined and is less effective. Generally speaking the messier the tar preparation the more effective it is, and the less cosmetically acceptable for the patient (Figure 119).

Tar is most useful when the patient has very numerous small plaques of psoriasis, particularly if they are fairly superficial (Figure 118). Although it is messy to use, it is quite safe to apply it to normal skin, so it can be rubbed in all over the skin without taking any special care.

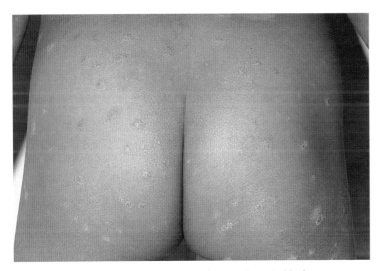

Figure 118 Widespread small plaques of psoriasis, suitable for treatment with a proprietary tar cream.

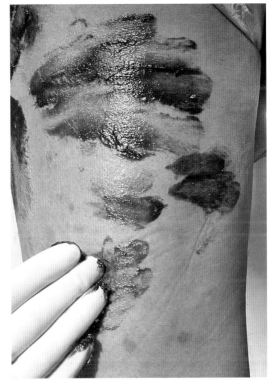

Figure 119 Very messy tar preparation. 5% crude coal tar in white soft paraffin. Not a very practical option for most patients because it is so messy.

For the patient shown in Figure 117, 2% or 5% crude coal tar in white soft paraffin or coal tar and salicylic acid ointment BP would be effective treatments but are not very practical because of the mess. For the patient shown in Figure 118, 2% crude coal tar in a water-miscible cream base like Unguentum Merck, so that it will rub in easily (at night or even twice a day) is quite practical because it is not too messy, although it does still smell of tar. The strength of the tar can gradually be increased if it does not work (up to 20% if necessary). Alternatively, one of the proprietary tars, containing coal tar solution rather than crude coal tar could be used, but these are less effective and only of use for very mild psoriasis.

Proprietary tar preparations containing coal tar solution

Alphosyl cream and lotion	Pragmatar cream
Carbo-Dome cream	Psoriderm cream
Clinitar cream	Psorigel
Gelcosal gel (+ salicylic acid)	Psorin cream (+ dithranol and salicylic acid)

Tar plus ultraviolet light is more effective than either on its own (providing a suberythema dose of UVL is given). If the patient has a secluded garden and can apply his tar ointment or cream and then go out into the sun, it is likely to work better than the ointment or cream alone. For the same reason, tar baths are recommended before treatment with ultraviolet light (*see* page 159). 20–30 ml of Polytar emollient, Balneum with tar or Psoriderm bath emulsion can be added to the patient's bath water. While soaking in the bath, the patient should gently rub off the psoriatic scales with a soft nail brush for maximum effect. It is unrealistic to expect tar baths to do much good on their own.

Extensive chronic plaque psoriasis

For patients with very extensive plaques of psoriasis the options for treatment are in-patient treatment, some kind of hospital day care treatment, including ultraviolet light or systemic therapy. 5% salicylic acid ointment or an emollient applied topically twice a day will keep the skin comfortable without actually clearing the psoriasis. Some such patients will be prepared to try a tar preparation for a while, but because the treatment is not a cure and they have to go on using it indefinitely, they will mostly get fed up with it.

In-patient treatment

Almost all patients with psoriasis can have their skin completely cleared in hospital over a period of 3 weeks. It is most worthwhile when the psoriasis has flared after a period of stress or after a bereavement. Once the stressful period is over, clearing the skin may result in a long period of remission. But it is also a useful treatment for any patient with extensive psoriasis (and occasionally a patient with less extensive disease) who finds that he cannot cope with it any longer. In hospital the patient relaxes in bed and is sedated with trimeprazine (10 mg three times a day and 20 mg at night; doubling the dose if necessary) to make sure that he rests.

It is essential to get the psoriasis completely cleared in hospital if it is to stay clear (although this cannot be guaranteed). Some patients will stay clear for years after a period of hospitalization, others will relapse almost as soon as they go home; there is no way of knowing which patient is likely to do which.

There are two standard treatment regimens employing either dithranol or tar as the active treatment.

1 Ingram regimen (dithranol) consists of:

(i) Tar bath. The patient soaks in a bath containing 20–30 ml of a tar emulsion (Polytar emollient, or Balneum with tar) for 10–15 minutes. While in the bath he rubs off the scales with a soft nail brush.

(ii) Short-wave ultraviolet light (UVB). Having got out of the bath and dried his skin, he is then exposed to a sub-erythema dose of UVB.

(iii) Dithranol in Lassar's paste is then applied carefully to each psoriatic plaque with a spatula or a gloved finger (Figure 120). The initial concentration of dithranol is 0.1% and this is increased daily by increments of 0.1% up to 1%, and then by 1% increments up to 10%. Talcum powder is applied on top of the dithranol in Lassar's paste to stop it being sticky, and the skin is covered with Tubegauz to prevent staining of the pyjamas and sheets (Figure 121). This is left in place for 24 hours. If the skin becomes very sore the dithranol will have to be stopped for a few days and white soft paraffin applied instead. It can then be restarted at a lower concentration and increased more cautiously perhaps every 2 or 3 days rather than every day. The next morning the dithranol in Lassar's paste is cleaned off with arachis oil or liquid paraffin because it does not come off with soap and water, and the whole process is repeated each day until the skin is clear.

When the psoriasis is better the skin where the psoriasis was will be stained brown (*see* Figure 122). When the treatment is stopped the brown colour will gradually fade over about 2 weeks. The brown stain can be removed more quickly by applying coal tar and salicylic acid ointment twice a day for 2–3 days.

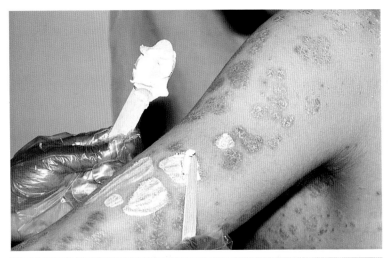

Figure 120 (*above*) Applying dithranol in Lassar's paste to plaques of psoriasis with a spatula.

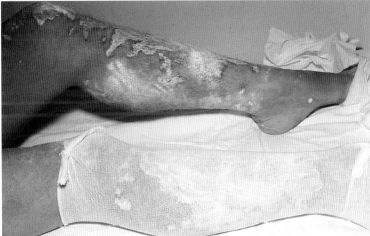

Figure 121 (*below*) Dithranol in Lassar's paste is covered with talcum powder and Tubegauz to protect the bedding and pyjamas.

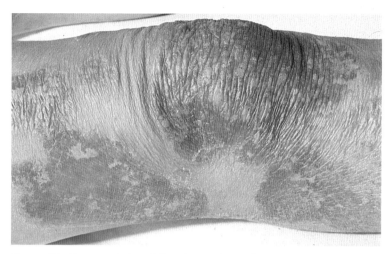

Figure 122 Brown staining of skin due to the oxidation products of dithranol retained in the skin as the epidermal cell turnover returns to normal as the psoriasis clears.

2   Goeckerman regimen (tar) consists of:
(i)   tar bath
(ii) UVB
(iii) 2% crude coal tar in Lassar's paste is applied to the psoriatic plaques and covered in Tubegauz to protect the patient's pyjamas and the sheets. The strength of the tar is raised twice a week, rather than every day, from 2% gradually up to 20%, until the psoriasis is clear. An alternative is to use crude coal tar in white soft paraffin rather than in Lassar's paste which is much quicker to apply because it does not have to be carefully applied to each plaque (*see* Figure 119, page 157).

Out-patient Ingram regimen

Some hospital dermatology departments run an out-patient Ingram regimen service either early in the morning or in the evening (so that patients can go before or after work). The treatment consists of:
(i)   tar bath. (The patient can have the bath at home before attending the hospital if there is no bath available in the out-patient department)
(ii) UVB
(iii) dithranol in Lassar's paste applied carefully to the plaques of psoriasis (by a nurse), covered with talcum powder and Tubegauz. The patient puts his own clothes on top of the Tubegauz and goes to work or goes home. The next day, the dithranol is cleaned off with oil and the process repeated.
It takes longer to clear psoriasis doing it like this than if the patient can be admitted to hospital (6 weeks rather than 3), but it means that they do not need to have time off work or time away from the family.

A few patients who are very well motivated to get their skin clear, who have previously been cleared in hospital, will want to use dithranol in Lassar's paste at home. This can be done if they have someone who can help to apply the dithranol to any inaccessible areas of skin, and if they are prepared to put up with the staining on their clothes and bedding.

Goeckerman day-care regimen

In the USA where in-patient beds are very expensive, day-care treatment is used instead. This is suitable for patients with psoriasis because they are usually otherwise well and not in need of expensive hospital facilities. The patient attends a clinic during the day and goes home at night.

The treatment consists of:

(i) The patient changes out of his normal clothes into pyjamas and is examined by the doctor or nurse.

(ii) Tar bath.

(iii) UVB at sub-erythema dose.

(iv) 2% crude coal tar in white soft paraffin is applied to the psoriasis and covered with Tubegauz.

(v) Coconut oil compound ointment is applied to the scalp.

(vi) The patient rests in a day care lounge for the rest of the day. During this time he can attend relaxation classes, counselling sessions, lectures, keep fit exercises etc. It is important that there is interaction with other patients so that he begins to understand that he is not alone in his suffering and learn something about the psoriasis itself.

(vii) In the afternoon he washes his hair to remove the coconut oil compound ointment and has a bath to remove the tar ointment.

(viii) UVB at sub-erythema dosage is again given.

(ix) Resistant plaques are treated with short contact dithranol therapy (*see* page 155), which is then washed off.

(x) Aqueous cream, white soft paraffin or some other emollient is then applied and the patient changes back into his normal clothes and goes home.

Treatment is given 6 days a week at the hospital and the patient just uses emollients on a Sunday. This kind of treatment will clear psoriasis in about 3 weeks, which is similar to conventional in-patient treatment.

Systemic therapy

For patients with very extensive psoriasis, systemic treatment may be much more effective than ointments or creams. Unfortunately all the systemic agents that are used have side effects which can be serious.

METHOTREXATE Methotrexate inhibits dihydrofolate reductase and therefore cell division. It is probably the most effective of the systemic agents in use for the treatment of psoriasis and it works very quickly, an effect being seen within 48 hours. Since its side effects are potentially lethal, there should be very strict criteria for its use.

Indications for the use of methotrexate

(i) Failure of in-patient treatment. This is extremely rare. Just because someone does not want to use an ointment or cream, or does not like using tar or dithranol, is not a reason for using a potentially lethal drug.

(ii) Early relapse after in-patient therapy. A patient whose skin clears in hospital but whose psoriasis returns just as badly almost immediately he returns home is a candidate for methotrexate. Unless something is done, he will be living in hospital instead of at home.

(iii) Generalized pustular psoriasis or erythrodermic psoriasis which does not settle on bed rest and emollients.

(iv) Bad psoriatic arthritis as well as extensive skin psoriasis. If a patient has bad psoriatic arthritis which does not respond to non-steroidal anti-inflammatory drugs, as well as awful skin, methotrexate may be the answer.

Dosage of methotrexate

It is given as a single dose of 10–25 mg orally, intramuscularly or intravenously once a week. It works just as well whichever route is used. It is excreted unchanged principally through the kidneys, so the dose needs to be reduced if renal function is impaired. Because there is a progressive deterioration in glomerular filtration rate as a patient gets older, the dose of methotrexate will need to be reduced accordingly. To work out what dose is safe to give to patients over the age of 50, the following formula* can be used:

$$\text{Predicted creatinine clearance} = \frac{(140\text{-age}) \times (\text{weight in kg}) \times (1.23 \text{ for men})}{\text{Serum creatinine in } \mu\text{mol/l}}$$

$$\text{Dose methotrexate} = 1.25 + (0.157 \times \text{predicted creatinine clearance})$$

In the elderly it is often possible to control psoriasis on as little as 2.5 mg or 5 mg methotrexate/week.

Side effects of methotrexate and ways of avoiding them

There are three serious side effects of methotrexate:

(1) Teratogeny. Methotrexate should not be given to women who are pregnant, who might become pregnant or who are breast feeding. In men it causes oligospermia; this is reversible when the drug is stopped. In both sexes conception should be avoided for 6 months after methotrexate is stopped.

(2) Bone marrow depression. A sudden fall in haemoglobin, white count or platelets can be fatal. A full blood count should be checked before methotrexate is started and repeated weekly for 1 month and then every 2–3 months. A rise in MCV may warn you that the blood count is about to fall and is an indication for reducing the dose and checking the blood count more frequently (start worrying when the MCV is more than 100).

If the blood count falls, methotrexate must be stopped. If the fall is profound, it can be reversed by giving folinic acid (the same dose as the dose of methotrexate) as a single dose orally or intramuscularly within 12 hours. If it is given more than 24 hours after the methotrexate it is unlikely to be of any use.

Certain drugs should be avoided in a patient taking methotrexate because of an increased risk of pancytopenia. They do this either by displacing methotrexate from its protein binding or by blocking its renal tubular secretion. The risk of pancytopenia is also increased if a patient's diet contains little folic acid.*

Drugs to be avoided in a patient taking methotrexate

Aspirin
Diuretics
Hypoglycaemics
Non-steroidal anti-inflammatory drugs
Phenytoin
Probenecid
Sulphonamides
Trimethoprim

---

(3) Fibrosis of the liver. Methotrexate should not be given to a patient with pre-existing liver disease or one who has a history of alcohol abuse. Before treatment is started he should have a liver biopsy to exclude pre-existing liver damage. Once on treatment, the liver biopsy is repeated once a year to check that fibrosis is not occurring. Measuring the ordinary liver function tests or even the gamma GT will not pick up liver damage until very late, so they are of no use in monitoring the patient. Alcohol is forbidden while the patient is taking this drug since alcohol enhances its liver toxicity.

---

*Formula devised by Drs Fairris, Dewhurst, White and Campbell in Southampton.

*Fruit, vegetables and cereals are the main source of folic acid in the diet.

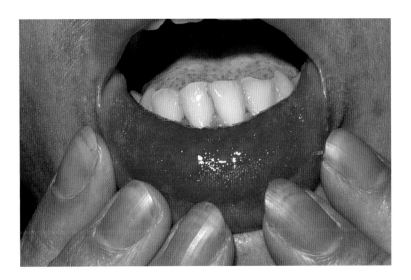

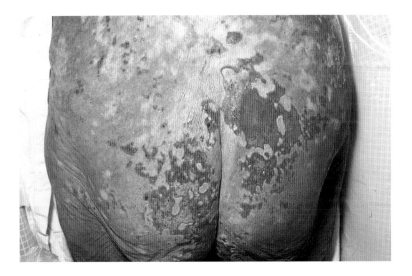

Figure 123 (*above left*) Stomatitis. Widespread erosions in the mouth after methotrexate therapy.

Figure 124 (*below left*) Ulceration of the skin in a 79-year-old woman after a single dose of 5 mg methotrexate.

Less serious side effects, which will not kill the patient but which may nevertheless be extremely unpleasant and necessitate withdrawal of the drug, are as follows.

1 Nausea, vomiting, diarrhoea and abdominal discomfort. These effects can often be avoided by changing from oral to intramuscular methotrexate.
2 Stomatitis and ulceration of the mouth (Figure 123).
3 General malaise. It is not at all uncommon for patients to feel generally unwell (headache, lethargy, irritability and depression) for about 24 hours after a dose of methotrexate.
4 Extensive ulceration of the skin. This usually occurs at the same time as a profound fall in blood count (Figure 124).
5 Hair loss. Theoretically this is possible but in practice it is extremely rare.
6 Lung problems. When methotrexate is used for treating neoplastic disease, acute pneumonitis or diffuse interstitial fibrosis can occur. With the doses used for treating psoriasis, these changes do not seem to happen.

Most of these side effects can prevented by giving 5 mg folic acid once a week with the methotrexate. The folic acid seems to block the adverse effects of methotrexate without stopping the therapeutic effect. But if you are going to do this, you must check the patient's B_{12} level first.

AZATHIOPRINE Azathioprine is an antimetabolite which is absorbed from the gastrointestinal tract and broken down to 6-mercaptopurine. It is not as effective as methotrexate in treating psoriasis and it takes longer to work (6–8 weeks). Its main advantages are that it can always be given by mouth and the

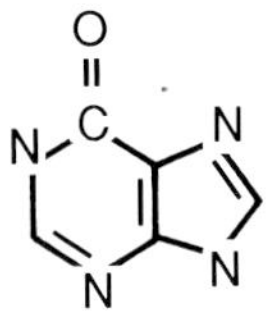

Figure 125
Hypoxanthine.

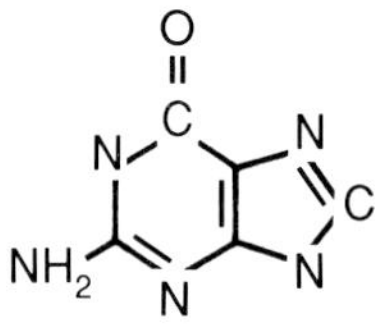

Figure 126
Guanine.

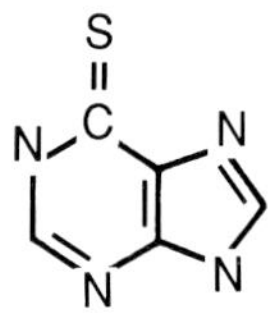

Figure 127
6-Mercaptopurine.

patient does not need to have a yearly liver biopsy. The dose is 2 mg/kg body weight/day. Except for very small individuals this means a dose of 50 mg three times a day.

Indications for use of azathioprine.

Because azathioprine interferes with the formation of nucleic acids and therefore cell division, it has the potential for causing lethal pancytopenia. For this reason, the criteria for use should be exactly the same as for methotrexate (*see* page 161).

Side effects

(1) Nausea, vomiting and diarrhoea. If this is going to occur it usually does so in the first week or two. It may be very severe and necessitate stopping the drug. Sometimes reducing the dose will stop the symptoms and the dose can later be increased safely. The gastrointestinal problems seem to be particularly serious in the elderly.

(2) Bone marrow depression. A full blood count should be checked before treatment is begun and then weekly for a month. After that once every 2–3 months is sufficient. If the blood count falls, the drug will need to be stopped or the dose reduced, depending on how great the fall.

(3) Teratogeny. It should not be given to pregnant women, those who want to become pregnant or those who are breast feeding.

There is no evidence that it affects spermatogenesis, so it is safe for a man to father a child while taking it.

(4) Mild cholestasis. This is not usually enough of a problem to warrant regular liver biopsy as for methotrexate.

(5) Hair loss. This is a theoretical problem but not one which we have seen.

HYDROXYUREA Hydroxyurea is an antimetabolite which inhibits the formation of DNA without any significant effect on RNA or protein synthesis. Its major toxic effects are on rapidly dividing cells, ie the fetus and the bone marrow. It must not be given to pregnant women or those who want to become pregnant. It is taken by mouth at a dose of 0.5 g twice a day. A full blood count should be done before treatment is begun, every week for a month and then every 2–3 months. Managing patients on this drug is difficult because they all have a high MCV and it is difficult to know when this heralds a fall in blood count.

The indications for using hydroxyurea are the same as for methotrexate, although it is unlikely that hydroxyurea will ever be the drug of first choice because it is not as effective as methotrexate and takes a lot longer to work (6–8 weeks before there is any noticeable effect on the skin and several months before a satisfactory clinical response is obtained).

PUVA (PHOTOCHEMOTHERAPY)
P = psoralen
UVA = long-wave ultraviolet light (320–400 nm)

PUVA involves the use of a photo-sensitizing drug, 8-methoxypsoralen (8-MOP) or 5-methoxypsoralen (5-MOP) followed by long-wave ultraviolet light. Neither the psoralen or the UVA alone have any effect on psoriasis, but together they cause specific photo-damage to the DNA in epidermal cells, inhibiting DNA replication and therefore cell division.

Strictly speaking the indications for PUVA should be the same as for methotrexate (*see* page 161) because of the potential long-term side effects. In practice the criteria which are used are:

1 widespread psoriasis which has not responded to topical therapy or UVB in a patient over the age of 18
2 rapid relapse after in-patient therapy (3–6 months)
3 patient cannot take time off work for in-patient therapy.

Treatment is contraindicated if the patient has:
- had a previous malignant melanoma
- Gorlin's syndrome
- xeroderma pigmentosa
- familial dysplastic naevus syndrome
- bullous pemphigoid
- pemphigus
- systemic lupus erythematosus
- dermatomyositis.

Relative contraindications include:
- the patient has had previous non-melanoma skin cancer
- the patient has malignant or premalignant skin lesions at present (basal cell carcinoma, squamous cell carcinoma, solar keratosis or Bowen's disease)
- the patient has had treatment with methotrexate or arsenic in the past
- the patient has had previous treatment with radiotherapy to the skin
- the patient is immunosuppressed
- there is clinically significant hepatic dysfunction.

Treatment is carried out twice a week since the erythema induced by PUVA takes 2 days to develop (further treatment should not be given until it is obvious that the previous treatment has not caused burning). The treatment involves:
(i) Taking 8-MOP tablets (0.6 mg/kg body weight), or 5-MOP tablets (1.2 mg/kg body weight).

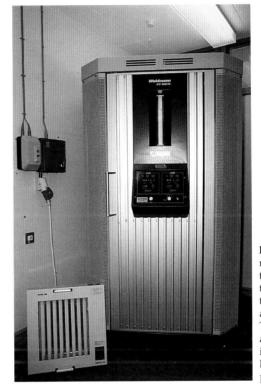

Figure 128 PUVA machine. Two hours after taking 8-MOP or 5-MOP tablets the patient is treated with UVA in a cabinet like this. Treatment is given twice a week and each dose is increased by 25% of the last dose given until the psoriasis is clear.

(ii) 2–3 hours later when blood levels of the psoralen are maximal the skin is exposed to UVA. The UVA is provided by banks of fluorescent lamps in a cabinet which allows the patient to stand and expose the whole of the skin to the UVA (Figure 128). Ordinary sunlight cannot be used because the patient would get sunburnt from the UVB in natural sunlight before he had had enough UVA to help his psoriasis (assuming you could guarantee sunshine on the day of treatment).

The dose of UVA is worked out in terms of light energy (joules/cm^2), and depending on the output of the machine (measured with a UVA meter), the time of exposure is calculated. The aim is to give the patient as much UVA as possible without producing more than a barely perceptible erythema.

(iii) The patient must protect his eyes against damage from ultraviolet light during and for 24 hours after the treatment, by wearing glasses which filter out both UVB and UVA (*see* box for those which are recommended).

Recommended protective sun glasses
Polarizing lenses manufactured by Polaroid
Boots polarizing lenses
Lenses treated with Orcolite UV 400
UV-Gard 400 lenses manufactured by Sola
Orma UVX lenses manufactured by Esrilor
Perfalit Lambda 400 by Rodenstock
Unispec/Histyle 6000 (with clear lenses)*

PUVA is a very popular treatment because it does not involve any messy ointments, and as a side effect the patient will get a tan! It has the disadvantage that it involves attendance at hospital twice a week. As far as clearing the psoriasis is concerned, it is just as successful as in-patient treatment but takes approximately twice as long.

Short-term side effects

1 Nausea. This can be prevented by taking the 8-MOP tablets with food or a glass of milk. Occasionally an anti-emetic is required; we usually give 10 mg metoclopramide hydrochloride (Maxolon) at the same time as the 8-MOP.

2 Dryness and itching of the skin. This is very common and may need an antihistamine such as chlorpheniramine 4–8 mg given with the 8-MOP. Rarely severe persistent itching makes the patient stop treatment; it can persist for several days or even weeks afterwards.

3 Erythema and tenderness. A few patients will get excessive erythema, oedema and tenderness of the skin 48–72 hours after treatment. This is the main reason why treatment is only given twice a week. If the patient gets burnt, the dose of irradiation is reduced for the next treatment. All patients are at risk of a phototoxic reaction after PUVA and should avoid direct sunlight for 8 hours after treatment (using a sunscreen which blocks out both UVB and UVA if necessary—*see* page 141).

4 PUVA pain. Severe skin pain is unusual but when it occurs patients cannot cope with it and it will often necessitate stopping the treatment. It can persist for several weeks after treatment is stopped.

Long-term side effects

1 Cataracts. The eyes are protected during treatment and for 24 hours afterwards to prevent cataract formation.

2 Skin cancer. There is an acceleration of the ageing process in the skin of patients who have been treated with PUVA and an increase in the incidence of basal and squamous cell carcinomas on the skin. There have also been some reports of malignant melanoma occurring.

In view of the long-term risks of PUVA, the amount of UVA that is given must be kept to a minimum. This is done by limiting the life time exposure to less than 200 treatments or 1000 joules/cm², not giving maintenance treatment, using topical rather than systemic psoralens (*see* page 167) and using RePUVA instead of PUVA alone (*see* page 170). Men must shield the genitalia during treatment because there is an increased risk of squamous cell carcinoma on the penis.

---

*Available from Arco Wessex, Omega Enterprise Park, Electron Way, Chandlers Ford, Eastleigh, Hampshire, SO5 3SE.

PUVA using topical psoralens

In out-patient departments where there are bathing facilities, 8-MOP can be put in the bathwater (at a concentration of 3.7 mg/l) instead of taken by mouth. The patient soaks in the bath containing the psoralen for 15 minutes, gets out and pats the skin dry and is **immediately** irradiated with UVA (the efficacy is lost if the UVA is not given immediately after the bath psoralens). Afterwards he showers it off with clean water. When used like this very little, if any, of the psoralen is absorbed, so there should be no need for protection of the eyes or skin afterwards. This form of PUVA is useful for patients who have a lot of nausea with oral 8-MOP, for those on haemodialysis and for those who do not absorb psoralens taken by mouth (who will not have responded to ordinary PUVA

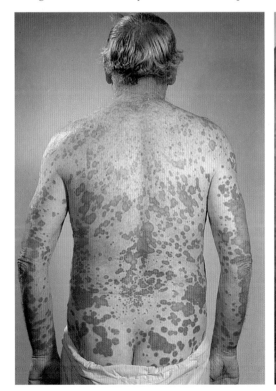 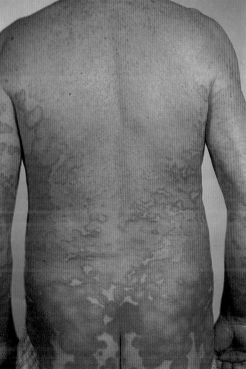 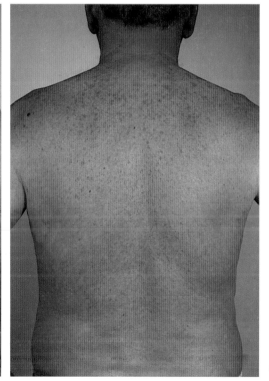

Figure 129 Widespread psoriasis in a man aged 58 years. Suitable for treatment with etretinate.

Figure 130 Same patient as Figure 129 3 months later. At this stage the dose can be reduced to decrease the side effects.

Figure 131 Same patient as Figures 129 and 130 6 months after starting treatment. Skin is now completely clear.

treatment). It also has the advantage that much less UVA is needed to clear the skin.

ETRETINATE Etretinate is an aromatic retinoid which inhibits cell division (although how it does this is poorly understood). In the UK it is only available on hospital prescription. It is not as good as methotrexate for the treatment of chronic plaque psoriasis, but it is not as hepatotoxic so is a useful alternative when methotrexate is contraindicated.

It is taken orally starting at a dose of 1 mg/kg body weight/day. It can be given as a single dose once a day or it can be divided into two or three doses, but it should be given with food. It takes 8–12 weeks before it works (Figures 129–131). Once the psoriasis has cleared the dose is reduced gradually until the patient is on the lowest dose that will control the rash.

Short-term side effects

1 Dry chapped lips (Figure 132a). This always occurs and you will be able to tell whether the patient is taking etretinate or not by whether his lips are dry, scaly or split. It is always enough of a nuisance to require something to be done about it. Vaseline or a lip salve stick will need to be applied frequently during the day.
2 Dryness of the nasal mucosa which sometimes leads to nose bleeds. A simple emollient like aqueous cream can be applied to the anterior nares two or three times a day to help.
3 Conjunctivitis and irritation of the eyes. If it is very bad the patient may need to use hypromellose eye drops several times a day to keep the eyes comfortable.
4 Itching of the skin ± an eczematous rash. This can be on any part of the skin and may need treatment with an emollient such as aqueous cream and very occasionally with 1% hydrocortisone cream or ointment.

5 Increased scaling of the psoriasis. This occurs when treatment is first begun and stops as soon as the psoriasis begins to clear.
6 Peeling of the palms and soles (Figure 132b). This only happens at the beginning of treatment. When it stops, the palms and soles feel very soft (always noticeable) and sometimes sticky.
7 Increased sweating. This does not usually cause any problems.
8 Poor wound healing. Most patients notice that they injure their skin more easily than they used to, and that cuts take longer to heal.
9 Hair loss (Figure 132c). Hair loss which is bad enough to be noticeable only occurs in a small proportion of patients on etretinate, but when it does, most people will not put up with it. Fortunately it is reversible when treatment is stopped.
10 Paronychia. Painful swelling around the finger and toenails occurs in a minority of patients; its appearance may be identical to that of an ingrown toenail (Figure 132d) and it may require surgical intervention to get it better.
11 Nausea, vomiting and abdominal pain. These are unusual complaints.

Long-term side effects

1 It is teratogenic and must not be given to females of reproductive age. After a single dose of etretinate, 70–80% is excreted in 5 days. After multiple doses, there is a slow elimination phase so that a small amount of the drug hangs around for a very long time. It is currently recommended that a woman should not get pregnant for 2 years after stopping it. Acetretin, the acid derivative of etretinate, has a shorter half life so it ought to be safer for women who want to become pregnant. Unfortunately some of the acetretin is converted to etretinate in the body so it is recommended that women who are on acetretin too should not become pregnant while taking it or for 2 years afterwards.

It has no effect on sperm counts or sperm mobility, so it is quite safe to use in men.

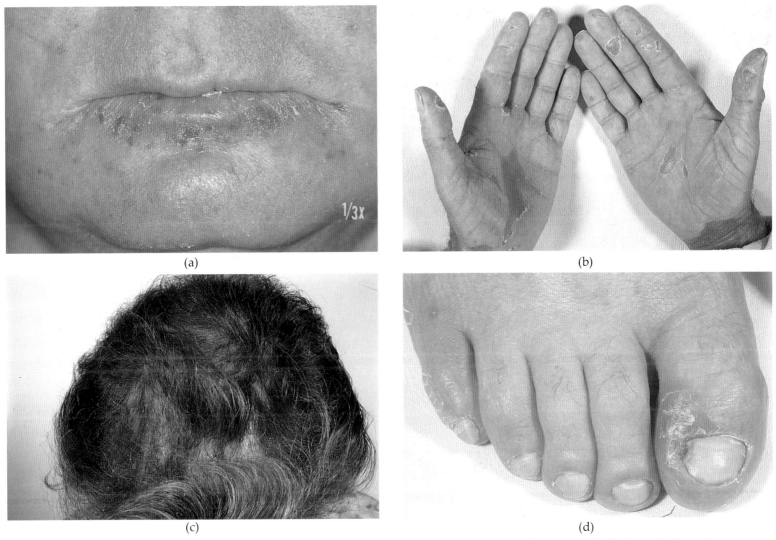

Figure 132 Side effects of etretinate. **(a)** Dry scaly lips extending onto the skin around the lips. **(b)** Peeling of the palms. **(c)** Hair loss. **(d)** Paronychia.

2 Musculoskeletal aches and pains. If patients are on long-term etretinate therapy, they can develop ossification of their ligaments. This can be seen on an X-ray or bone scan. It is recommended that an annual X-ray of the spine and long bones be carried out to pick this up before symptoms occur, because once it has happened it is irreversible.

3 Increase in liver enzymes and rarely hepatitis.

4 Increase in triglycerides due to decreased extra hepatic breakdown and increased secretion by the liver.

Patients should have their liver enzymes and fasting lipids measured before starting treatment, after 2 months and then every 6 months. If they become abnormal, a low-fat diet may help or the dose will need to be reduced or stopped depending on how abnormal they are.

RePUVA

Re = retinoid (etretinate or acetretin)
PUVA = photochemotherapy
A few patients who do not respond to either PUVA or retinoids will respond when they are given together. The retinoid is started 2 weeks before the PUVA. Then both treatments are given until the skin is clear. Once the psoriasis is clear, the PUVA is stopped, and the patient continues on the retinoid alone. It is usually possible to clear the skin more quickly with the combination treatment than with PUVA alone and therefore reduce the dose of UVA that the patient is exposed to. It is also usually possible to use a lower dose of the retinoid (25–50 mg etretinate/day or 25–50 mg acetretin daily) and thus reduce the side effects. Retinoids can also be used in conjunction with topical PUVA.

CYCLOSPORIN A This is an effective treatment for psoriasis, but it is very expensive and has a lot of side-effects. We currently use it only when we have run out of other options. It is an immunosuppressive drug which has no direct effect on epidermal growth, but it increases the production of interleukin 2 from activated T-helper lymphocytes and thus suppresses their further production. It can be given as a tablet or a liquid which is mixed in milk or a fruit juice once a day. It takes 6–8 weeks before there is any effect. The starting dose is 3–4 mg/kg body/weight/day depending on the severity of the psoriasis.

Side effects

1 The major problem with cyclosporin A is its **toxic effect on the kidneys**. The risk of permanent renal damage is minimized if the dose is kept below 5 mg/kg/day and the dose adjusted so that the serum creatinine does not rise more than 30% above the pretreatment level.

The patient needs to have his urine checked for blood and protein and his blood urea and creatinine measured before treatment is begun, after one month and then every 2–3 months. If the creatinine rises the dose must be reduced.

2 Hypertension. A rise in both systolic and diastolic blood pressure can occur and it should be checked when the patient is having his blood taken for urea and creatinine. If the blood pressure increases above 160/95 the calcium channel blocker, nifedipine can be given to reduce it (start with a dose of 10 mg three times a day). This usually works well; if it does not, the dose of cyclosporin A must be reduced. The changes are reversible as the dose is reduced or stopped.

3 Nausea, vomiting and gingivitis. In patients with poor dental hygiene gingival hypertrophy can occur. These effects are reversible if the dose is reduced.

4 Tiredness, headaches, parasthesiae, tremor, and rarely convulsions may occur. They will improve if the dose is reduced.

5 Hypertrichosis. This occurs all over but is a problem mainly on the face in women (men will either not notice the increased hairiness or not mind it). Once it occurs the patient will usually want to stop the drug; it then takes about a year to disappear.

6 In the long term there is an **increased risk of lymphoma, malignant melanoma and non-melanoma skin cancer.**

7 Other biochemical abnormalities which can occur are an increase in liver enzymes, serum uric acid and cholesterol and a fall in serum magnesium.

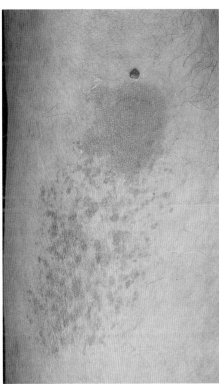

Figure 133 Side effects of arsenic: raindrop pigmentation.

ARSENIC Arsenic is an effective treatment for psoriasis which is not used very much these days because it causes multiple skin cancers 10–15 years later. We think that it still has a useful place in the treatment of extensive psoriasis in the elderly and are prepared to use it in patients over the age of 70. It is given as Fowler's solution (1% arsenic trioxide solution), beginning with a very small dose (0.06 ml three times a day) and gradually increasing it until it works. The effective dose is usually in the region of 0.3–0.4 ml three times a day. It is not possible for the patient to reliably take such small amounts of Fowler's solution, so it is mixed by the pharmacist in equal parts of double strength chloroform water and distilled water, so the patient takes a 5 ml dose.

Side effects

1 Burning of the lips, constriction of the throat, dysphagia, abdominal pain, vomiting and diarrhoea. These occur within minutes of taking the arsenic and can be very severe. They can be avoided by starting with a very small dose and gradually increasing it until a therapeutic level is reached. It should not be a problem in practice.

2 Raindrop pigmentation (Figure 133). Small brown macules appear around the plaques of psoriasis within the first few weeks of starting treatment. Once treatment stops the pigmentation disappears.

3 Keratoses on the palms and soles (Figure 135). These look a bit like warts and develop between 5 and 10 years after a patient has taken arsenic. They are of no significance in themselves although occasionally they stick out like a cutaneous horn and get in the patient's way, and need to be curetted off. Their main importance is in confirming that a patient has taken arsenic in the past when he presents with multiple skin cancers.

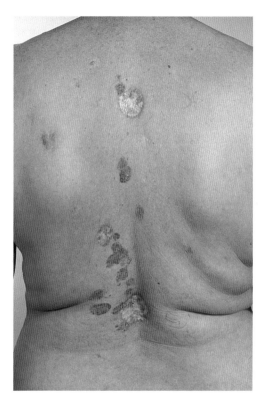

Figure 134 Side effects of arsenic: multiple basal cell carcinomas on covered parts of the skin.

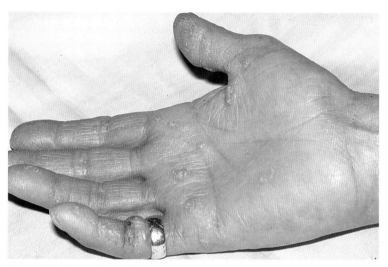

Figure 135 Side effects of arsenic: arsenical keratoses on the palm.

4   Multiple skin tumours—Bowen's disease, basal cell carcinomas and squamous cell carcinomas occur 15–20 years after taking arsenic. They are often very numerous on the trunk and limbs and go on developing for years (Figure 134). They can be removed by excision or curettage and cautery as and when they occur.

Extensive small plaques of psoriasis

If a patient has very numerous small plaques of psoriasis (not guttate psoriasis), the options for treatment are:

1   Calcipotriol ointment applied twice a day. This is suitable if the psoriasis is not too extensive and the patient would not be using more than 100 g of the ointment a week.

2   A tar cream such as 2% crude coal tar in Unguentum Merck, or one of the proprietary tar preparations containing coal tar solution (*see* page 158) applied at night. The patient cannot usually use this in the daytime because of the smell. These mild tar preparations work well if the plaques are fairly superficial.

3   Short-wave ultraviolet light—UVB (this is different to PUVA). Giving a sub-erythema dose of UVB two or three times a week for

Hospital UVB treatment is usually given in a stand-up unit which looks very like a PUVA cabinet (*see* Figure 128, page 165). The dose is worked out by measuring the patient's minimal erythema dose (MED) first. Treatment is started just below this; generally this is just a few seconds to begin with (*see* below).

	Skin type I	**Skin type II**	**Skin type III and IV**
Week 1	5 seconds	10 seconds	10 sec for 2 R_xs
Week 2	10 seconds	20 seconds	20 sec for 2 R_xs
Week 3	15 seconds	30 seconds	30 sec for 2 R_xs
Week 4	20 seconds	40 seconds	40 sec for 2 R_xs
Week 5	25 seconds	50 seconds	50 sec for 2 R_xs
Week 6	30 seconds	1 minute	1 min for 2 R_xs. Up 10 sec every 2nd R_x

Ordinary sunlight is even better than artificial UVB but cannot be relied upon in this country. A holiday abroad in a sunny climate will often improve psoriasis and some patients will choose to have a sunny holiday once or twice a year simply to keep their skin clear. **4** If the skin is very bad, in-patient treatment can be considered (*see* page 158), but the Goeckerman regime will need to be used because it would be too time-consuming to apply dithranol to very numerous small plaques.

Guttate psoriasis

This is an acute eruption which occurs 10–14 days after a streptococcal infection (usually of the throat) and clears spontaneously after 2–3 months. Dithranol and strong tar preparations should be

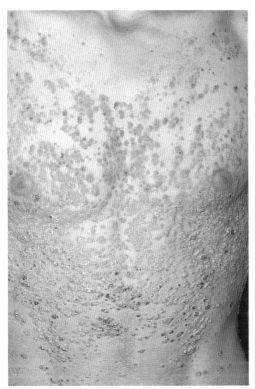

Figure 136 Extensive small plaques of psoriasis in a 17-year-old man. He was successfully treated with UVB.

6–8 weeks is an ideal treatment for very widespread small plaques of psoriasis because it saves the patient having to apply messy ointments to a large area of the skin. It means that the patient will have to go to the local hospital to have it done, which is a disadvantage. The kind of sun-bed that can be bought for use at home, and which can be found in some hairdressing salons and beauty parlours, is of no use because it emits mainly UVA which has no effect on psoriasis. This treatment is not suitable for patients with a very fair skin who burn rather than tan in the sun.

avoided because they will make it worse (the skin will become red, inflamed and sore). Since it is usually asymptomatic, no treatment is needed other than an explanation about what has happened and reassurance that it will clear completely. If it is itchy, an emollient such as aqueous cream or a very mild tar preparation such as 2% liquor picis carbonis in Ung. aquosum or Unguentum Merck can be applied to the skin once or twice a day.

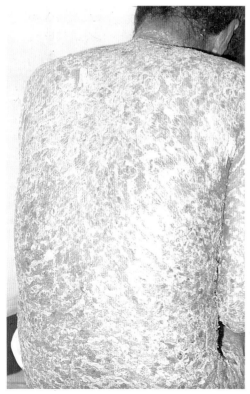

Figure 137
Erythrodermic psoriasis in a man aged 49 years. Although the psoriasis is universal, it is not unstable and therefore not as dangerous as that shown in Figure 139.

Erythrodermic psoriasis

On no account should tar or dithranol be applied to psoriasis when it is universal or it will get even worse. The patient should be admitted to hospital urgently where he will be kept warm (with a space blanket if necessary to prevent hypothermia), rested in bed and sedated with trimeprazine to keep him there. Only simple emollients will be applied to the skin twice a day to keep it comfortable. If it does not clear with these simple measures he will need methotrexate, etretinate or PUVA (*see* pages 161, 164 and 168).

Generalized pustular psoriasis

This is a true dermatological emergency. The patient should be admitted urgently to hospital where he will be rested in bed, sedated and covered with white soft paraffin (either pure or mixed in equal parts with liquid paraffin). Tar and dithranol must not be used because they will make it worse, and if he has been using topical steroids, these must be stopped. He can easily become hypothermic and may need nursing under a space blanket to keep him warm. He is likely to have a fever (Figure 138) but this is not due to infection and he does not need antibiotics. If he does not get better with bed rest and emollients, he will need methotrexate (*see* page 161). It is a very slow process to get the patient better and there is no way of rushing it. He is likely to be in hospital for at least 6 weeks and maybe quite a lot longer than that. Although methotrexate works well, it is easy to give too much, causing ulceration of the skin (*see* Figure 124, page 163) and pancytopenia. Treating this condition is like walking on a knife edge, and even with expert care some patients will die.

Generalized pustular psoriasis is often caused by withdrawal of steroids (either a potent topical steroid or systemic steroids). For

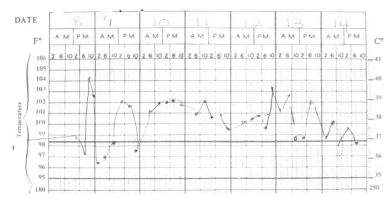

Figure 138 Temperature chart of a patient with generalized pustular psoriasis.

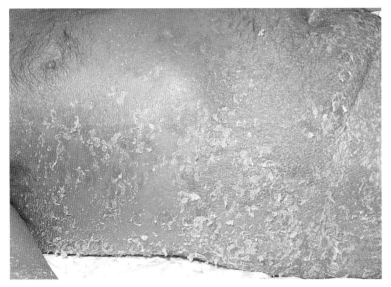

Figure 139 Erythrodermic psoriasis on the edge of becoming pustular in a man aged 46. Compare with Figure 137; this is much more unstable.

this reason systemic steroids should be avoided in psoriasis unless they are absolutely essential, and topical steroids should be used in the flexures only where there is no alternative.

Treatment of psoriasis at special sites

Psoriasis on the face

Both tar and dithranol can be used on the face. We suggest starting with 0.1% Dithrocream as a short contact treatment (rubbing it carefully onto the affected skin, leaving it for 30 minutes and then washing it off with soap and water; *see* also page 155). It is important not to get it into the eyes, as this will make them very sore. This can easily be avoided by applying the Dithrocream on a cotton wool bud so that its application can be very accurate. A cotton wool bud is also useful at other sites if the plaques are very small, so that the Dithrocream is kept off normal skin. If 0.1% Dithrocream is not effective, the concentration can be increased every 2 weeks until it is (from 0.1% to 0.25% to 0.5% to 1% to 2%).

2% crude coal tar in Lassar's paste is also very effective on the face and will stay where it is put. It is too messy to use in the daytime but can be used successfully at night. If the psoriasis is very mild, one of the proprietary tar creams containing coal tar solution can be used twice a day (for a list of these *see* page 158).

Psoriasis in the scalp

If there are thick plaques of psoriasis in the scalp, the most effective treatment is coconut oil compound ointment (Ung cocois co.). The hair is parted and the ointment rubbed onto the scalp; it is then parted again a little further along, and more ointment applied; this is continued until the whole scalp has been treated. It is done every

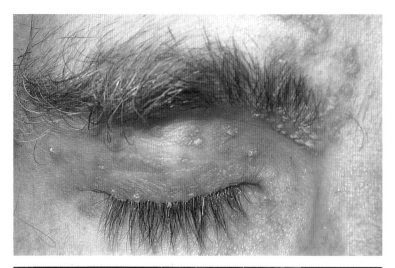

night before the patient goes to bed and washed off the following morning with Polytar shampoo or whatever shampoo the patient likes. Because it makes a mess, the head should be covered over-night with a scarf or shower cap to keep the ointment off the pillow (*see* Figure 106, page 144). The treatment is repeated each night and washed off each morning until the scalp is clear. This usually takes 7–10 days. Once it is clear, the treatment can be done once a week or once a fortnight to keep it clear. Alternatively, once it is clear, the scalp can be washed with Capasal shampoo (which contains 1% distilled coal tar, 0.5% salicylic acid and 1% coconut oil) once a week to keep it clear.

Coconut oil compound ointment* can be made up by the chemist, in which case it must be kept in the refrigerator when it is not being used, otherwise it becomes very runny and makes a mess everywhere (*see* Figure 105, page 143).

Formula of coconut oil compound ointment (Ung cocois co.)	
Emulsifying wax BP	65 g
Yellow soft paraffin BP	45 g
Precipitated sulphur BP	20 g
Salicylic acid BP	10 g
Coal tar solution BP	60 ml
Coconut oil BP	300 g

If coconut oil compound ointment does not work (which is unusual), Ung pyrogallol co., dithranol pomade or oil of Cade ointment can be used instead. Ung pyrogallol co. is used in exactly the same way as Ung cocois co., ie it is rubbed in at night and washed off the next morning. It is extremely difficult to remove when the hair is washed; the patient may have to rub Ung cocois co. in to loosen the Ung pyrogallol co. enough to shampoo it out!

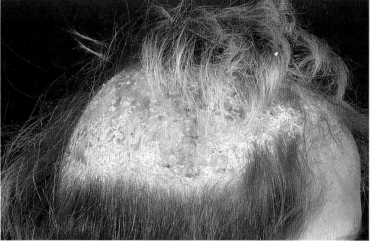

Figure 140 (*above*) Psoriasis around the eyes. This can be treated with 0.1% Dithrocream applied on a cotton wool bud.
Figure 141 (*below*) Alopecia due to psoriasis. The hair loss is not due to the psoriasis itself, but to constant rubbing and scratching causing the hairs to break off.

*Available also as a proprietary ointment, Cocois ointment made by Bioglan Laboratories.

Formula for Ung pyrogallol co.

Pyrogallol	5 g
Salicylic acid	8 g
Phenol BP	5 g
White soft paraffin	182 g

Dithranol pomade must not be used in patients with blond or very fair hair because it stains it mauve! It is massaged into the scalp, making sure that it does not get into the eyes. It is washed off again after 2–4 hours so that it does not burn the scalp.

Formula for dithranol pomade

Dithranol	2 g
Salicylic acid	0.8 g
Mineral oil (coconut oil or liquid paraffin)	149.2 g
Emulsifying wax	45 g

Oil of Cade ointment is also rubbed in at night and washed off the next morning.

Formula for oil of Cade ointment

Cade oil	6 g
Precipitated sulphur	3 g
Salicylic acid	2 g
Emulsifying ointment	89 g

Psoriasis should not cause hair loss, but if it is very itchy the hairs can break off due to constant rubbing and scratching (Figure 141).

In this situation, use Ung cocois co. until the psoriasis is clear. Once the patient stops scratching the hair will regrow normally.

For mild scalp psoriasis, where the scales are not very thick, shampooing the scalp twice a week with Capasal shampoo may be all that is needed. If that is not enough, or if the scalp is very itchy, a topical steroid lotion or gel can be applied every night until it is clear (0.1% hydrocortisone 17-butyrate [Locoid] lotion, 0.1% beta-methasone valerate [Betnovate] lotion or 0.025% fluocinolone acetonide [Synalar] gel). Topical steroid lotions contain alcohol, so the patient should be warned that it will sting if the skin is broken. The gel is water miscible and will not sting. Both are completely ineffective if there is thick scaling; they are very popular, however, because they do not make a mess and do not smell.

Psoriasis of the flexures and genitalia

Tar and dithranol are likely to make the skin sore in the flexures and on the genitalia, so they should not be used. Topical steroids are the treatment of choice at these sites. The weakest possible steroid to clear the skin is required, but 1% hydrocortisone is ineffective and is not worth trying. Start with either 0.05% clobetasone butyrate (Eumovate) or 0.1% hydrocortisone 17-butyrate (Locoid) cream or ointment applied twice a day. One or other is likely to be effective. Whether the patient will prefer a cream or ointment you will have to discover by trial and error.

Psoriasis on the palms and soles

There are three patterns of psoriasis that occur on the palms and soles. The treatment of each is slightly different so they will be dealt with separately.

1 Ordinary plaque psoriasis on the palms and soles. The treatment of this is the same as treatment of plaque psoriasis anywhere else. Use one of the following:

(i) calcipotriol ointment applied twice a day

(ii) 0.1% Dithrocream rubbed carefully into the plaque, left in place for 30 minutes and then washed off with soap and water. If it does not clear in 2 weeks, increase the strength of the Dithrocream to 0.25%, and then to 0.5%, 1% and 2% every 2 weeks until it works. When the psoriasis is gone, the skin will be brown instead of red. The cream is then stopped and the brown colour will clear within 10–14 days

(iii) coal tar and salicylic acid ointment BP at night (under a pair of cotton gloves on the hands or a pair of old socks on the feet so that it does not make a mess on the bedding) and white soft paraffin in the morning.

2 Thick hyperkeratotic psoriasis. The first thing is to get rid of the thick scale (Figure 142). This is done by:

(i) applying 2% salicylic acid in lanolin (as salicylic acid ointment BP) or 5% salicylic acid in white soft paraffin twice a day

(ii) applying 50% propylene glycol in water at night covered with polythene (gloves on the hands, bags on the feet). It usually takes about a week to get most of the scale off

(iii) soaking the feet in 40% urea solution for 10 minutes at night. Whichever of the keratolytic agents are used, the patient will also need a specific anti-psoriatic treatment. We suggest you use one of the above treatments at night and coal tar and salicylic acid ointment in the morning. The tar will make a mess and the patient will need to wear a pair of cotton gloves and/or a pair of old socks to keep the ointment on the skin and off other things. If a tar ointment is completely impracticable because of the patient's work, he can

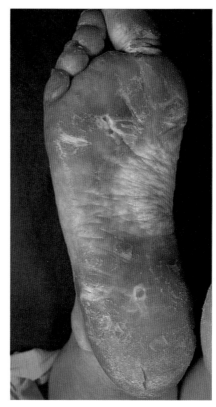

Figure 142 Thick hyperkeratotic psoriasis on the soles. The fissures cause a lot of pain.

use white soft paraffin in the daytime until the thick scale is gone and then use calcipotriol ointment twice a day.

3 Pustular psoriasis of the palms and soles. This is a very difficult condition to help. Start by trying one of the following:

(i) coal tar and salicylic acid ointment applied at night with a pair of cotton gloves over it on the hands, or a pair of old socks over it on the feet, to keep the tar off the bedding. Most patients will find it helpful to apply white soft paraffin in the morning to keep the skin supple

(ii) 0.1% Dithrocream rubbed carefully into the psoriasis at night and covered with gloves and/or socks to keep it off the sheets. The strength can be increased to 0.25% or 0.5% if the 0.1% does not work, provided the skin does not burn

(iii) a topical steroid ointment or cream applied twice a day, eg 0.025% betamethasone valerate (Betnovate RD) or the equivalent (see page 8). Alternatively a mixture of a topical steroid with salicylic acid can be tried, eg 5% salicylic acid in quarter strength betamethasone valerate ointment, or for a short time something stronger like 0.05% betamethasone dipropionate and 3% salicylic acid (Diprosalic ointment). Alternatively, the steroid and salicylic acid may be used at different times of the day, eg the topical steroid in the morning and the salicylic acid at night. When a topical steroid cream or ointment is applied to the palm or sole, some of it inevitably gets onto the thinner skin on the dorsum of the hand or foot where it can cause atrophy. It is important therefore not to go on using a potent topical steroid for too long.

Sometimes none of these treatments help. A patient may be prepared to put up with it and just use white soft paraffin to keep the skin comfortable. Another will be disabled by it, being unable to use his hands, or walk because of painful feet. In these circumstances you will have to consider using one of the systemic treatments.

(i) Etretinate at a starting dose of 1 mg/kg body weight/day works well. Once the skin is better the dose can be reduced to a maintenance dose which is just enough to keep the hands and feet clear (often only 25 mg daily or on alternate days). For the problems with the use of etretinate see page 168.

(ii) PUVA. There are special hand and foot machines for PUVA with small banks of light tubes (emitting long-wave ultraviolet light) about the size of an X-ray viewing box. The patient takes the 8-methoxypsoralen as he would for ordinary PUVA treatment and 2 hours later puts the hands or feet on the box emitting the UVA. He will still need to protect both his eyes and his skin in the same way as if he had been irradiated all over, because of the circulating psoralens. For details about the precautions to be taken with PUVA and the side effects see page 164.

Topical PUVA can also be used. The hands and/or feet are soaked in a 1% solution of 8-methoxypsoralen for 15 minutes, patted dry and then irradiated with UVA using a hand and foot machine (see above).

(iii) One of the cytotoxic drugs—methotrexate, azathioprine or hydroxyurea. Obviously the disease will need to be seriously interfering with the patient's life to consider using a drug like this. For details of how to use these drugs and the problems associated with them, see pages 161, 163 and 164.

Psoriasis of the nails

There is no topical treatment which will help psoriatic nail changes (pitting, salmon patches onycholysis or subungual hyperkeratosis). Coloured nail varnish will hide onycholysis in a woman, and keeping the nails cut short will stop onycholysis getting worse because of trauma. Fortunately patients do not often ask for treatment for their nails. If the skin psoriasis is bad enough to be

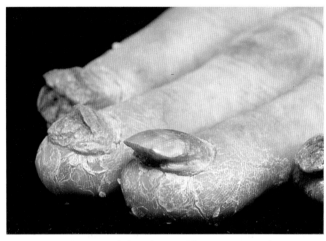

Figure 143 Very unsightly subungual hyperkeratosis due to psoriasis. To improve this change in the nails, the patient would need some form of systemic therapy (methotrexate, azathioprine or etretinate).

treated with a systemic agent, the nails will improve as the skin does. If it is just the nails which are involved, it is hard to justify using a systemic agent just for them unless they are so unsightly that it prevents the patient from mixing socially or keeping a job. If they are as bad as shown in Figure 143, etretinate, methotrexate or azathioprine will probably be needed, but obviously the pros and cons will need to be discussed with the patient so that he can make an informed decision about whether or not he wants to have treatment.

Psoriasis in children

The treatment of psoriasis in children is not very different from the treatment in adults except that none of the systemic agents are safe to use. Psoriasis often begins in childhood, but the pattern of disease may be quite different to that in adults. There are three common patterns in children.

1 Guttate psoriasis. This usually does not require any treatment since it does not itch and gets better spontaneously in 2–3 months (*see* page 173).

2 Psoriasis begins on the scalp or genitalia. On the scalp there is often thick scale which grows out along the hairs (pityriasis amantacea, *see* page 143); it is unsightly and may itch. Treatment is with Ung cocois co. (*see* page 143). If it is not too extensive, simply washing the hair with Capasal shampoo may be sufficient.

When it is on the genitalia, boys in particular, may be embarrassed about showing it to you. Parents too may be anxious about where it is. It is best to simply explain that psoriasis often begins on the penis in boys and that it usually clears up. It may of course later appear elsewhere. Treatment is the same as for adults with a moderately potent topical steroid (*see* page 177).

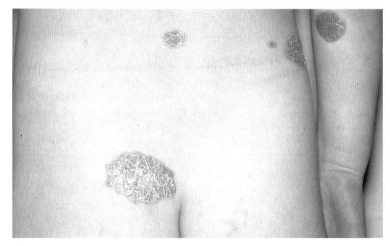

Figure 144 Psoriasis in a child.

3 The adult pattern with plaques predominantly on the elbows, knees and sacrum (Figure 144). In the summer, children can be encouraged to get out into the sunshine as much as possible unless they are very fair. On the skin they can use either tar or dithranol. Children do not like the smell of tar any more than adults do, so unless the plaques are very widespread, Dithrocream is the treatment of choice (*see* page 155).

If a child is getting frequent sore throats followed by guttate psoriasis, he may need to have a tonsillectomy. Sometimes psoriasis begins after a traumatic experience (bereavement or sexual abuse). If that is the case the child and the family may need some help but there is not always an obvious reason why the psoriasis begins when it does.

Some patients with psoriasis and some parents of children with psoriasis, will want to be put in touch with others with the disease. The Psoriasis Association provides information and literature and arranges meetings for sufferers and their families all over the country. Their address is:

THE PSORIASIS ASSOCIATION
7 Milton Street
Northampton, NN2 7JG
Tel: 0604 711 129

Typical prescription for adult with psoriasis

R$_x$ calcipotriol ointment	**30 g**
Apply to psoriasis twice a day	
Do not use it on the face	
Wash your hands after applying it so that it does not get onto the face accidentally	
Coconut oil compound ointment	**80 g**
Massage into the scalp at night before you go to bed	
Cover with a scarf or shower cap to keep the ointment off the pillows	
Polytar shampoo	**150 ml**
Use in the morning to wash off the coconut oil compound ointment	

Typical prescription for child with psoriasis

R$_x$ 0.1% Dithrocream	**50 g**
0.25% Dithrocream	**50 g**
Start with the 0.1% cream	
Rub it carefully into the psoriasis taking care not to get it onto the normal skin	
Leave it for 30 minutes	
Wipe it off with cotton wool or a tissue	
Wash thoroughly with soap and water	
After 2 weeks, if the psoriasis is not gone and if the skin is not sore, change to the 0.25% cream	
Eumovate ointment	**30 g**
Apply to the genitalia twice a day	

Table 15 Summary of topical treatments used in psoriasis

Drug	When and how to use it	When not to use it
Calcipotriol	Drug of first choice for ordinary plaque psoriasis. Apply twice a day until skin is clear (*see* page 154).	If the patient will require more than 100 g ointment a week in case it causes a rise in serum calcium.
Dithranol	1 In a cream base, useful in ordinary plaque psoriasis providing the patient can see the plaques to apply the cream accurately. Apply just to the psoriasis, rub it well in; leave in place and wash off 30 minutes later (short contact therapy, *see* page 155). 2 In Lassar's paste it is the mainstay of in-patient treatment; used for patients with extensive plaque type psoriasis (*see* page 159). 3 Pustular psoriasis of the palm or sole. Rub well into affected skin and wash off 30 minutes later (*see* page 179).	1 In any kind of eruptive psoriasis, guttate psoriasis, erythrodermic psoriasis or generalized pustular psoriasis. 2 In the flexures and on the genitalia. 3 Do not use on the scalp in patients with blond or white hair because it will stain it mauve.
Tar	1 Most patients do not like tar because of its brown colour and the smell. It is useful in a cream or ointment base, if there are too many small plaques for the patient to be able to apply dithranol to accurately (*see* page 157). It is usually used at night and covered with old clothes. 2 As an alternative to dithranol in in-patient treatment (*see* page 160). 3 Tar baths (Polytar emollient) as part of in-patient therapy or before treatment with UVB (*see* page 159). 4 As coal tar and salicylic acid ointment for pustular psoriasis on the palms and soles. Use at night and cover the hands with cotton gloves and the feet with a pair of old socks to keep it off the bedding (*see* page 178). 5 In Lassar's paste on the face. Apply at night and clean off with arachis oil in the morning (*see* page 175). 6 As Ung cocois co., it is the mainstay of treatment for psoriasis on the scalp. Rub into the scalp at night and wash off the following morning (*see* page 175). 7 Tar shampoos for washing the hair (tar alone or mixed with salicylic acid and coconut oil, *see* page 176).	1 In any kind of acute erupting psoriasis, eg generalized pustular psoriasis or erythrodermic psoriasis (a weak concentration of coal tar solution can be used for guttate psoriasis). 2 In the flexures.

(Table continues opposite)

Table 15 Summary of topical treatments used in psoriasis (continued)

Drug	When and how to use it	When not to use it
UVB	Extensive small plaques of psoriasis that it would be difficult to apply ointments to. As an in-patient, a sub-erythema dose is given daily; as an out-patient it is given twice a week for 6–8 weeks (*see* page 172) or as part of day care therapy (*see* page 160).	1 In patients with very fair skin, who burn rather than tan in the sun. 2 In eruptive psoriasis, erythrodermic psoriasis or generalized pustular psoriasis.
Emollients (aqueous cream, WSP or a mixture of WSP and liquid paraffin)	1 On any acute erupting psoriasis, erythrodermic psoriasis or generalized pustular psoriasis, apply two or three times a day to keep the patient comfortable (*see* page 174). 2 Some patients will use an emollient rather than an active treatment simply because it is less messy. 3 In the bath mixed with tar to stop the skin drying out too much with the tar alone (*see* page 159).	It has no effect on psoriasis itself and will not clear the rash. It may make the patient feel more comfortable simply by keeping the skin greasy.
Keratolytics	1 Ordinary plaque-type psoriasis when the patient does not want to use tar or dithranol because of the mess. Salicylic acid ointment, usually 2% or 5%, is applied once or twice a day (*see* page 158). 2 Some patients with extensive psoriasis will use a keratolytic ointment once or twice a day to reduce the amount of scaling. 3 On hyperkeratotic psoriasis on the palms and soles. Use at night with an emollient in the daytime (*see* page 178).	In the flexures.
Topical steroids	1 In the flexures. Use one of the moderately potent group, because hydrocortisone does not work, applied twice a day (*see* page 177). 2 On the scalp if there is only mild scaling. Use as a lotion or gel at night (*see* page 177). 3 Pustular psoriasis on the palms and soles if tar and dithranol do not work. Use a steroid from the moderately potent group alone or mixed with salicylic acid twice a day (*see* page 179).	Anywhere except the flexures, scalp, palms and soles. Ideally would not be used at all because of the risk of generalized pustular psoriasis occurring when the steroid is stopped.

Table 16 Summary of systemic treatments used in psoriasis

Drug	When and how to use it	When not to use it
Methotrexate	1 Failure of in-patient treatment. 2 Frequent relapse after clearing with in-patient treatment. 3 Generalized pustular psoriasis or erythrodermic psoriasis not responding to bed rest and emollients. 4 Extensive skin psoriasis and bad psoriatic arthropathy. Given as a single dose orally, intramuscularly, or intravenously once a week (*see* page 161).	1 Woman of childbearing age, or man who wishes to father a child. 2 Patient has pre-existing liver disease. 3 Patient has been a heavy drinker. 4 Patient likes to drink alcohol and is not prepared to stop completely. 5 Patient needs to take aspirin, diuretics, hypoglycaemics, NSAIDs, phenytoin, probenecid, sulphonamides or trimethoprim.
Azathioprine	Same indications as for methotrexate (*see* page 161). Use instead of methotrexate in patient with methotrexate-induced liver disease, or in a patient who is not prepared to stop drinking or have a yearly liver biopsy. Given orally at a dose of 2 mg/kg body weight/day in three divided doses (*see* page 163).	1 Women of childbearing age. 2 Patient who is unreliable about taking tablets and/or is not prepared to have his blood checked regularly. 3 If patient has had severe gastrointestinal upset with azathioprine in the past.
Hydroxyurea	1 In a patient who has failed to respond to methotrexate and azathioprine. 2 In a patient who has had to stop methotrexate or azathioprine because of side effects. Given orally at a dose of 0.5–1.5 g/day in two or three equally divided doses (*see* page 164).	1 In a woman of childbearing age. 2 In a patient who has previously had pancytopenia from the drug.
Etretinate	1 Patient with extensive small plaques of psoriasis. 2 Patient needing frequent hospital admissions to control his psoriasis. 3 Pustular psoriasis of the palms and soles unresponsive to topical treatment. 4 Occasionally in erythrodermic or generalized pustular psoriasis in a patient who cannot have methotrexate. Given orally with food, at a dose of 1 mg/kg body weight/day as a single dose or three equally divided doses (*see* page 168).	1 Women of childbearing age, unless they are sure they have finished having a family and are taking adequate contraception. It is safe for men. 2 Elderly patients of either sex do not cope well with the side effects, so probably not suitable over the age of 60. 3 Patients with pre-existing liver disease. 4 Patients with raised serum lipids. 5 Patients with a history of myocardial infarction.

(Table continues opposite)

Table 16 Summary of systemic treatments used in psoriasis (continued)

Drug	When and how to use it	When not to use it
PUVA	1 Patient with plaque-type psoriasis which is too extensive for him to apply tar, dithranol or calcipotriol. 2 Patient needing frequent hospital admissions to keep his psoriasis at bay or who cannot take time off work for in-patient treatment. 3 Occasionally in a patient with erythrodermic psoriasis or generalized pustular psoriasis who cannot have methotrexate. 4 Pustular psoriasis of the palms and soles which has not responded to topical treatment. Patient takes 8-methoxy psoralen (8-MOP) 2 hours before a visit to the hospital to be irradiated with long wave ultraviolet light (UVA), twice a week. He needs to protect his eyes with glasses which filter out both UVA and UVB for 24 hours after taking his 8-MOP (*see* page 164).	1 Woman of childbearing age unless she has completed her family and is taking adequate contraceptives. It is safe for men. 2 Patient with type I skin or a coexistent photosensitive disease (eg SLE). 3 Patient has or has had skin cancer. 4 Patient has had previous treatment with radiotherapy to the skin. 5 Patient is immunosuppressed. 6 Patient has a cataract.
RePUVA	When a patient has failed to respond to either PUVA or etretinate separately. Etretinate at a dose initially of 1 mg/kg body weight/day is taken every day. 8-methoxy psoralen is taken by mouth 2 hours before exposure to UVA on 2 days a week. The patient needs to protect his eyes with polarizing lenses for 24 hours after taking the 8-MOP (*see* page 170).	See contraindications for etretinate and PUVA.
Cyclosporin A	When you have run out of all the other options. The minimum requirements are those enumerated for methotrexate, but because of its exorbitant cost it is not used as a first line systemic agent. It is given as a single daily dose, either as a tablet or as a liquid which needs to be mixed with milk or fruit juice (*see* page 170).	1 Pre-existing renal disease or hypertension. 2 Females will not usually tolerate the hypertrichosis which occurs. 3 Young adults because of the long-term risk of neoplasia.
Arsenic	In patients over the age of 70 with extensive psoriasis. Given as a small dose of Fowler's solution (arsenic trioxide) mixed in chloroform water three times a day. The dose is gradually increased until it is effective (*see* page 171).	Under the age of 70 years because of the risk of skin cancer 10–20 years later.

PTERYGIUM OF THE NAILS

Scarring of the nails due to lichen planus (pterygium) can be switched off by giving a large dose of systemic steroids. Start with 60 mg prednisolone daily for about 2 weeks and then rapidly reduce the dose every 2–3 days from 60 mg to 50 mg, to 40 mg, to 30 mg, to 20 mg, to 15 mg, to 10 mg, to 5 mg, to 0 mg. Once stopped it does not usually recur. It is effective only if treatment is started as soon as the nail changes begin. If it looks as if the cuticle is beginning to grow over the nail, urgent referral to a dermatologist is required. Once scarring has occurred, the changes are permanent and cannot be reversed.

PURPURA

If the patient has widespread purpura, the first thing to do is to check a full blood count and clotting screen. If the platelet count is low or there is an abnormality in the clotting process, the treatment will be of the underlying cause. The patient should be referred to a haematologist, oncologist or general physician.

If the blood count and clotting screen are normal, it is worth also doing the auto-immune profile, and looking for cryoglobulins, immunoglobulins and cold agglutinins. Again if any abnormality is found, the treatment will be of the underlying cause.

If the patient has a vasculitis rather than straight purpura (red macules and papules, vesicles and necrotic lesions as well as purpura), treatment will be directed to the cause of that (*see* page 248).

Most other kinds of purpura need no specific treatment. Almost all rashes on the lower legs can be purpuric due to hypostatic pressure, and its presence has no sinister implications.

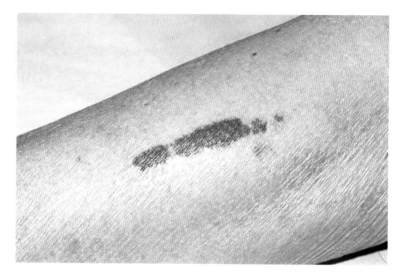

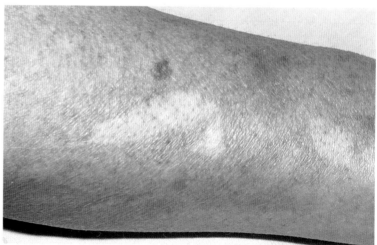

Figure 145 (*above*) Senile purpura.

Figure 146 (*below*) Scar due to tearing of skin in elderly patient.

Senile purpura on the backs of the hands and forearms does not need any treatment other than an explanation to the patient about its cause. It is due to loss of dermal collagen which acts as a support for the blood vessels (due to getting older or the use of topical or systemic steroids). Without proper support, the slightest knock results in bleeding into the skin (Figure 145). If the trauma is more substantial, the skin can tear giving rise to stellate scars (Figure 146). Obviously the patient should take care not to injure his skin but it is impossible to avoid doing so altogether. Individual tears should be covered for protection against further injury or stuck together with butterfly plasters.

PYODERMA GANGRENOSUM

Patients with pyoderma gangrenosum should be referred to the hospital for investigation of the underlying cause.

Causes of pyoderma gangrenosum
Ulcerative colitis
Crohn's disease
Multiple myeloma
Rheumatoid arthritis

In patients with ulcerative colitis, the activity of the pyoderma gangrenosum reflects the activity of the bowel problem, but with the other diseases the two conditions seem to behave independently of each other. In a patient with ulcerative colitis, the priority is to treat the bowel, and when that is done the rapidly spreading ulcer of pyoderma gangrenosum will heal.

In a patient without ulcerative colitis, the underlying disease will still need treating, but you should not expect that to heal the skin.

The pyoderma gangrenosum is treated with large doses of systemic steroids, beginning with 60 mg prednisolone daily. Usually that is sufficient, but occasionally 120 mg prednisolone is needed. Once the ulcer is healed the dose can gradually be reduced, and eventually the patient will be able to come off the steroids.

Topical treatment will not heal the ulcer, but nevertheless some kind of dressing will be needed to cover the open area. The alternatives are:
- eusol and paraffin dressings applied once a day (*see* page 232).
- 0.05% clobetasol propionate (Dermovate) cream applied once or twice a day (occasionally this is used as the only treatment, in a patient for whom systemic steroids are contraindicated).

Both will need to be covered with a dry dressing and a pad.

If systemic steroids do not work, azathioprine, clofazimine, dapsone, minocycline or salazopyrine can all be tried. The patient needs to be under the care of a dermatologist, gastroenterologist or general physician with some experience of managing this difficult condition.

PYOGENIC GRANULOMA

A pyogenic granuloma can be removed by curetting it off under a local anaesthetic (you will need a ring block if it is on the finger). It bleeds a lot when you do this. A useful tip is to rotate a silver nitrate stick in the hole, this will stop most of the bleeding and a cautery can be used to stop the rest. Curettage and cautery usually gets rid of it once and for all, but occasionally the original lesion recurs almost immediately, surrounded by satellite lesions

(Figure 147). If that happens it is best to leave well alone and wait for it to sclerose up and disappear by itself.

Excision of a pyogenic granuloma often results in recurrence, so curettage and cautery is the treatment of choice; freezing with liquid nitrogen or cautery alone are usually ineffective.

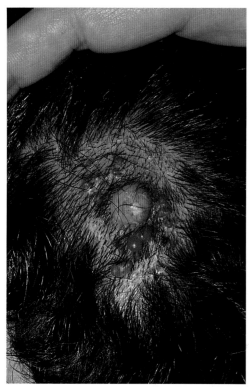

Figure 147 Pyogenic granuloma with satellite lesions.

ROSACEA

Broad spectrum antibiotics are the mainstay of treatment of rosacea. How they work is not known. Oxytetracycline 250 mg twice a day for 6 weeks is cheap and effective. It must be given on an empty stomach (half an hour before a meal or 2 hours after) as it chelates with calcium in milk and food, and with iron and antacids. In most patients the rash will be gone in 6 weeks. If it is improved, but not completely clear, it is worth persevering with the oxytetracycline for a further 6 weeks. At the end of the course of treatment (6–12 weeks) the patient can stop the tablets and usually the rash will not recur. If it does recur, a further 6 week course of oxytetracycline can be given.

There are a few patients who seem to need long-term treatment with oxytetracycline to keep the rosacea at bay; every time they stop the tablets the rash recurs. There is no harm in continuing oxytetracycline indefinitely if necessary.

If oxytetracycline does not work (unusual if it is taken properly on an empty stomach), a different antibiotic can be tried instead. The options are:
- erythromycin 250 mg twice a day
- Septrin 1 tablet twice a day
- minocycline 50 mg twice a day
- minocycline 100 mg modified release capsule once a day
- metronidazole 200 mg three times a day.

They are all given initially for 6 weeks, and if they are going to work, they should certainly have done so by the end of 12 weeks.

For patients in whom you do not want to use an oral antibiotic, 0.75% metronidazole gel (Metrogel) can be applied as a thin film to the skin twice a day. It seems to work as well as oral antibiotics and is particularly useful for women who develop candidiasis with oxytetracycline.

There are a few patients for whom none of these will work. Most of them will have telangiectasia rather than papules and pustules. Sometimes clonidine (Dixarit) 25–50 µg twice a day will help. For others cosmetic camouflage may be all that can be realistically offered. Some patients with classical rosacea simply do not respond to treatment. They should be referred to a dermatologist. Sometimes 13-*cis*-retinoic acid will work, and occasionally radiotherapy is used as a last resort.

Steroid-induced rosacea

The topical steroid must be stopped or the rash will not get better. Unfortunately when the steroid is stopped, the rash will get worse initially, and you should warn the patient that this will happen. It is a good idea to see the patient 2–3 days later to reassure her. If you do not, she will simply go back to applying the topical steroid. Once the steroid is stopped, the rash will gradually clear, but it may take several months. The process can be speeded up by taking oxytetracycline 250 mg twice a day for 6 weeks (half an hour before food). The patient may want to use some kind of topical preparation for dryness or itching, so prescribe a simple moisturizer, such as aqueous cream, which can be used as often as she likes.

Eye changes in rosacea

The eye changes will all clear when the skin is treated with oxytetracycline 250 mg twice a day for 6 weeks (*see* page 188).

Rhinophyma

The first thing is to treat any active rosacea which is present with oxytetracycline 250 mg twice a day for 6 weeks (*see* page 188). Once

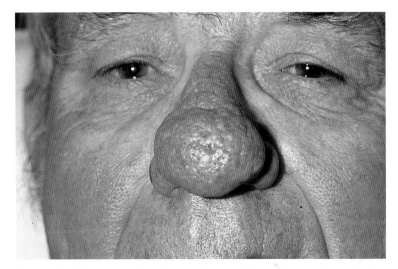

Figure 148 Rhinophyma in a 68-year-old man before the excess tissue was shaved off under local anaesthetic using an electrosurgical cautery. Compare with Figure 149.

the rosacea is quiescent, the excess tissue on the nose can then be shaved off; this can be done under a regional local anaesthetic block of the nose or under a general anaesthetic. The excess sebaceous tissue is literally planed off with a knife, carbon dioxide laser or bendable loop radio surgical cautery, to give a flat, smooth surface which will then re-epithelialize from the hair follicles. The shaved area is covered with 3% chlortetracycline hydrochloride ointment (Aureomycin) and a non-stick dressing for 5 days, after which it is best left open. Healing occurs in about 2 weeks (Figures 148 and 149).

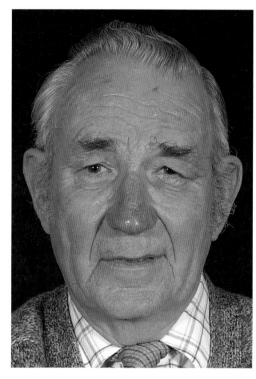

Figure 149 Same patient as Figure 148 5 months after the rhinophyma was shaved off.

SARCOID

What treatment to use in sarcoid depends on which organs are involved. It is never enough to diagnose sarcoid of the skin without a full investigation for sarcoid elsewhere. The patient should be referred to a chest physician so that this can be done. Patients with symptomatic lung disease, hypercalcaemia or uveitis need systemic steroids and if the skin is involved, that will improve as the rest does.

If the skin alone is affected, the decision about whether or not to offer treatment will depend on the variety of involvement and how disfiguring it is. There are three main patterns to be considered.

1 Erythema nodosum. The patient will be acutely ill with a fever and arthralgia, and will almost certainly have bilateral hilar lymph-adenopathy on a chest X-ray. The immediate management involves the patient resting in bed and taking analgesics (paracetamol 1 g every 4 hours) or non-steroidal anti-inflammatory drugs (indomethacin 25 mg twice a day) for the pain. The skin problem is an acute one which should resolve without any specific treatment over a period of 4–6 weeks.

2 Lupus pernio. This is extremely unsightly and the patient will want something done about it. The options are:

(i) Triamcinolone hexacetonide, 5 mg/ml (Ledercort) injected intradermally into the abnormal skin. This can be repeated every 4–6 weeks until a satisfactory response is obtained. It is best to err on the side of caution because if too much steroid is injected, there will be atrophy of the dermis which may be irreversible. Sometimes this works very well. If it does not consider one of the other options.

(ii) Systemic steroids. If the patient has symptomatic multi-system disease as well as lupus pernio, this will be the first line of treatment. If it is just the skin which is causing problems, it is more difficult to decide to use steroids because at least 30 mg prednisolone will be needed to improve the skin initially. Once the skin has improved, the dose of prednisolone can be reduced, but the rash is likely to recur once the dose is reduced to a reasonable maintenance dose.

(iii) Methotrexate 10–25 mg orally or intramuscularly once a week, or azathioprine tablets 2 mg/kg body weight/day or chlorambucil tablets 2–4 mg/day. The risks of treatment will have to be weighed up against the problems of having a disfiguring facial rash.

(iv) An antimalarial such as chloroquine 250 mg twice a day or hydroxychloroquine 200 mg twice daily. If these are going to be used the patient will need to be under regular scrutiny by an ophthalmologist.

(v) Etretinate 1 mg/kg body weight/day. For information about the side effects of this, *see* page 168.

None of these treatments can be guaranteed to work. It is often a matter of trial and error to try and find something which helps.

3 Papular, nodular or plaque sarcoid. Topical steroids do not help but systemic steroids work well to clear this type of sarcoid. Since the treatment may have to be given long term, the side effects may outweigh the benefits. If the rash is not on a part of the body which shows, and if it does not itch, the patient may be prepared to put up with it. If systemic steroids do not work or too big a maintenance dose is needed an alternative is methotrexate 10–25 mg intramuscularly once a week (for side effects of methotrexate and precautions to be taken when using it, *see* page 162).

SCABIES

Scabies is transmitted by prolonged physical contact (eg holding hands, lying in the same bed all night, cuddling children). Once the diagnosis has been made, it is essential to treat not only the patient but anyone else who has been in close contact with him. In practice this means all individuals living in the same house and any sexual partner(s). The rash itself does not occur for 6–8 weeks after infestation, so other members of the family must be treated whether or not they are itching. If there are children in the family, grandparents, aunts and uncles, baby-sitters, neighbours and anyone else who has been holding the children will also need treating.

The idea of treatment is to kill all stages of the life cycle of the scabies mite (eggs, larvae, nymphs and adults) at the same time. Five drugs are effective in doing this:

- 1% lindane lotion or cream (Quellada)
- 25% benzyl benzoate emulsion (Ascabiol)
- 25% monosulphiram (Tetmosol) in an alcoholic solution (it needs to be diluted with 4 parts of water before use)
- 0.5% malathion lotion (Derbac-M)
- 5% permethrin cream (Lyclear).

Lindane is the cheapest and should probably be used routinely (except in young children); it is more pleasant for the patient to use than benzyl benzoate which stings the skin (especially on the genitalia). It works by destabilizing ion exchange across nerve membranes leading to abnormal nerve impulses; in the mites this causes convulsions and death. The lotion or cream is applied to the whole body surface except the face and scalp (including the skin between the fingers and toes, the genitalia and the soles of the feet). This means that the patient will need some help to put it on, since there will be parts of his back that he cannot reach. Treatment is applied at night before the patient goes to bed and repeated once more 24 hours later. The whole family should be treated at the same time. 24 hours after the second treatment the patient can have a bath and wash the scabicide off. He should then change his underwear, pyjamas and the sheets on his bed. The clothes should be washed and ironed to kill any wandering acari, although in practice it is very unlikely that any will be left alive at this stage. There is no need to go to elaborate means to fumigate the house or bedding.

In infants it is probably better to use permethrin cream. It is applied to the whole of the skin, including the face, neck, scalp and ears, but avoiding the skin immediately around the mouth (because it could be licked off!). It is washed off 8 hours later. Do not use in patients who are allergic to chrysanthemums.

75 ml of lotion or 15 g of cream will be needed for a single application (for an adult), so you can work out how much to prescribe for the whole family.

The itching will usually stop immediately after a single application of the scabicide but may occasionally go on for up to 7 days. Any itching that is left can be treated with calamine lotion or crotamiton (Eurax) cream twice a day. Rarely the patient will be left with **scabetic nodules** (Figure 150). These are itchy papules, particularly around the axillae, which go on itching for months. They are best treated with a dilute topical steroid such as 1% hydrocortisone cream or ointment. Their presence does not mean that the infestation has not been eradicated and there is no reason to use the anti-scabies treatment again.

Reasons for treatment failure

- Wrong use of the scabicide. If the cream or lotion has been applied only where the patient is itching rather than all over (except on the face and scalp), some mites and immature forms may not have been killed and the infestation not completely eradicated.
- The patient's contacts were not treated at the same time and the patient has been re-infected.
- The diagnosis is wrong. If the patient has eczema and not scabies, anti-scabies treatment is likely to make the rash worse.

Animal scabies (sarcoptic mange)

Animal scabies due to the mite, *Sarcoptes scabei* var *canis*, is a common infestation in dogs (rare in cats). In the UK most of it originates in foxes. The creature looks identical to the human

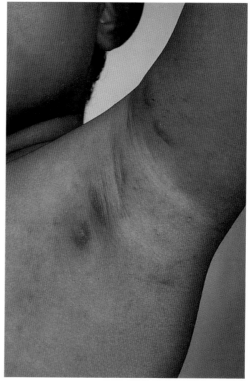

Figure 150 Scabetic nodule in an 18-month-old child.

scabies mite but is in fact host-specific and will not breed on people. The life cycle is exactly the same as in the human variety. The animal scratches, gnaws or rubs the sites of infestation causing the skin to become thickened, crusted and infected and the fur to fall out (Figure 151). It is often just localized around the ears or elbow joints and there may not be much in the way of symptoms—chronic thickening of the skin, minimal crusting or persistent mild itching.

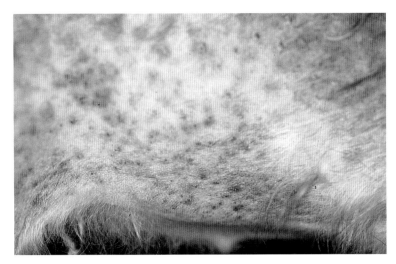

Figure 151 Sarcoptic mange in a dog. Courtesy of Dr Ian Mason.

The human in contact with such an animal will develop a rash that looks identical to human scabies but without the presence of burrows. The diagnosis is made by taking brushings from the dog (*see* page 97 for method) and identifying the scabies mite. The animal with scabies may not be the family pet but belong to a relative or friend (the owner's skin may be unaffected!).

For long standing infestations, the pet and the surrounding environment will need treating (carpets, armchairs etc). If it is a recent infestation, only the dog will need treating. The dog can be washed with 1% lindane lotion or with monosulphiram (Tetmosol) soap. Carpets should be vacuumed, soft furnishings washed and floors washed with lindane emulsion.

The patient is treated with crotamiton (Eurax) cream twice a day until the itching stops.

Norwegian scabies

Norwegian scabies is so called because it was first described in lepers in Norway in the late 19th century. It is an infestation with *Sarcoptes scabei* var *hominis* in an individual who for some reason does not scratch normally (patients with sensory loss [diabetes, leprosy, syringomyelia, hemiplegia, paraplegia], those who are mentally handicapped or who are immunosuppressed [lymphoma, leukaemia, AIDS, on systemic steroids or cytotoxic drugs]). It is the same organism that causes ordinary scabies but a different host response.

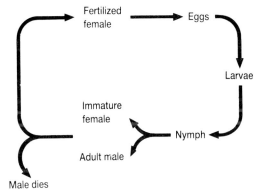

Figure 152 Life cycle of scabies mite. In normal individuals scratching removes mites mechanically and allows 2° infection which kills them. In patients with Norwegian scabies, there is no scratching and the thick hyperkeratosis allows the reproductive cycle to continue unabated, leading to enormous numbers of creatures at all stages of the life cycle.

There are thousands, or even millions of mites in the skin. Thick hyperkeratotic scale occurs on the palms and soles, in the flexures and under the nails. There may or may not be a widespread scaly rash on the rest of the body including the face and scalp. Usually the rash is misdiagnosed as eczema, (Figure 153) but if you look carefully you will see lots of burrows, particularly on the palms and soles.

Rash in those in contact with the patient with Norwegian scabies

The diagnosis usually comes to light, not because the patient with Norwegian scabies is complaining of a rash, but because those in contact with him (relatives, friends, other residents in an old people's home, hospital or residential school), or those caring for him (nurses, doctors, home helps, teachers etc) get an itchy rash. It may take weeks or months before the diagnosis is made. When there are just immature mites on the skin there may only be a few itchy papules on the forearms. Several weeks later there are enough mature mites in the skin to produce the ordinary scabies rash, including the typical burrows.

Diagnosis. Remove some of the thick scale from the patient and/or collect up scales and other skin debris from his bed and examine under a microscope; numerous eggs, larvae, nymphs and adult mites will be seen.

Treatment in an old people's home

1 Identify the patient with Norwegian scabies.
2 Identify a single room where he can be isolated.
3 Empty that room of all furniture and soft furnishings apart from a bed. Clean the room thoroughly and wash the floor and walls with 1% lindane emulsion. Make up the bed with freshly washed and ironed bedding.

4 Treat the patient with 1% lindane emulsion or cream as a single application all over (including the face and scalp).
5 After treatment put the patient into the cleaned single room.
6 The home should be closed to new residents and visitors until stages 7–10 have been carried out.
7 Explain to the staff what is happening (all staff whether or not they have had direct physical contact with the patient). Explain that the patient has Norwegian scabies and that whether or not they are itching, they will almost certainly have caught it and will need treatment. Explain that the variety they have caught is ordinary scabies and not the very infectious kind that the patient has. Explain that they are only infectious to very close contacts, ie immediate family or those who share a bed.
8 Explain what is happening to the other residents and tell them that will not be able to go out or have visitors until they have been treated. Treat them by painting 1% lindane emulsion over the whole of the skin except the face and scalp on two successive nights.
9 Removal of mites from the environment: wash and iron all bedding, curtains and other soft furnishings in the patient's bedroom and any public rooms that he has used. Wash or spray the floors, walls and other hard surfaces in all the rooms where he has been with 1% lindane emulsion.
10 All staff and their husbands, wives, boyfriends, girlfriends and children must be treated with 1% lindane emulsion or cream applied over the whole body surface from the neck to the toes on two successive nights.
11 Once **9** and **10** above have been done the home can be reopened to visitors.

If the infestation has arisen in a children's home, rather than an old people's home, the procedure is basically the same. But, since children from a single home may attend a variety of schools and be in different classes, help from the local medical officer of health will

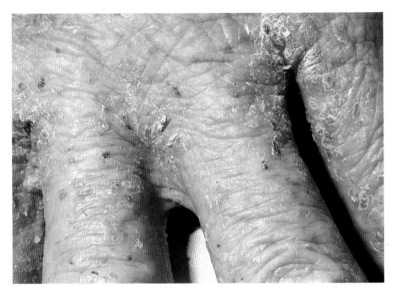

Figure 153 Norwegian scabies. Rash on back of hand looks very like eczema.

be needed to ensure that all the relevant individuals are identified and treated. As well as the children and staff in the children's home, the children, teachers and school helpers in all the classes which have children from the home in them will need treatment, as will their families.

SCARLET FEVER

Oral phenoxymethylpenicillin (penicillin V) 62.5–125 mg every 6 hours for a week depending on the child's age. The sore throat may be helped by gargling with paracetamol suspension (120 mg/5 ml) every 4 hours and then swallowing it.

SCARRING ALOPECIA

Once the hair follicles have been replaced by scar tissue the hair loss will be permanent, so prevention of further hair loss is the immediate priority. Since there are many different causes of scarring alopecia, referral to a dermatologist is required to make a diagnosis and advise on any possible treatment.

SCLEROSING LYMPHANGITIS OF THE PENIS

This condition gets better on its own so no treatment is needed other than reassuring the patient that this will occur.

SEBACEOUS GLAND HYPERPLASIA

If the patient wants it removed, it can be curetted off under a local anaesthetic. It is perfectly harmless, however, and it is quite safe to leave alone. The only problem is that it can sometimes be mistaken for a basal cell carcinoma.

SKIN TAGS

These are completely harmless and can safely be left alone. If the patient finds them very unsightly or they catch on her clothes, they can be cut off with a pair of fine sharp scissors or a scalpel, having first injected a little local anaesthetic underneath each one. Cautery of the cut surface will stop any bleeding.

Very small ones can be cauterized with a Hyfrecator, or cut off with a pair of sharp scissors without any anaesthetic. If bleeding occurs this is easily stopped by dabbing the surface with a cotton wool bud soaked in 20% aluminium chloride hexahydrate solution.

SOLAR KERATOSIS

For a single lesion or for a few lesions the simplest treatment is to freeze them with liquid nitrogen on a cotton wool swab or with a cryospray (Figure 154). The idea is to freeze just enough to produce a blister at the dermo–epidermal junction (Figure 156), not to cause necrosis of the skin. This means that you freeze it until the whole lesion goes white and there is a white rim about 2 mm around it (about 5–10 seconds). The patient should be warned that a blister may occur and that this is nothing to worry about. The solar keratosis should drop off after 7–10 days.

If the solar keratosis does not fall off after freezing, or if it is very large or has a lot of keratin on the surface, it may be better to curette it off.

If the patient has too many solar keratoses to freeze or curette off, they can be treated with topical 5% 5-fluorouracil cream. This is applied to the whole of the face (and bald scalp) twice a day for 4 weeks. For the first 2 weeks not a lot will happen. After that any solar keratoses will start to become red and sore. The treatment should be continued for a full month however sore the skin is. At the end of that time, all the solar keratoses will be red and eroded (Figure 155). The patient should be warned in advance that they will look very unsightly for the second 2 weeks of treatment. The 5-fluorouracil cream is then stopped and 1% hydrocortisone cream applied twice a day for 7–14 days until the inflammatory reaction has subsided. All the solar keratoses will have been treated

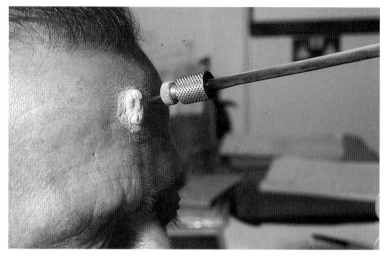

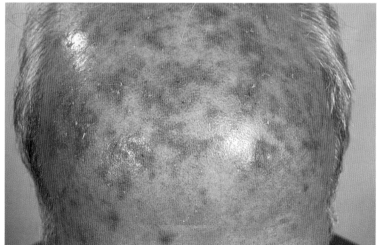

Figure 154 (*above*) Freezing a solar keratosis with liquid nitrogen using a cryospray.
Figure 155 (*below*) Multiple solar keratoses treated with 5% 5-fluorouracil cream twice a day for a month. All the affected areas of skin are now red and sore.

on only 1 day a week for 12 weeks. The solar keratoses should be gone without all the redness and soreness that occurs with conventional treatment. It may be kinder to use it this way.

SPIDER NAEVUS

The central feeding arteriole can be cauterized using the cold point tip of a cautery (or a fine looped end of an electrocautery). Rest the cautery point on the centre of the spider naevus until the whole thing blanches. Turn on the cautery until there is a tiny burn on the surface (Figure 157). It takes about 1 second. For small lesions this can be done without local anaesthetic.

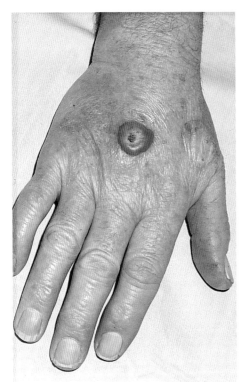

Figure 156 Two days after solar keratosis was treated with liquid nitrogen: a large haemorrhagic blister. The patient should be warned that this might happen so that he will not be anxious.

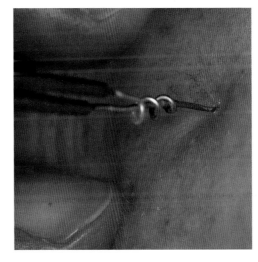

Figure 157 Spider naevus being treated with the cold point cautery. Put the tip of the cautery on the central arteriole until the whole spider naevus disappears, then heat it up.

whether or not they had been identified before treatment was begun. This is a good treatment on the face or bald scalp but it does not work on the hands or forearms.

For patients who would not be able to cope with the normal treatment with 5% 5-fluorouracil cream, it can also be used once a week which produces much less inflammation. The cream is applied to the whole of the face (and/or bald scalp) twice a day but

SQUAMOUS CELL CARCINOMA

Local excision or radiotherapy are probably equally effective. Which is used depends on which will give the best cosmetic result at the particular site involved. If radiotherapy is going to be used, a biopsy to confirm the diagnosis should be performed before treatment is begun. The local lymph nodes should be checked before embarking on any kind of local treatment but metastases are unusual, and if they do occur are a late finding.

Local excision

Surgical removal with an excision margin of 2–3 mm is all that is needed. If the tumour is too large for primary closure, a skin flap or full thickness skin graft can be applied.

Radiotherapy

Radiotherapy is suitable for tumours which are too large for excision, those which would need grafting in patients who are too frail for this to be carried out, those which would be technically difficult to remove or those which would involve amputation or major reconstructive surgery afterwards (Figure 158).

Radiotherapy treatment is fractionated in the same way as it is for basal cell carcinomas and the total dose is the same (37.5 Gy). It is usually given as 10 daily fractions of 3.75 Gy or in patients who are very frail, 10 weekly fractions of 3.75 Gy. Electrons rather than standard X-rays are very useful on the nose and ears, where they are less likely to damage cartilage. Here treatment will probably be given daily for 2–3 weeks.

How to manage the local reaction after treatment

Nearly all patients will get some local reaction on the skin after radiotherapy treatment, but they should not get any systemic upset. Depending on the technique used, erythema, scaling,

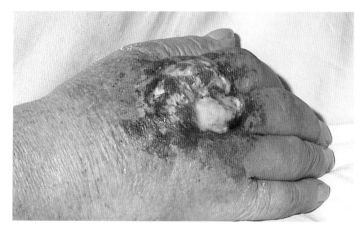

Figure 158 Squamous cell carcinoma on the back of the hand. Surgery here would involve amputation, so radiotherapy would be the treatment of first choice.

weeping and the formation of a scab will begin towards the end of treatment or shortly afterwards. It lasts for a variable time, but generally for up to 3–4 weeks.

Most patients do not need any treatment for the reaction. The area should be left open because covering it increases the risk of secondary infection. If it becomes wet, it can be bathed twice a day with bicarbonate of soda (a pinch of bicarbonate of soda in a tumbler of water), or with potassium permanganate (made up to a pale pink solution, *see* Figure 47, page 62). Some people use 1% hydrocortisone ointment topically twice a day, but most reactions settle without this.

Curettage and cautery

In some elderly patients squamous cell carcinomas are very well differentiated and slow-growing, and if they are difficult to remove surgically can be treated perfectly satisfactorily by curettage and cautery (Figure 159).

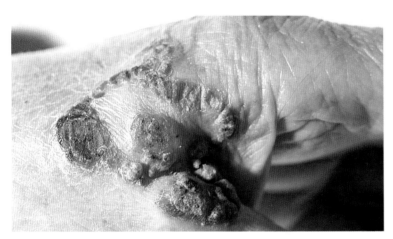

Figure 159 Large well differentiated squamous cell carcinoma treated with curettage and cautery in a 94-year-old man.

Treatment of advanced disease

Large fungating tumours should be treated by excision if at all possible (even if there is widespread disease) because it is difficult for the patient and his relatives to put up with the mess and smell of the exudate. If it is not possible to operate, the smell can be lessened by bathing the area in a weak solution of potassium permanganate (*see* Figure 47, page 62) and applying 0.75% metronidazole gel topically.

Involvement of local lymph nodes can be treated by block dissection. Widespread metastases are not treatable.

STRAWBERRY NAEVUS

The parents should be told the natural history of this lesion, that it will grow for about 12–15 months and then gradually shrink up and disappear completely, probably by the time the child is about 7. It is helpful to have a series of photographs to show the parents (and grandparents) of a naevus that has disappeared completely in order to reassure them (Figure 160).

Problems with strawberry naevi

1 Cosmetic. If the naevus is on the trunk or a limb there is not usually any cosmetic problem; if it is on the face there will be. Then the problem is whether to initiate some kind of active treatment rather than waiting for nature to take its course. The possibilities for treatment are surgical removal, injection of intralesional steroids or systemic steroids. The size of the naevus (most parents can cope with a small one providing they know that it will eventually go away), and whether or not there is a deep component to it, will determine whether active treatment is a viable proposition. Surgical removal is most successful in a naevus with a deep (cavernous) component to it (Figure 162). Injection of intralesional steroids directly into the naevus may cause it to shrink, but there is a risk of permanent atrophy if too much is injected. Systemic steroids are usually reserved for naevi that are covering the eye or interfering with feeding or breathing. Parents should be in no doubt that without treatment the naevus will disappear without leaving a scar; any kind of intervention may leave a scar.

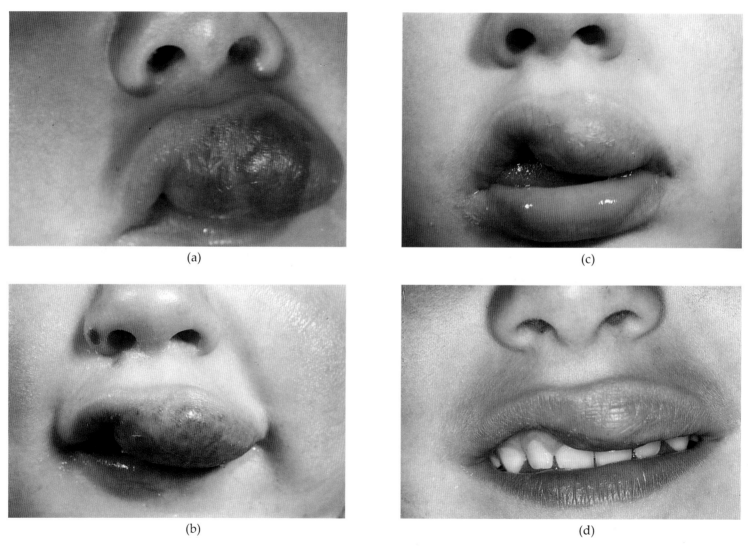

Figure 160 Enlargement and disappearance of a strawberry naevus. **(a)** Age 7 months. **(b)** Age 14 months. **(c)** Age 3 years. **(d)** Age 4 years.

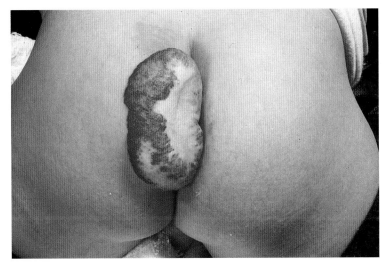

Figure 161 Large strawberry naevus on buttock causing a problem with bleeding.

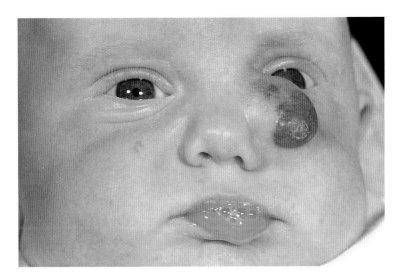

2 Bleeding. The parents should be instructed to press firmly until the bleeding stops. This will be a particular problem if the naevus is in the nappy area (Figure 161).

3 Thrombocytopenia. Extremely rarely a naevus will enlarge so rapidly that it consumes large numbers of platelets causing thrombocytopenia. Systemic steroids in the form of prednisolone 40 mg on alternate days will stop it immediately. They should be given for 1–2 weeks.

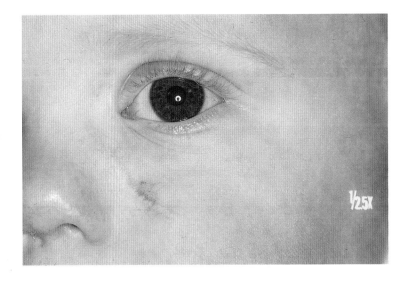

Figure 162 (a) (*above right*) Strawberry naevus with a large cavernous component: the parents were worried that it would soon obstruct the child's vision. **(b)** (*below right*) 4 months after surgical removal by a plastic surgeon: good cosmetic result.

4 Interference with the child's sight. If the naevus covers the eye, vision will not develop on that side. It is imperative to get the eye open as soon as possible and this can be done by giving oral steroids in the form of prednisolone 40 mg on alternate days until the eye is open and then gradually reducing it. Once started, steroids will need to be given until the naevus begins to regress spontaneously at about 15 months of age (the only alternative is to remove it surgically if that is practical).

5 Interference with any other vital function. Large naevi on the neck, lip or nose can interfere with breathing and eating. They should be treated in the same way as those covering the eye.

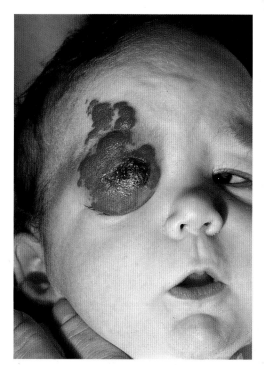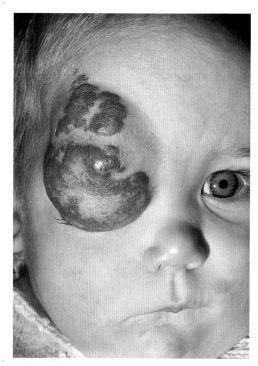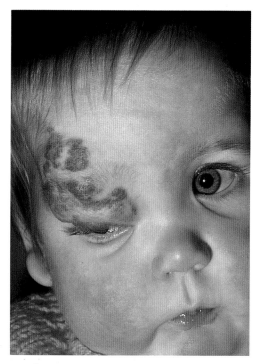

Figure 163 (a) Strawberry naevus of right upper eyelid obstructing the child's sight (female aged 2 months).

(b) Enlarged at age 6 months.

(c) After 1 month's treatment with oral prednisolone the naevus has shrunk and the eye is now open. It was in fact too late to prevent her losing her sight in that eye.

STRIAE

Nothing can be done about striae although the colour tends to fade with time. The parents of teenage children who develop them on the thighs and lumbosacral area need reassurance that this is a normal thing to happen at this age.

SUBUNGUAL EXOSTOSIS

If it is causing pain by lifting up the nail or pressing on the shoe, the abnormal bone can be sawn off, preferably by an orthopaedic surgeon. An X-ray of the digit will show the exostosis (Figure 164).

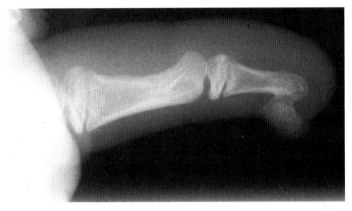

Figure 164   X-ray showing subungual exostosis.

SUBUNGUAL HAEMATOMA

If the patient attends the surgery immediately it has occurred, open out a paper clip and heat it to red heat in a flame (Bunsen burner, spirit burner or gas ring). Apply the red-hot end to the nail over the centre of the haematoma; blood will spurt out, giving immediate relief of pain. If the patient comes to see you once the blood has clotted, there is nothing that can be done apart from recommending analgesics for the pain.

SUBUNGUAL MALIGNANT MELANOMA

Amputation of the digit usually at the metacarpophalangeal joint is required. The prognosis should be excellent because amputation will give a good clearance margin; in practice it may not be good because the diagnosis is often not thought of until late in the course of the disease.

SUBUNGUAL SQUAMOUS CELL CARCINOMA

Surgical excision is needed, probably amputation of the terminal phalanx.

SUNBURN

Topical calamine lotion will produce symptomatic relief if the skin is just red and oedematous. If it is very severe a single application of a very potent topical steroid, 0.05% clobetasone propionate (Dermovate) ointment, will reduce the redness and bring almost instant relief. On no account should it be used more than once. If there are blisters, soaking in a bath containing a few crystals of

potassium permanganate (so that the water is a pale pink colour—
see Figure 47, page 62) will help to dry them up.

For the future, the patient should be advised to use a high
protective factor sunscreen (see page 140) so that burning is avoided
and the risk of developing a malignant melanoma is reduced.

SYCOSIS BARBAE

Before treatment is begun the diagnosis should be confirmed by
taking swabs for bacteriology culture from one of the pustules and
from the anterior nares. Start with flucloxacillin 250 mg four times
a day orally for 7 days (or erythromycin 250 mg four times a day if
the patient is allergic to penicillin). If *Staphylococcus aureus* is grown
from the nose as well as the skin, neomycin ointment or mupirocin
ointment should be applied to the anterior nares four times a day
for 2 weeks.

In some patients it will keep recurring. If so, treatment may need
to be continued long term for a minimum of 6 months and
sometimes for several years. If that is the case, long-term low-
dose antibiotics using erythromycin, 250 mg twice a day, or co-
trimoxazole 480–960 mg twice a day, work better than flucloxacillin.

Pseudo-sycosis barbae

There are only two ways of dealing with this condition.
1   The patient can be encouraged to grow a beard. As the hairs get
longer, they uncurl themselves and free themselves from the skin,
so curing the condition.

2   If the patient does not want to grow a beard, he will need to
persuade someone to take a fine needle or pin and uncurl each of
the hairs individually for him (very time-consuming and tedious,
but some wives and girlfriends may be prepared to do it).

SYPHILIS

All patients with syphilis should be seen in a department of genitourinary medicine so that other sexually transmitted diseases can
also be screened for and the patient's sexual contacts traced.

Primary syphilis

Procaine penicillin 1.2 g by intramuscular injection daily for 10
days. If the patient is allergic to penicillin, the treatment is
erythromycin 250 mg every 4 hours (six times a day) for 21 days.

Secondary syphilis

Procaine penicillin 1.2 g by intramuscular injection daily for
14 days. If the patient is allergic to penicillin, use erythromycin
250 mg every 4 hours (six times a day) for 21 days.

Tertiary syphilis

Procaine penicillin 1.2 g by intramuscular injection daily for
14 days. In order to prevent a Herxheimer reaction from
developing, the patient is also given prednisolone 15 mg daily,
starting the day before the penicillin is started and continuing until
1 day after the penicillin is stopped. If the patient is allergic to
penicillin, erythromycin is given instead at a dose of 250 mg six
times a day for 21 days.

SYRINGOMA

These small sweat-gland tumours are perfectly harmless and the patient can be reassured. Usually they are best left alone. If the patient is very keen to have them removed, and if they are <2 mm in diameter, they can be cauterized under local anaesthetic; if they are >2 mm in diameter they can be removed by curettage and cautery.

SYSTEMIC LUPUS ERYTHEMATOSUS

The diagnosis should first be confirmed by finding a high titre of anti-nuclear antibody and antibodies to double-stranded DNA. What is then done depends on the severity of the illness and which organs are affected. To ensure optimal treatment, referral to a specialist with some expertise in this condition is necessary; this may be a general physician, a rheumatologist or a dermatologist.

If there is involvement of the kidneys (proteinuria or renal failure), the pleura (pleuritic chest pain), the pericardium (pericarditis), the central nervous system (epilepsy or psychosis), or a haemolytic anaemia, treatment will be started with high doses of systemic steroids in the form of oral prednisolone, 60 mg daily or intravenous methyl prednisolone 1 g once a week until the disease is controlled. The idea is then to reduce the steroids to the lowest possible maintenance dose to control the disease. Sometimes azathioprine or cyclophosphamide will be added so that the dose of steroids can be reduced.

If the skin is involved, the patient should be advised to avoid excessive exposure to the sun and to use a high protective factor sun screen—Factor 15 or above (*see* page 141). A very potent topical steroid, 0.05% clobetasone propionate (Dermovate) ointment or cream applied twice a day, can be very helpful in actually getting rid of the rash.

If the joints are the main problem, non-steroidal anti-inflammatory drugs will be the treatment of choice.

If it is only the skin and joints involved, one of the antimalarials may be the treatment of choice. The options are:
● hydroxychloroquine 200 mg twice a day
● chloroquine phosphate 250 mg daily
● mepacrine 200 mg twice a day.

If either hydroxychloroquine or chloroquine is used, the eyes will need checking by an ophthalmologist every 6 months to check the visual acuity and visual fields to make sure that no damage is done to the retina. Both drugs may also stain the nails a greyish–blue colour and chloroquine can bleach the hair, eyelashes and eyebrows especially in patients with red hair. If mepacrine is used the patient's skin will go yellow (*see* Figure 32, page 47) and there may be vomiting and diarrhoea.

Patients who develop recurrent thromboses (deep vein thromboses, cerebral thromboses or placental thromboses leading to repeated abortions) form a small sub-group who have cardiolipin antibodies. They will need long-term anticoagulants.

During pregnancy there is no increased risk of an exacerbation of the disease (other than the normal pattern of exacerbations and remissions of the disease) although there is often a post-partum flare. If cardiolipin antibodies are present there is an increased risk of spontaneous abortion.

There is a self-help group for patients and their families:

LUPUS UK
Queens Court
9–17 Eastern Road
Romford
Essex, RM1 3NG
Tel: 0708 731 251
      0708 731 252

TATTOOS

Problems with tattoos

1 It is illegal in the UK to tattoo someone under the age of 18, but this is largely ignored.

2 There is a risk of infection (hepatitis and HIV) because tattooing needles are not disposable.

3 Individuals may later regret that they had the tattoo(s) done because they simply do not like it, because they had a name tattooed on their skin which is now an embarrassment, because they cannot get the job they would like or because they were drunk at the time and were not fully aware of what was happening.

4 The patient becomes allergic to one of the pigments in the tattoo causing a red lump to develop (Figure 165).

Removal of tattoos

If tattoos are going to be removed it is important for the patient to understand that it is not possible to remove them so that there will be no mark left; there will always be a scar left behind. How big the scar will be depends on the size of the original tattoo and whether it was done by a professional tattooist (the pigment will all be at the

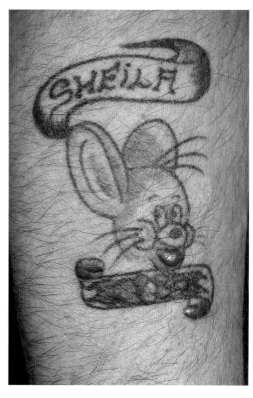

Figure 165 Allergic reaction to the mercury in a tattoo (the red part).

same depth in the dermis) or an amateur (the pigment will be scattered throughout the dermis).

Possible methods of removal are:

1 **Surgical excision** with or without a skin graft.

2 **Excision using a carbon dioxide laser** rather than a scalpel.

3 **Salabrasion.** This involves applying common salt to the skin over the tattoo and rubbing it firmly into the skin with a gauze swab soaked in normal saline. Rubbing should continue until the whole of the epidermis has been removed (it is extremely tedious to do

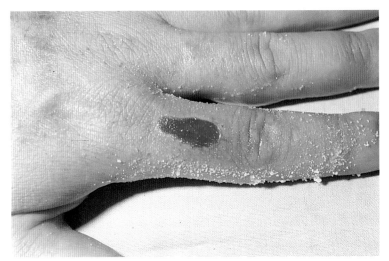

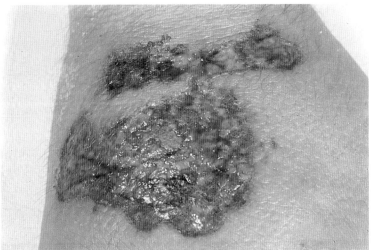

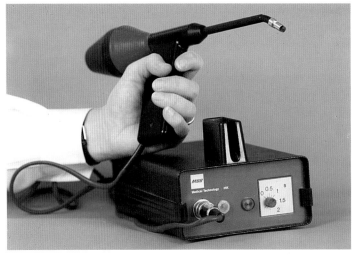

Figure 168 Infra-red coagulator. Infra-red heat is transmitted through the skin to cause a localized burn.

Figure 166 (*above*) Salabrasion—rub the skin over the tattoo with common salt until a uniform red bleeding surface is produced.

Figure 167 (*below*) Four days after salabrasion to a larger tattoo: much of the pigment has been extruded through the open wound.

and the operator's wrist will ache long before the desired result occurs) and a uniform red base appears (Figure 166). The open wound is then covered with a dry dressing which is left in place for 10 days. When the dressing is removed, much of the pigment will have come out of the skin onto the dressing. If it has not all been removed, the process can be repeated one or more times. Salabrasion works quite well for small tattoos, particularly those done by amateur tattooists.

4 Dermabrasion. The epidermis and upper part of the dermis are removed with sandpaper on a high speed rotating drill. The effect is very similar to that produced by salabrasion. The disadvantage is that skin is sprayed everywhere; the operator needs to protect himself from the risk of infection with hepatitis or HIV infection.

5 Infra-red coagulation. This is a good method for removing small tattoos on the hands and forearms—letters, words or a small picture up to about 4 cm in diameter (tattoos on the upper arms and trunk do not do well, tending to end up with hypertrophic or keloid scars). The tattoo is anaesthetized with a local anaesthetic (2% lignocaine mixed with adrenaline) and an ice pack applied for 5–10 minutes. A test area (about a quarter of the tattoo) is treated by firing 0.75 second pulses of infra-red heat at it from the coagulator using a special sapphire tip. The ice pack is then re-applied for a further 5–10 minutes. The patient is instructed to apply 0.05% clobetasone propionate (Dermovate) ointment twice a day for 2 weeks but not to cover the area with a dressing. The wound should be kept clean and dry and away from oils. The ice before and after the procedure and the topical steroid afterwards are meant to cut down the inflammatory reaction and so reduce the possibility of scarring. The wound will take 6–10 weeks to heal. If the patient and the operator are happy with the result, the rest of the tattoo can then be treated in stages using the same time setting. If the pigment was not totally removed, then a longer pulse time will be needed (1–1.25 seconds). Small tattoos will usually need two treatments; larger ones may require up to six treatments over a period of several months. If tattoos are present on both hands, only one hand should be done at a time so that the patient is not incapacitated during the 6–10 weeks it takes the wound to heal (*see* Figures 168 and 169).

6 **Other lasers.** For blue/black tattoos, the ruby laser gives the best combination of pigment removal and lack of residual scarring (but there are very few centres in the UK where these lasers are available).

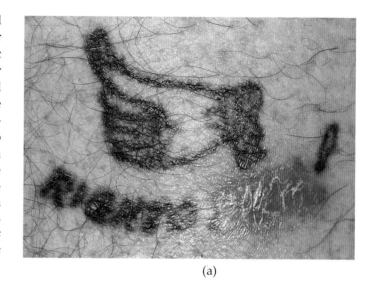

(a)

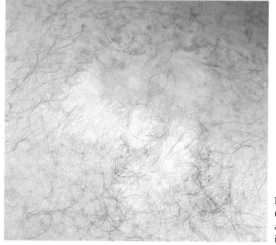

(b)

Figure 169 Tattoo **(a)** before, and **(b)** after treatment with infra-red coagulator.

TINEA (RINGWORM)

Treatment of the superficial fungal infections of the skin (called tinea or ringworm) depends on the fact that these fungi (dermatophytes) only invade the stratum corneum (keratin). In most instances it will be better to treat with a topical agent which will get directly into the keratin than with a systemic agent. The exception to this will be if it is not possible to get a topical drug to the place where it is required, eg:

- nails (difficult to get topical drugs into nail keratin)
- scalp (cannot get a topical agent into the hair below the scalp surface).

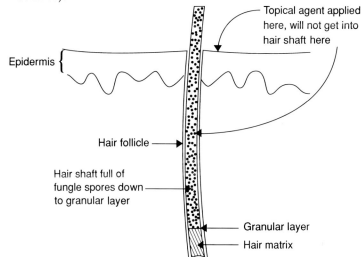

Figure 170.

Topical treatments will either remove the keratin on which the fungi live or harm or kill the fungus itself (Figure 172). Systemic treatments all aim to inactivate or kill the fungus. The major groups of drugs available to treat tinea are shown in Table 17.

Table 17 Main drugs available for treating tinea

TOPICAL		SYSTEMIC	
Group of drugs	**Individual drugs**	**Group of drugs**	**Individual drugs**
Keratolytic	Whitfield's ointment	Antibiotic*	Griseofulvin
Thiocarbamates*	Tolnaftate	Triazoles*	Fluconazole Itraconazole
Imidazoles*	Bifonazole Clotrimazole Econazole Fenticonazole Isoconazole Ketaconazole Miconazole Oxyconazole Sulconazole Terconazole Tioconazole***	Imidazoles*	Ketaconazole
Morpholines*	Amorolfine		
Allylamines**	Terbinafine	Allylamines**	Terbinafine

*Fungistatic.   **Fungicidal.   ***Only used on nails, not on the skin.

How do these drugs work?

1   Keratolytic agents. These remove the keratin on which the fungi live. They are just as effective as the various fungistatic agents and a lot cheaper. The one most commonly used is Whitfield's ointment which contains:

6% benzoic acid   } in emulsifying ointment
3% salicylic acid   }

2 Griseofulvin. Griseofulvin is an antibiotic produced by certain species of *Penicillium*. It has a fungistatic effect by:

- making the cell wall abnormally soft or abnormally rigid causing distortion of the hyphae (curling effect)
- impairing cell division (arrest of mitosis in metaphase)
- inhibiting formation of microtubules. It has to be taken up actively into the cell in order to be active on the tubules (some fungi are not able to transport much of the drug into the cells and these will be resistant to treatment).

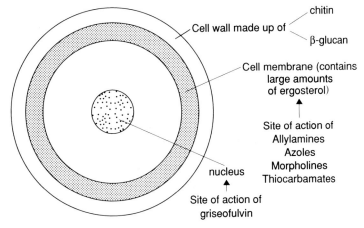

Figure 171 Griseofulvin.

chitin

Cell wall made up of

β-glucan

Cell membrane (contains large amounts of ergosterol)

Site of action of
Allylamines
Azoles
Morpholines
Thiocarbamates

nucleus

Site of action of
griseofulvin

Figure 172 Site of action of antifungal drugs.

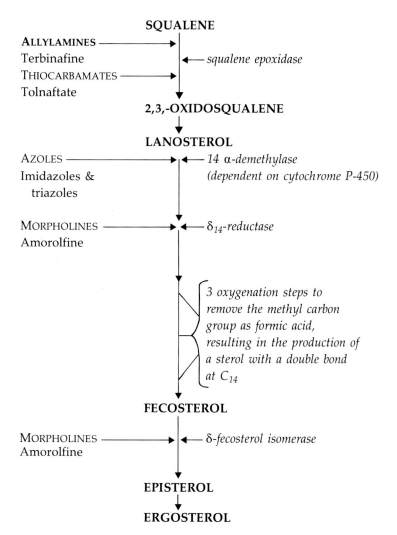

SQUALENE

ALLYLAMINES ⟶
Terbinafine ⟵ *squalene epoxidase*
THIOCARBAMATES ⟶
Tolnaftate

2,3,-OXIDOSQUALENE

LANOSTEROL

AZOLES ⟶ ⟵ *14 α-demethylase*
Imidazoles & *(dependent on cytochrome P-450)*
   triazoles

MORPHOLINES ⟶ ⟵ δ_{14}-*reductase*
Amorolfine

3 oxygenation steps to remove the methyl carbon group as formic acid, resulting in the production of a sterol with a double bond at C_{14}

FECOSTEROL

MORPHOLINES ⟶ ⟵ δ-*fecosterol isomerase*
Amorolfine

EPISTEROL

ERGOSTEROL

Figure 173 Sterol synthesis in fungal cell membrane and site of action of anti-fungal drugs.

3 Azoles. Azoles (imidazoles and triazoles) bind to cytochrome P-450 and therefore interfere with the enzymatic steps involved in the complicated synthesis of ergosterol (Figure 173). These enzymes are not specific to fungi, being present also in the host cells. The drugs which are the safest and most effective are those which react strongly with fungal cytochrome P-450 and have only weak or no activity against the human enzyme. When less ergosterol is produced, there is a concomitant increase in the C_{14}-methylated sterols, causing impairment of the barrier function of the fungal cell membrane, leaking out of low molecular weight components from the cell and cell death.

4 Allylamines. Terbinafine is a broad spectrum anti-fungal drug which is fungicidal. It acts by inhibition of squalene epoxidase in the fungal cell membrane (Figure 173). This causes depletion of ergosterol and accumulation of squalene which leads to cell death. Squalene epoxidase in the fungal cell membrane is 30,000 times more sensitive to the action of terbinafine than the enzyme in human cells, making the drug safe to use in humans (it does not suppress the adrenal axis or affect the gonadal hormones).

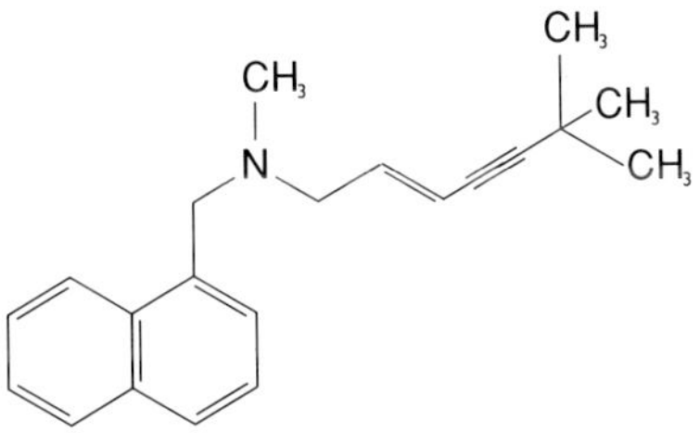

Figure 174 Terbinafine.

Imidazoles

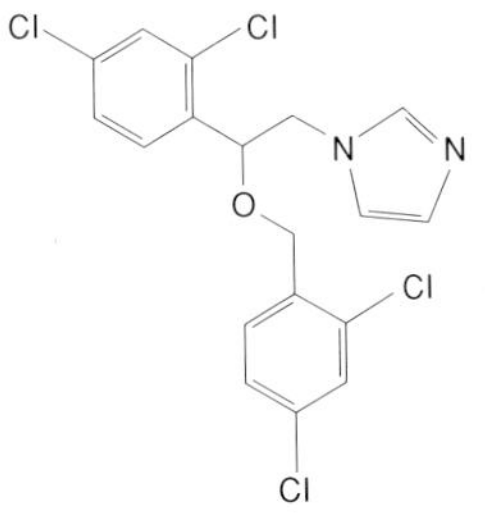

Figure 175 Miconazole. 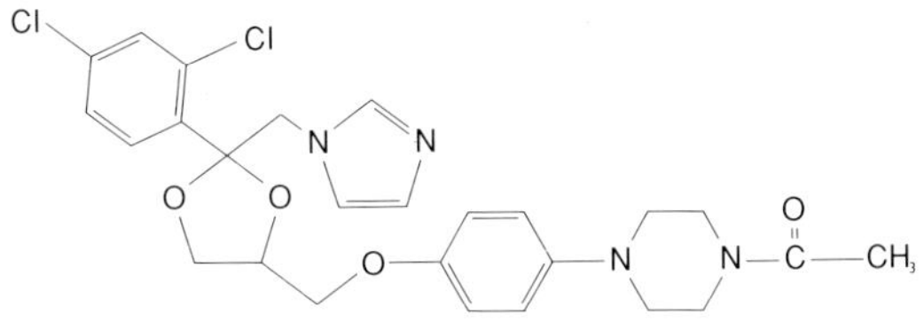   **Figure 176** Ketaconazole.

Triazoles

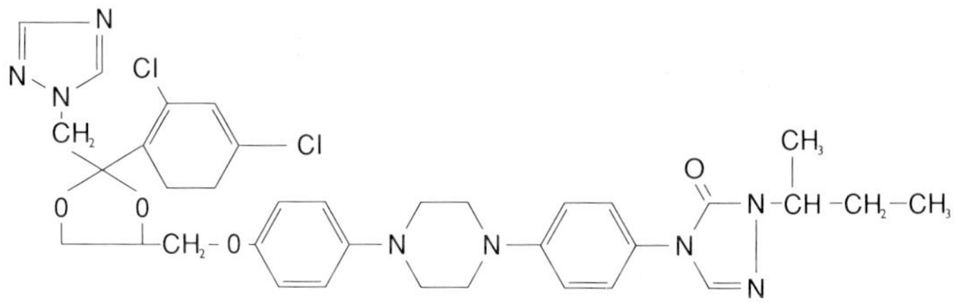

Figure 177 Itraconazole.

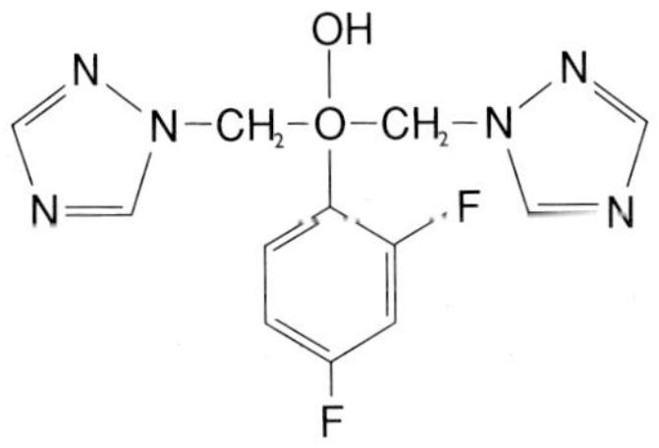

Figure 178 Fluconazole.

5 Thiocarbamates. Tolnaftate, like the allylamines, interferes with fungal sterol biosynthesis at an early stage (*see* Figure 173), leading to deficiency of ergosterol and accumulation of squalene in the cell membrane. This has a drastic effect on fungal cell growth and may cause cell death.

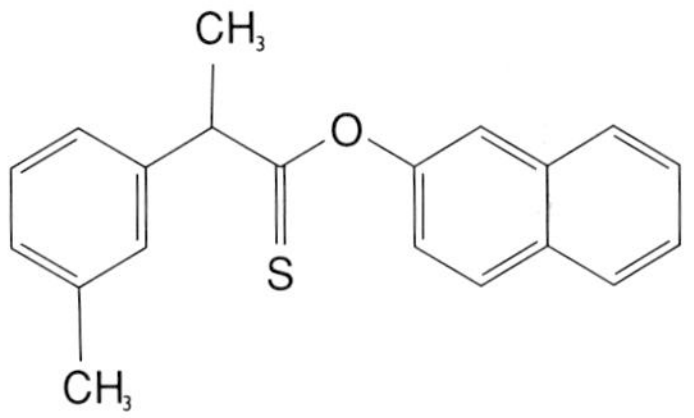

Figure 179 Tolnaftate.

6 Morpholines. Amorolfine has a broad spectrum of anti-fungal activity by interfering with both δ_{14}-reductase and δ-fecosterol isomerase in the fungal sterol pathway (*see* Figure 173). This causes a drastic fall in the amount of ergosterol that is produced and instability of the fungal cell membrane.

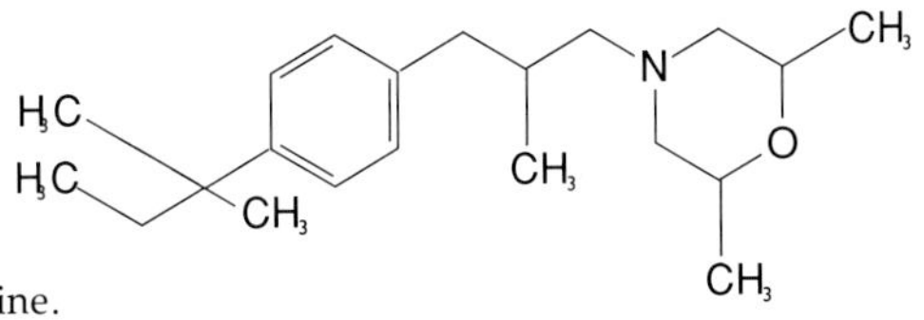

Figure 180 Amorolfine.

7 Ideal anti-fungal drugs. Theoretically the best type of anti-fungal drug would inhibit cell wall synthesis. This would be highly specific because only fungal cells build their wall of chitin and β-glucan. So far none of the drugs which have been developed do this.

Deciding what to do

Before deciding on which treatment to use, it is important to confirm the diagnosis by direct microscopy and/or culture of skin scales from the edge of the rash, from broken-off hairs or from nail clippings. Treatment can be begun before the results are available providing the investigation has been sent off. Most public health laboratories provide a mycology culture service; scales, hairs or nail clippings can be sent in small opaque envelopes (obtainable from HMSO, code no. 27–67). Tinea is usually classified according to the site of the body involved. The fungi come from humans or animals and belong mainly to three genera of fungi imperfecti: *Microsporum*, *Trichophyton* and *Epidermophyton*.

Table 18 Most common organisms causing tinea in the UK

Site	Organism
Scalp	*Microsporum canis* (animal—cat or dog) *Microsporum audouinii* (human)
Beard	*Trichophyton verrucosum* (animal–cow) *Trichophyton mentagrophytes* var *granulare* (animal—cow or horse)
Face and body	*Microsporum canis* (animal—cat or dog) *Trichophyton rubrum* (human) *Trichophyton erinacei* (animal—hedgehog)
Feet, hands and groin	*Trichophyton rubrum* (human) *Trichophyton interdigitale* (human) *Epidermophyton floccosum* (human)
Nails	*Trichophyton rubrum* (human) *Trichophyton interdigitale* (human) *Epidermophyton floccosum* (human) *Hendersonula toruloidea* (saprophytic mould) *Scopulariopsis brevicalis* (saprophytic mould)

Table 19 Treatment of tinea

Site of infection	Treatment	Comments, side effects and precautions
Scalp (tinea capitis)	Griseofulvin 10 mg/kg body weight/day as a single dose, with food, daily for 6 weeks. Approximate dosage would be 125 mg/day for a child under 1 year; 187 mg/day for a child aged 1–5; 250–375 mg/day for a child aged 6–12 years. It can be given as tablets (125 mg each) or as a suspension (125 mg/5ml). Alternatively it can be given as a single large dose (5 g) in ice-cream. There is no need for topical treatment too. If it is due to *Microsporum canis*, the affected pet (kitten or puppy) must be treated with griseofulvin too. The pet should be taken to the local vet to get the treatment. If the child has a kerion, the crusts should be softened with arachis oil and then removed. It is worth taking a bacteriology swab from under the crust or from a pustule; if *Staphylococcus aureus* is grown, treat with flucloxacillin as well.	Griseofulvin is long acting and is best absorbed with food. It is therefore given as a single daily dose taken at the end of a meal. Ringworm on the scalp only occurs in children in the UK, so it should not be diagnosed after puberty. If it is due to *Microsporum audouinii*, the child must be kept off school until better because it is very infectious. If it is due to *Microsporum canis*, the child can go to school because it is only infectious from animal to child.
Beard (tinea barbae)	Griseofulvin 1 g daily as a single oral dose with food for 4–6 weeks.	Side effects are unusual. Headaches, irritability and nausea are the most common. Occasionally causes photosensitivity or a drug-induced LE. If the patient is taking warfarin, the INR will need to be checked more frequently because the anticoagulant effect of warfarin is diminished when taken in conjunction with griseofulvin. Do not use in patients with acute intermittent or variegate porphyria because it can induce acute attacks.
Face (tinea corporis)	An imidazole cream applied twice a day for 2 weeks. All the imidazoles work equally well, so use whichever is the cheapest. The choice is between clotrimazole, econazole, ketaconazole, miconazole and sulconazole. Whitfield's ointment can also be used, twice a day for 2 weeks.	There are no problems with these unless the patient is allergic to the base or the preservative in the base. They are more expensive than Whitfield's ointment. It may be a little harsh on the face and make it sore.
Trunk and limbs (tinea corporis)	Whitfield's ointment applied twice a day for 2 weeks is cheap and effective. An imidazole cream applied twice a day for 2 weeks is an alternative. Choose whichever is the cheapest from clotrimazole, econazole, ketaconazole, miconazole and sulconazole*.	Greasy, but otherwise no problems with its use. Expensive to use if there are large areas of the body involved. There are no other problems unless the patient is allergic to the base or the preservative in the base.

*If the infection is very extensive or the lesions are slow to clear, consider using griseofulvin 500 mg–1g orally/day for 4 weeks in adults or 10 mg/kg body weight/day in children.

(Table continues over)

Table 19 Treatment of tinea (continued)

Site of infection	Treatment	Comments, side effects and precautions
Feet (tinea pedis)	**For the common pattern of tinea between the toes or for blisters on the instep,** Whitfield's ointment can be applied twice a day for 3–4 weeks or until it is better, or An imidazole cream can be rubbed in twice a day until the itching and rash have gone and for a further 2 weeks (use clotrimazole, econazole, ketaconazole, miconazole or sulconazole, whichever is the cheapest), or 1% terbinafine cream applied once a day for 2 weeks, or Tolnaftate cream applied twice a day until it is better and for another 2 weeks after that. For recurrent infections which do not seem to get better with topical agents, oral griseofulvin 500 mg–1g/day as a single dose with food for 6 weeks, or terbinafine 250 mg/day as a single dose for 2 weeks should clear it. **For the white scaling on the soles which occurs with some infections with** *Trichophyton rubrum*, terbinafine 250 mg orally once a day for 2 weeks should clear it up.	Effective and cheap. It is not suitable for the white scaling on the soles which occurs with some infections due to *Trichophyton rubrum*. A lot more expensive than Whitfield's ointment. Not usually any problems with using it unless the patient has become allergic to one of the ingredients (unusual). More expensive than Whitfield's ointment, but only needs applying once a day. A lot more expensive than Whitfield's ointment. Not as effective as the imidazoles. Always check the toenails too. If they are involved terbinafine is likely to be more effective in clearing it, but treatment should be for 3 months instead of 2 weeks (see under nails). Always check the toenails too. If they are involved terbinafine should be for 3 months instead of 2 weeks. Do not use during pregnancy or lactation.
Hands (tinea manuum)	Whitfield's ointment applied twice a day for 2–3 weeks, or an imidazole cream (clotrimazole, econazole, ketaconazole, miconazole or sulconazole) applied twice a day for 2 weeks.	Check the feet and nails too; if they are involved they will also need treating. Whitfield's ointment is a lot cheaper than the imidazoles, but it might be too greasy on the hands.
Groin (tinea cruris)	An imidazole cream (clotrimazole, econazole, ketaconazole, miconazole or sulconazole, whichever is the cheapest) should be applied to the affected area of the groin and/or buttock and to the toewebs twice a day for 2–3 weeks or until it is clear.	Whitfield's ointment is not recommended for the groin because it tends to sting. Almost all groin infections have been acquired from the patient's own feet, so they must always be examined and treated at the same time if they are involved.
Tinea incognito (any site—due to application of topical steroids)	Stop topical steroids. Apply Whitfield's ointment or one of the imidazole creams (clotrimazole, econazole, ketaconazole, miconazole or sulconazole, whichever is the cheapest) twice a day until it is clear.	It will not get better unless the topical steroids are stopped. Otherwise the treatment is the same as for ordinary tinea at the same site.

(Table continues opposite)

Table 19 Treatment of tinea (continued)

Site of infection	Treatment	Comments, side-effects and precautions
Toenails (tinea unguium)	If there are only one or two nails involved, paint with 5% amorolfine nail lacquer once or twice a week. Amorolfine also works for toenail infections with the saprophytic moulds, *Hendersonula toruloidea* and *Scopulariopsis brevicalis*. An alternative is 28% tioconazole solution painted onto the nails daily (it has only an approximately 22% success rate).	The surface of the nail is first filed down with a nail file, then degreased with a presoaked alcohol swab, then the lacquer applied with a spatula (all included with the lacquer from the manufacturers) and allowed to dry (it takes about 3 minutes). May occasionally cause a burning sensation in the nail immediately after applying.
	If there are more than two or three nails involved, it is better to use terbinafine 250 mg daily as a single dose by mouth for 3 months.	Expensive but effective. It has replaced oral griseofulvin as the treatment of choice because it is much more effective and does not need to be given for such long periods of time. Side effects: mild gastrointestinal upsets, anorexia, nausea, diarrhoea, abdominal fullness. Do not use during pregnancy or lactation.
	Alternatives to terbinafine are: Itraconazole 100 mg orally/day for 7 months.	Side effects include nausea, abdominal pain, dyspepsia and headache.
	Griseofulvin 1 g daily as a single dose with food for 18 months or more, until the nails have grown out normally (may be as long as 5 years). Removal of the affected toenail(s) plus griseofulvin 1 g/day until the nails have regrown. 28% tioconazole solution applied topically to the nails each day together with oral griseofulvin, 1 g/day until the nails are back to normal.	Side effects are unusual—headaches, irritability and nausea are the most common. Occasionally causes photosensitivity or a drug induced LE. If the patient is taking warfarin, the INR will need to be checked more frequently because the anticoagulant effect of warfarin will be diminished. Do not use in patients with acute intermittent or variegate porphyria because it can induce acute attacks. Do not use oral ketaconazole because of the risk of liver disease (1 in 50,000 risk).
Fingernails (tinea unguium)	Oral terbinafine 250 mg daily for 3 months.	Always examine the toenails too; it is extremely rare for the fingernails to be involved on their own. The treatment will deal with both, but it is important to ensure that treatment is continued until the toenails are also clear.

TOXIC EPIDERMAL NECROLYSIS

The term toxic epidermal necrolysis is used for two quite distinct diseases which happen to have the same clinical appearance.

Staphylococcal scalded skin syndrome

This disease is due to a toxin produced by phage type 71 *Staphylococcus aureus* which causes necrosis in the upper half of the epidermis resulting in it shearing off (Figure 181a). It occurs almost entirely in infants and young children under the age of 5. The source of the staphylococcus is often an older child in the family with impetigo, infected eczema or scabies.

Treatment is with oral flucloxacillin elixir, 62.5–125 mg every 6 hours for 7 days (62.5 mg for children under the age of 2; 125 mg for children over the age of 2). The pain will stop almost immediately, causing the child to stop screaming. Erythromycin is an alternative for children who are allergic to penicillin. Topical antibiotics should not be used because applying them will cause the skin to be rubbed off. Other children in the family with impetigo should have that treated at the same time—*see* page 94.

Toxic epidermal necrolysis

The problem here is necrosis of the lower half of the epidermis giving a histological picture very like that of erythema multiforme (Figure 181b). It occurs in adults rather than children and is much more serious than staphylococcal scalded skin syndrome, having a considerable mortality. It is not due to infection; it can be due to drugs (particularly sulphonamides, NSAIDs and barbiturates), carcinomas or lymphomas, or there may be no obvious cause.

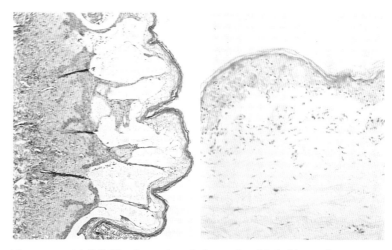

Figure 181 **(a)** (*left*) Histology of staphylococcal scalded skin syndrome. **(b)** (*right*) Histology of toxic epidermal necrolysis.

If it is due to a drug, obviously the drug must be stopped. If it is due to a neoplasm that will also need treating, but the immediate need is the care of large areas of skin loss. The effects are very similar to those of extensive burning of the skin (although it is not due to a burn) and the management is the same. Patients need to be admitted urgently to hospital, preferably to a burns unit because the main problems are:
- fluid and electrolyte loss through the eroded skin
- infection of the skin ± septicaemia
- problems with nursing patients whose skin comes away on the hands of those touching them.

TOXIC ERYTHEMA

There is no difference clinically between a toxic erythema due to a drug and one due to infection, be it viral or bacterial. There is also no test that can be applied which will distinguish between the various causes. If a drug is suspected, it should be stopped. If the drug is essential for some life-threatening condition, it is better to continue with the drug and for the patient to put up with the rash. Often this rash looks awful but is completely asymptomatic; if so, no treatment is needed. If it is itchy, calamine lotion may be soothing.

TRACTION ALOPECIA

You must explain to the patient that the hair loss is due to constant pulling of the hair either because the hair has been pulled back into a pony tail or the patient has used hot combs. They must stop these things and leave the hair loose. If they do so, the hair will usually regrow normally. Remember that hair grows at about 1 cm/month so the regrowth will not be instantaneous.

TRICHOEPITHELIOMAS (EPITHELIOMA ADENOIDES CYSTICUM)

This rather uncommon condition with multiple translucent papules on the face is inherited as an autosomal dominant trait. The number of papules can be very variable from half a dozen to a hundred or more. If the lesions are small and not too unsightly they are best left alone, but if they are larger or very numerous they are best treated by curettage and cautery under a general anaesthetic (Figure 183).

TRICHOMYCOSIS AXILLARIS

If the patient is complaining of it, the axillary hair should be shaved off and the patient told to wash the axillae with soap and water at least once a day.

Figure 182 Trichomycosis axillaris: concretions of propionibacteria along the axillary hairs.

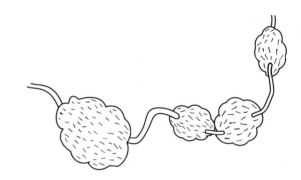

TRICHORRHEXIS NODOSA

In most instances nothing can be done for this. In a few patients it is due to a congenital abnormality of copper metabolism (Menke's syndrome), or arginosuccinicaciduria. It is worth sending the patient to see a dermatologist with an interest in hair problems in case there is a treatable cause. This goes for the other structural abnormalities of the hair shaft too.

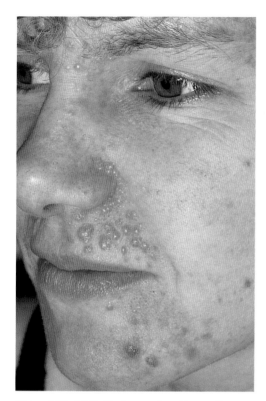

Figure 183 **(a)** Epithelioma adenoides cysticum pre-operatively.

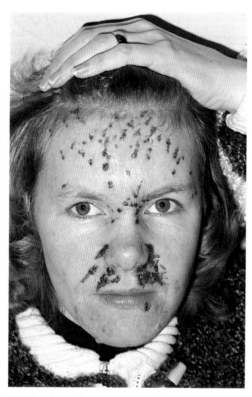

(b) Five days after curettage and cautery.

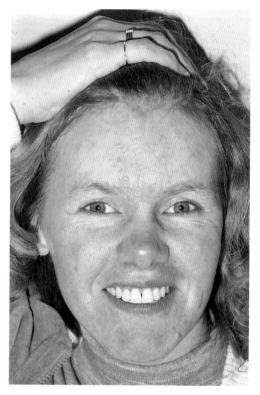

(c) Four months after curettage and cautery.

TRICHOSTASIS SPINULOSA

Most elderly patients who have this on the nose have not noticed it and do not want any treatment for it (Figure 184). If they do complain about it, a 0.025% solution of tretinoin (Retin-A) applied at night for 6–8 weeks will give a fairly dramatic improvement. It can be kept clear by using it twice a week.

A similar condition on the trunk (Figure 185), with multiple hairs present in each follicle can present with itching. The best treatment here is removal of the hairs by waxing or sugaring. The patient can get this done by a beautician.

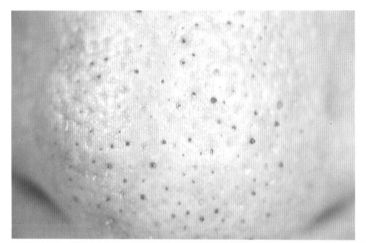

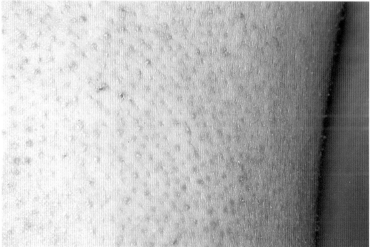

Figure 184 (*above*) Trichostasis spinulosa on the nose. This is due to a failure of shedding of vellous hairs in the hair follicles of the nose in the elderly.

Figure 185 (*below*) Trichostasis spinulosa on the trunk causes an itchy follicular rash.

TRICHOTILLOMANIA

In a young child there is usually an obvious reason why he or she has started pulling the hair out—one of the parents has left home or died, or some other major area of stress has occurred. Often the parent(s) have not noticed the child twisting the hairs around one of the fingers or pulling it out, but will do so once you tell them what is happening. It is best for them not to make a big thing of it, particularly not to punish the child for it, and to give them as much love and security as they can during the difficult time. Once the time of trauma is over, the child will nearly always stop pulling the hair out and the hair will regrow normally.

In teenagers who pull out their hair the cause is often less obvious, but most will need psychiatric help to resolve the problem. If there is any doubt as to the diagnosis (it can sometimes be confused with alopecia areata), a biopsy of the scalp will help. In trichotillomania there are usually lots of catagen hairs visible histologically; there is no other condition where this is so. It can be important to be sure of the diagnosis if long-term psychiatric help is contemplated.

TUBERCULOSIS OF THE SKIN

The treatment of tuberculosis of the skin is the same as tuberculosis elsewhere with 9 months of chemotherapy; the first 2 months with triple therapy (three drugs):

1 Isoniazid 300 mg/day as a single dose.

2 Rifampicin 450–600 mg/day dependent on body weight (10 mg/kg/day up to a maximum dose of 600 mg/day) as a single dose before breakfast.

3 Pyrazinamide 20 mg/kg body weight/day in 3–4 divided doses, or ethambutol 15 mg/kg body weight/day as a single dose.

For the next 7 months two drugs are used, generally isoniazid and rifampicin in the same doses as above. Treatment is best supervised by a chest physician who is familiar with the drugs being used and all the side effects which can occur.

Side effects of anti-tuberculous chemotherapy

Isoniazid

(1) Common problems in patients who are slow acetylators, helped by pyridoxine:

- acne
- peripheral neuropathy
- mental disturbances
- pellagra-like rash on face, neck and hands.

(2) Allergic reactions:

- agranulocytosis
- hepatitis.

Rifampicin

- red urine
- hepatitis
- thrombocytopenia
- psychosis
- interferes with the effectiveness of the pill
- decreases effectiveness of systemic steroids.

Pyrazinamide

- hepatitis
- hyperuricaemia.

Ethionamide

- nausea and vomiting
- metallic taste in the mouth.

Rarely:

- peripheral neuropathy
- optic neuritis causing blurred vision and red/green colour blindness

- hepatitis
- hypothyroidism
- hypoglycaemia
- gynaecomastia.

TUBEROSE SCLEROSIS

Nothing can be done, or needs to be done, for the white patches on the skin. The angiofibromas on the face (adenoma sebaceum) can be very unsightly and many patients would like to be offered treatment for them (Figure 186). Curettage and cautery under a general anaesthetic works quite well. It is no good trying to remove them under a local anaesthetic because you have to pull hard with the curette to get them off and that is much easier with the patient asleep (the procedure is identical to that used for trichoepitheliomas, *see* Figure 183, page 218). For very small lesions cautery alone can be used. If it is available locally, the argon laser also works quite well and that can also be used on the similar lesions around the nails.

TYLOSIS

The patient should be referred to a dermatologist so that the diagnosis can be confirmed since there are many different types of palmar and plantar hyperkeratosis. 5% salicylic acid ointment applied at night may keep the hyperkeratosis down. Regular chiropody will almost certainly be needed. If it is very severe it may be necessary to use etretinate by mouth. This is only available in hospitals. The dosage is the same as in psoriasis, *see* page 168.

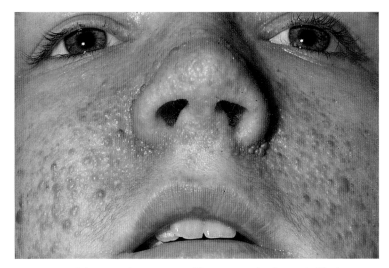

Figure 186 Tuberose sclerosis: angiofibromas on the face suitable for treatment with curettage and cautery (*see* Figure 183).

ULCERS ON THE LEGS AND FEET

Venous ulcers

Venous ulceration is due to loss of the valves in the deep or perforating veins of the leg. If a single valve is lost from a perforating vein, tying off that vein surgically will put the whole system back to normal. However such a scenario is rare because usually many of the valves have disappeared. It is theoretically possible to replace the valves in the deep veins with valves from veins in the arms, but this is not usually a practical option (although there are vascular centres where it is being done).

What can be done is to:

- reduce tissue pressure due to oedema
- reduce venous hypertension
- clean the ulcer so that it can heal
- apply a dressing that will promote rather than hinder healing.

Reduction of tissue pressure and reduction of venous hypertension can both be achieved by the patient wearing graduated compression bandages from the toes to the knees and keeping the calf muscles moving by taking exercise. Compression counteracts the high pressure in the superficial veins, allowing the calf muscle pump to aid the return of blood to the heart (Figure 187), and it counteracts the increased tissue pressure due to oedema, particularly around the ankle where the ratio of bone to soft tissue is higher. If a bandage is applied at a constant tension, it will provide graduated compression if it is shaped to fit accurately at both the ankle and the calf. Graduated compression means that the greatest pressure is exerted at the ankle, progressively decreasing to a lower pressure at the calf.

1 Bandages. There are different ways of applying graduated compression to the leg (*see* Table 20). Bandaging is by far the most popular method, but it is a skill that requires a lot of practice to do well. The simple spiral method using a 10 cm wide bandage is the easiest to use (Figure 188). Bandaging is started on the medial side of the foot at the base of the toes and secured by making one or two turns. The patient may find it easier to sew the end of the bandage into a loop which can be hooked over the foot to start the bandaging, so that it is secure and will not come undone. The bandage is then wrapped around the foot, including the heel, and up the leg to the knee, each turn overlapping the previous one by half (Figure 188). At the knee any surplus bandage is cut off, otherwise there will be a tourniquet effect.

There is a choice of bandages available. They should have enough elasticity to provide compression of the superficial veins and they should not lose their elasticity after washing or use. Blue line, Red line or Molastic forte bandages are best. Crêpe bandages

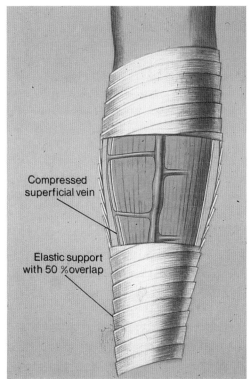

Compressed
superficial vein

Elastic support
with 50 % overlap

Figure 187 Elasticated bandages are applied so that the superficial veins are compressed.

Table 20 Ways of applying graduated compression to the leg

Support	Technique
1 Bandages	1. Simple spiral method using 10 cm width bandages, eg Molastic forte, Blue line, Red line (**not** crêpe bandage) 2. Paste bandages covered with a an elastic cohesive bandage
2 Secondary compression	Foam pad over the ulcer or to pad out an awkward shape
3 Circular support bandage	Shaped Tubigrip, preferably two layers
4 Graduated support stockings	Class II (18–24 mmHg pressure), or Class III (25–35 mmHg pressure)
5 Intermittent sequential compression pump	Flowtron boot (Figure 88, page 112) to reduce oedema

or elastocrêpe bandages do not provide adequate or sustained compression and have no place in the treatment of venous ulcers (Table 21).

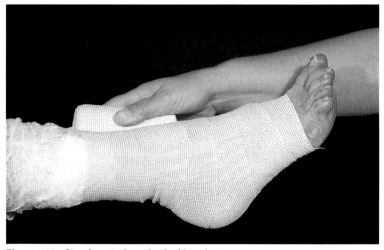

Figure 188 Simple spiral method of bandaging.

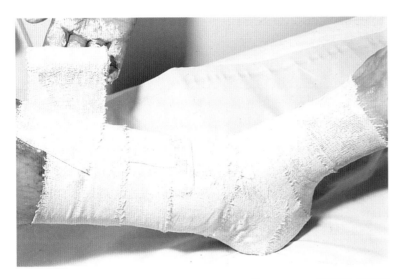

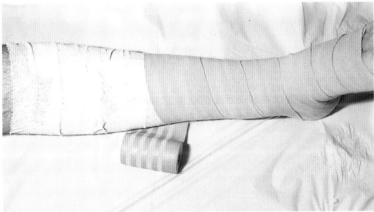

Figure 189 (*above*) Applying Calaband (paste bandage). The bandage is folded back on itself after each turn, to prevent it cutting into the skin if oedema occurs.

Figure 190 (*below*) Applying Lestreflex, an elasticated sticky bandage over a paste bandage: this sticks to itself and can be left in place for 7–14 days.

Table 21 Bandage and compression stocking classification (Pressure = mmHg at ankle)

Bandage	British stocking	European stocking
Class IIIa (14–17 mm Hg) J-Plus, K-crêpe	Class I (14–17 mmHg)	Class I (18–21 mmHg)
Class IIIb (18–24 mm Hg) Molastic light, Veinopress, Granuflex adhesive compression bandage	Class II (18–24 mmHg)	Class II (25–32 mmHg)
Class IIIc (25–35 mm Hg) Setopress, Tensopress, Molastic medium	Class III (25–35 mmHg)	Class III (36–46 mmHg)
Class IIId (up to 60 mmHg) Blue line, Red line, Molastic forte		Class IV (over 59 mmHg)

Bandages should be applied first thing in the morning before the patient gets out of bed, and worn all day, only being taken off when she goes back to bed at night. Some bandages are easier to apply than others. For example, Blue line bandages are difficult to apply, particularly around the heel, and once applied they have a tendency to fall down. A Red line bandage looks similar, gives the same amount of compression but is easier to apply and has less tendency to fall down.

If the patient is not able to apply her own bandages and has no one at home who is able to do them for her, paste bandages which can be applied by the district nurse and left on for a week at a time are an alternative. The paste bandages have no value in themselves for the treatment of venous ulcers, being non-stretchy, but they enable a sticky elasticated bandage (giving graduated compression)

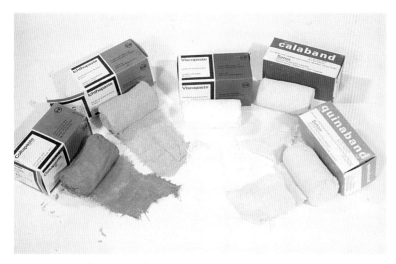

Figure 191 Different kinds of paste bandages.

it should be cosmetically acceptable to the patient and enable her to wear ordinary shoes on top.

Table 22 Types of paste bandages

Constituents of bandages	Name of bandage	Allergens they contain
Zinc paste and ichthammol	Ichthopaste Icthaband	Parabens Parabens
Zinc paste and calamine and chloroquinol	Calaband Quinaband	None None
Zinc paste and tar	Coltapaste Tarband	Lanolin and parabens Lanolin and parabens
Zinc oxide	Viscopaste PB7 Zincaband	Parabens Parabens

to be applied over the top (Figures 189 and 190). When applying the paste bandage, it should be cut off after each turn, or the bandage folded back on itself, so that there is some room for the skin to stretch without the bandage cutting into the skin (Figure 189). When first applied, these bandages are very comfortable for the patient, but they tend to dry out after about 48 hours. To keep them moist, so that they will stay supple and not cut into the patient's skin, they should be moistened each day by soaking a flannel in tepid water, wringing it out, and then putting it over the bandage to allow the moisture to soak through.

The main disadvantage of the paste bandages is that they nearly all contain parabens as a preservative to which the patient can become allergic after a period of time (Table 22). Shaped Tubigrip can be applied over the paste and elasticated bandages to give better graduated compression. Whatever type of bandage is used

2 Secondary compression. Silicone or foam padding applied over the ulcer itself will increase the amount of compression. Chiropody foam is useful for applying over bony prominences to prevent injury from pressure bandages.

3 Circular support bandages. Circular support bandaging is a useful way of gradually building up compression levels, for patients who do not think they can tolerate compression bandages. Initially just one layer is applied, but this is increased to two when the patient can manage it. The leg circumference should be measured over dressings at both the ankle and the calf to ensure that the correct size is prescribed. Two layers of shaped Tubigrip provide graduated compression. The straight variety should not be used because it does not provide graduated compression. A single

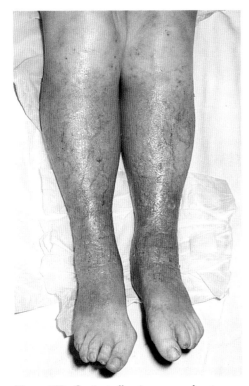

Figure 192 Contact allergic eczema due to parabens in paste bandage. Note the sharp cut off of the rash at the toes and knees.

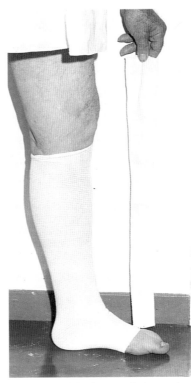

Figure 193 Wearing single layer of tapered Tubigrip.

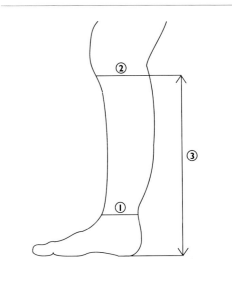

① Circumference of ankle above malleoli

② Circumference of leg 2cm below bend of knee

③ Length from heel to 2cm below bend of knee

Figure 194 Measurements required for fitting shaped Tubigrip or graduated compression stockings.

layer of shaped Tubigrip over other bandages is a useful addition to provide increased pressure and to prevent slipping of the bandage. The life-span of shaped Tubigrip is limited because of the need to wash them; they will need replacing every 3–4 weeks.

Table 23 Sizes of below knee tapered Tubigrip

Size	Leg circumference 2 cm below bend of knee
Small B/C	32–36 cm
Medium C/D	35–39 cm
Large D/E	38–42 cm

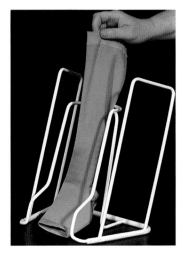 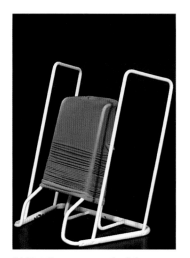 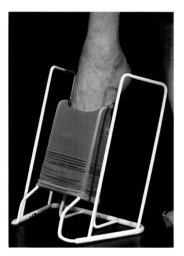 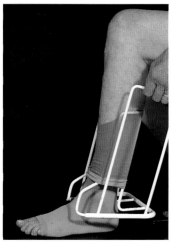

Figure 195 Using the Medi stocking valet. **(a)** Put the stocking in the half circle with the toe pointing forward.

(b) Put the upper end of the inside of the stocking over the top of the half circle and stroke it down until the heel appears at the top.

(c) Put the foot into the stocking and push the foot down to the floor.

(d) Take hold of the stocking valet and pull it firmly up over the leg to the knee. This gadget can be used with the patient either sitting or standing, whichever is easiest.

4 Graduated compression stockings. These are classified according to the amount of compression produced (Table 21, page 223):
Class I Light support for early varicose veins and prevention of varicosities during pregnancy.
Class II Medium support in severe varicose veins, mild oedema and healed venous ulcers.
Class III Strong support for marked oedema and venous ulceration. Do not use in patients with arterial insufficiency.

A correctly fitted below knee elastic support stocking will give sustained compression levels adequate to cause healing of a venous ulcer. Their advantages are that they do not rely on good bandaging technique, generally they are more cosmetically acceptable than most of the bandages and they only need replacing every 6 months. The disadvantages are that they are not suitable for an ulcer with a lot of exudate and they require quite a lot of strength to pull them on. For patients who cannot bend down to pull them on there is a stocking valet available* (Figure 195). When an ulcer is healed the patient will need to wear a Class II or Class III compression stocking for the rest of her life.

---

*From Medi UK Ltd, Hereford, HR4 0EL. Tel: 0432 351 682.

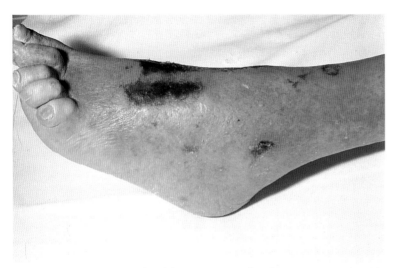

Figure 196 Ischaemia produced by compression bandaging in a patient with arterial disease.

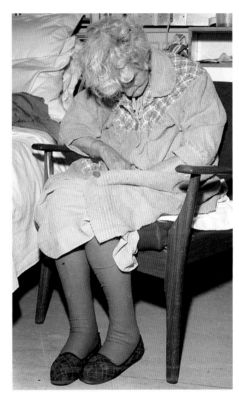

Figure 197 Patients with venous disease should not be allowed to sit like this at home or in hospital. If sitting, the feet should be elevated on a stool and the ankles flexed several times every half hour.

Hazards of compression

If the patient has arterial disease as well as a venous problem, compression bandaging can impede the blood supply further, causing ischaemia. If the leg is grossly oedematous, compression bandaging can cut into the leg. The oedema should first be controlled with diuretics, with an intermittent or sequential compression pump or by putting the patient to bed and raising the foot of the bed by about 6 inches.

5 Intermittent sequential compression pump. The Flowtron boot can be used by the patient for 1–2 hours/day to reduce the swelling of the leg. This is most useful in patients with gross oedema in whom a period of bed rest is not practical (*see* Figure 88, page 112).

Other ways of reducing tissue pressure and venous hypertension

Venous hypertension can be reduced by lifting the leg so that it is level with the heart, ie going to bed. This works well but is an inappropriate treatment for most patients because it is severely disruptive to their lives, has a considerable morbidity (DVTs, pressure sores, loss of mobility in the elderly and depression associated with bed rest and elevation of the leg) and is an expensive use of hospital beds. It can be used as a last resort when

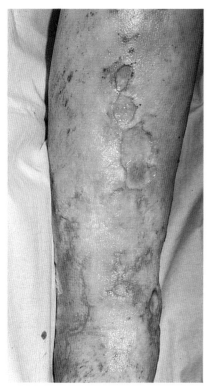

Figure 198 Cellulitis is easily recognized clinically. The leg is red, hot and swollen due to infection with a group A beta haemolytic streptococcus.

long as the patient is wearing adequate elastic compression. When the patient is sitting the feet should be put up on a stool and again the ankle kept moving by wiggling the toes up and down to keep the muscle pump working.

Cleaning the ulcer and dressings

The large numbers of dressings which are available show that the ideal dressing is yet to be found. It is a mistake to think that the choice of dressing will have a major influence on the rate of healing of an ulcer. What matters is whether or not the patient is wearing graduated compression bandages or stockings.

Cleaning the ulcer

Sterility is not a prerequisite for healing an ulcer. Colonization with moderate numbers of pathogenic bacteria does not delay healing, unless the organisms are group A beta haemolytic streptococci. You will know if they are present without doing a bacteriology culture by the fact that the patient has cellulitis (Figure 198). With this one exception, the use of systemic antibiotics does not speed up the rate of healing. Likewise there is no point in using topical antibiotics on a venous ulcer; the only likely outcome of doing so will be that the patient develops a contact allergic eczema. Cleaning the ulcer with normal saline before applying a clean non-adhesive dressing is usually all that is required. Alternative cleaning agents are shown in Table 24.

The presence of slough (Figure 200), the viscid yellow layer of fibrin, pus and dead tissue, will delay healing because of the presence of proteolytic enzymes within it, so it should be removed. Black necrotic tissue should be removed by surgical debridement. This does not necessarily mean sending the patient to hospital but simply cutting it off with a pair of sharp scissors or a scalpel. Superficial slough will be removed by cleaning with normal saline or one of the other cleaning agents, but thicker slough will need the help of a debriding agent (Figures 201 and 202).

an ulcer just will not heal with graduated compression bandaging which has been expertly applied. For all patients it is helpful to raise the foot of their bed by about 6 inches by putting the end of the bed up on blocks so that at night the legs are raised above the level of the heart. Sleeping in a chair with the legs hanging down should be forbidden (Figure 197).

Long periods of standing still should be discouraged. If patients are standing they must be using their calf muscles by walking or at least flexing the toes as they stand. Exercise is to be encouraged as

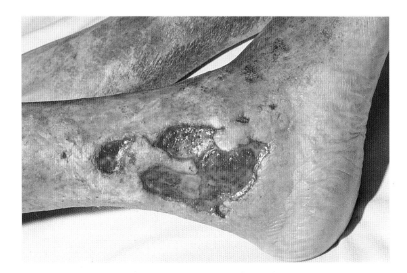

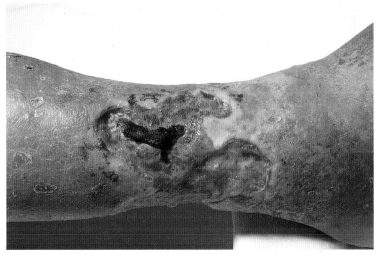

Figure 199 (*above*) Ulcer without slough. Needs only to be cleaned with normal saline before application of a non-adhesive dressing.

Figure 200 (*below*) Ulcer containing slough. The black area in the centre can be removed with a pair of sharp sissors. The yellow areas will be removed with a chemical debriding agent.

Table 24 Types of cleaning agents

Cleaning agents	When to use
Normal saline (0.9% sodium chloride solution)	For cleaning most ulcers
0.05% aqueous chlorhexidine	For cleaning dirty ulcers containing slough
Potassium permanganate solution diluted to a pale pink colour (Figure 47 page 62)	For soaking off dressings and for soaking the leg in if eczema is present
Acetic acid (5%)	If the ulcer is green and smelly due to pseudomonas
Hypochlorites, eg 0.3% sodium hypochlorite solution	Probably no indication for these today
Hydrogen peroxide (3% or 6%)	Probably no indication because it is rapidly broken down by the enzyme *catalase*; therefore very limited antibacterial action

Debriding agents and how they are used

1 Enzymes—Varidase

This comes in a Topical Combi-Pack containing:

1 vial of Varidase—dry sterile powder containing

- streptokinase 100,000 units
- streptodornase 25,000 units

1 vial of diluent (20 ml sterile normal saline)

1 transfer needle

It must be stored in a fridge at a temperature between 2–8°C. Once it has been mixed it must be used within 24 hours. Streptokinase activates fibrinolysis and streptodornase liquefies pus. It can be used in one of two ways.

(i)   The diluent is mixed with the powder. A piece of gauze is cut to the size of the ulcer; it is then soaked in the liquid and

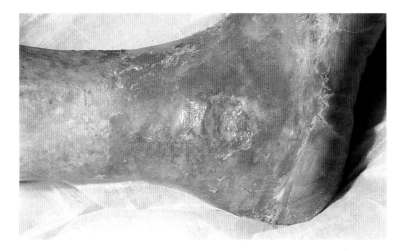

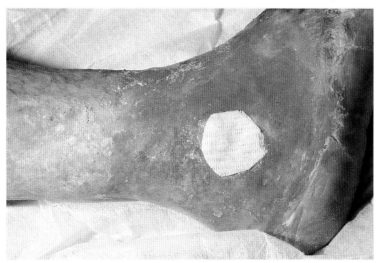

Figure 201 (*above*) Use of Varidase: ulcer before treatment.

Figure 202 (*below*) Same patient as Figure 201. Ulcer with Varidase applied. Note the dressing is cut to the exact size of the ulcer.

applied to the ulcer (Figure 202). A polythene dressing is applied on top (Melolin or a polythene bag or glove) to stop the ulcer drying out. On top of this is put the ordinary dressing consisting of:

- dry dressing
- 9″ × 9″ pad
- cotton bandage
- graduated compression bandage.

(ii) Add 5 ml of sterile water (rather than the supplied diluent) to the sterile Varidase powder. Put 15 ml KY jelly (lubricating jelly) into a small galley pot. Mix the two together with a spatula and apply to the ulcer. This combination is useful for deep ulcers. Again cover with polythene, a dry dressing, a 9″ × 9″ pad, a cotton bandage and a graduated compression bandage. The dressing is changed once a day until all the slough is removed when a simple non-adhesive dressing is used instead.

2 Capillary and osmotic absorbents. These debride slough by their physical properties. There are three substances which work in this way:

(i) Debrisan. Debrisan consists of small spherical beads of dextranomer (dextran cross linked with epichlorohydrin). It works by being able to absorb up to four times its own weight of fluid, including dissolved and suspended material of molecular weight up to 5000. It comes in two forms as single use sachets (4 g) or as 6 × 4 cm pads.

Using the sachets. Clean the ulcer with normal saline, pour the beads straight onto the ulcer and cover with Jelonet immediately so that none of the beads fall out of the hole. On top of that apply a dry dressing, a 9″ × 9″ pad and a graduated compression bandage. They can be changed daily or every 2 days depending on how much exudate is being produced; the more the exudate, the more frequently it will need changing. Before putting new beads onto the ulcer the old ones must be removed by thoroughly cleaning out the wound with normal saline on a cotton wool swab. It is important to do this because otherwise, if the ulcer is full of beads, it will look as if it is nearly healed when it is not. Also be careful not to let the beads fall on the floor or people will slip over on them.

Using the pads. These look a bit like tea bags! They contain a paste consisting of 90% dextranomer beads and 10% polyethylene glycol and water in a textile bag. The pads are applied directly over the ulcer. They are easier to use than the beads because there is no cleaning out needed before or after the dressing and there is no risk of the beads falling out of the ulcer or onto the floor.

(ii) Iodosorb (cadexomer iodine = 2-hydroxy-trimethylene cross linked (1-4)-α-D-glucan carboxymethyl ether containing 0.9% iodine). This comes as a single use sachet (3 g) containing a powder of microbeads, or as an ointment (10 g). Use in exactly the same way as Debrisan for the powder; the ointment is squirted onto the ulcer to fill it completely. When it is applied it looks brown; when the dressing is changed the brown colour will have disappeared because the iodine will have gone into the serous exudate. Do not use in patients who are allergic to iodine.

(iii) Sugar paste. If you can get this made up locally it is a cheap, comfortable and easy to use preparation. The paste is applied to the ulcer cavity so that it fills it; cover with Jelonet, a dry dressing, a 9″ × 9″ pad and a graduated compression bandage. When you come to change the dressing, the sugar paste will have dissolved, so it is just a case of refilling the cavity with some more of the paste.

Formula for sugar paste	
Caster sugar	400 g
Icing sugar	600 g
Glycerine BP	480 ml
Hydrogen peroxide solution (30% BP)	7.5 ml

3 **Hydrocolloids.** These are both debriding agents and a dressing at the same time. They consist of a hydrocolloid matrix backed with a waterproof polyurethane foam. When applied to an ulcer, the hydrocolloid interacts with the ulcer exudate to form a soft moist gel which provides an acid environment causing self-digestion of any necrotic material. It is also said to aid the formation of granulation tissue. They allow colonization of the ulcer with both aerobic and non-aerobic organisms which produces an unpleasant smell but does not otherwise seem to matter. Several hydrocolloid dressings are currently available; these include:

- Granuflex
- Comfeel
- Tegasorb

The hydrocolloid dressing is applied to the ulcer. It is meant to overlap by ¼″ all around, but in practice it needs to overlap by quite a bit more than this or it will not hold in the exudate which is produced. The dressings stick onto the skin so do not need anything else on top other than a 9″ × 9″ pad and a graduated compression bandage. The dressing is changed as soon as it begins to leak (approximately once or twice a week). There is a tendency for the exudate, when it accumulates, to force its way out of the dressing and run down the patient's leg particularly when she is

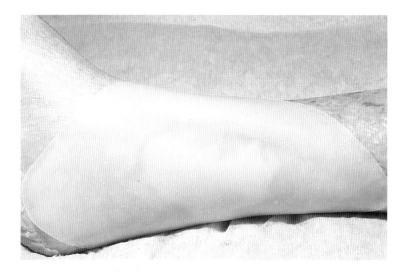

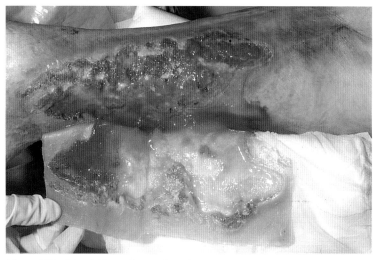

Figure 203 (*above*) Granuflex on leg ulcer.
Figure 204 (*below*) Taking off Granuflex dressing: lots of exudate and smell.

walking about. It smells and makes the skin sore, so it is best to change the dressing as soon as this begins to happen. When the dressing is changed, there will be a lot of exudate (Figure 204) and an unpleasant smell. It is cleaned off with normal saline, the skin around the ulcer is dried and a fresh dressing applied. These dressings are most suitable for large mucky ulcers which are fairly superficial. They are not suitable for patients with any associated arterial insufficiency.

4 Acids. Aserbine is the one most frequently used; it contains malic acid, benzoic acid and salicylic acid. It comes as a cream and as a solution:

Aserbine cream	**Aserbine solution**
Propylene glycol 1.7% v/w	Propylene glycol 40% v/v
Malic acid 0.36% w/w	Malic acid 2.25% w/v
Benzoic acid 0.024% w/w	Benzoic acid 0.15% w/v
Salicylic acid 0.006% w/w	Salicylic acid 0.0375% w/v

Clean the ulcer with Aserbine solution, fill the ulcer with the cream and cover with Jelonet, a dry dressing and a graduated compression bandage. The dressing will need changing every day. Some patients are allergic to propylene glycol, in which case Aserbine is not a suitable debriding agent.

5 Hypochlorites. Eusol (Edinburgh University Solution Of Lime) has for years been the standard debriding agent for leg ulcers, but it has gone out of favour because of experimental evidence that it is toxic to fibroblasts, endothelial cells and white blood cells in culture. It is however a good debriding agent, possibly because of the damage it causes to the superficial layer of granulation tissue which loosens any slough. It should only be used until an ulcer is clean; if used after that it is likely to delay healing.

A 25 ml sachet of sodium hypochlorite solution (Sterets Chlorosol) containing 0.3% available chlorine is mixed with an equal volume of liquid paraffin (the liquid paraffin will stop the dressing sticking to the ulcer). A piece of gauze is cut to the same size and shape as the ulcer, soaked in the mixture and applied to the ulcer so that it does not overlap onto normal skin (Figure 202). If there is any surrounding eczema it is wise to apply a topical steroid ointment around (but not on) the ulcer before putting the gauze containing the hypochlorite solution on the ulcer itself. The dressing is covered with Jelonet, a dry dressing, a 9″ × 9″ pad and a graduated compression bandage. The dressing is changed daily or on alternate days, depending on how much slough there is. The hypochlorite must be stored at a temperature below 25°C and out of the light.

6 Hydrogen peroxide. 1.5% hydrogen peroxide stabilized as a cream (Hioxyl) is used as a last resort because it stings a lot and patients do not like it.

7 Maggots! Both patients and doctors are usually horrified to see an ulcer crawling with maggots, but maggots are actually extremely efficient debriding agents, feeding on the necrotic debris.

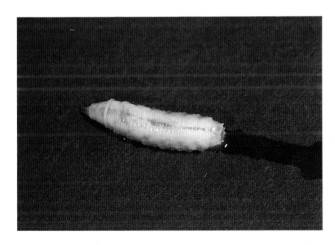

Figure 205 Maggot found on an ulcer.

Dressings

People all seem to have their favourite dressings, but which one is used will not have any influence on how quickly an ulcer heals. One that is comfortable for the patient and keeps the ulcer moist while it heals is what is required.

Table 25 Types of dressing and when to use them

Type of dressing	When to use it
1 Simple non-adherent dressing	Clean ulcer or on top of debriding agents
2 Hydrocolloid	Superficial but dirty ulcer with moderate amount of exudate
3 Alginate (seaweed based dressing)	Ulcer with a lot of exudate; only apply to wet surfaces
4 Silastic foam	Deep cavities
5 Activated charcoal dressing	Very smelly ulcer

1 Simple non-adherent dressings

(i) Paraffin gauze dressing (Jelonet). A cotton fabric impregnated with white soft paraffin. This is suitable for applying over an ulcer which does not have a lot of exudate, to keep it moist, or over one of the debriding agents. Do not use if the skin around the ulcer is soggy.

(ii) Melolin. A sterile cotton and acrylic fibre pad with a polyester film on one side. Applied with the shiny film side down on the ulcer. Useful for clean, lightly exuding ulcers, particularly if the skin around the ulcer is wet.

(iii) N-A Dressing. A sterile knitted acrylic coated viscose dressing can be used as an alternative to Melolin if the patient finds Melolin uncomfortable.

(iv) Lyofoam. A sterile polyurethane foam with an inner hydrophilic (absorbent) layer and an outer hydrophobic (non-absorbent and protective) layer. This is useful for a mildly exuding ulcer when you want the dressing to be left in place for maybe a week at a time but you want the exudate to be absorbed. It can also be used over one of the other dressings as a pressure pad.

(v) Hydrogels (Geliperm, Scherisorb and Vigilon). These all contain a starch polymer matrix which swells to absorb moisture although the dressing itself does not increase in size. They are transparent so have the advantage that you can see through them to the ulcer underneath to see what is happening. They are used on lightly exuding ulcers and can be left in place for a week at a time.

2 Hydrocolloid dressings (Granuflex, Comfeel, Tegasorb). These dressings are most suitable for large mucky ulcers which are fairly superficial (*see* also page 231). The hydrocolloid dressing is applied to the ulcer, overlapping onto normal skin by about ½″ all around and sticking to it. The dressing must be changed as soon as it begins to leak—usually once or twice a week. The exudate, when it accumulates, has a tendency to force its way out of the dressing and run down the patient's leg. Since it smells and makes the skin sore, it is best to change the dressing as soon as this begins to happen. Every time the dressing is changed, there will be a lot of exudate (Figure 204) and an unpleasant smell. It will need to be cleaned off with normal saline, the skin around the ulcer is dried and a fresh dressing applied.

3 Alginate dressings. Alginates are naturally occurring polysaccharides found only in brown seaweeds (*Phaeophycae*). The alginic acid is usually converted to calcium or sodium salts. Calcium alginate is insoluble in water; sodium alginate is very soluble in water. The two preparations most commonly used are:
- Kaltostat
- Sorbsan.

They are both calcium alginate dressings. On contact with an exuding ulcer, the calcium ions in the alginate fibre exchange with sodium ions in the exudate to form a fibrous gel which creates a moist, warm environment. They cannot be used on dry ulcers, and are most suitable for use when there is a lot of exudate.

The alginate dressing is cut to the exact size and shape of the ulcer, soaked in normal saline and applied to the ulcer (it must not be applied dry). It is left in place for several days or up to a week at a time. When the dressing is changed, Sorbsan is removed by squirting a syringe full of normal saline onto it; Kaltostat is removed by cleaning off with normal saline.

4 Silastic foam dressings. The foam is made by mixing a liquid silicone base with a stannous octoate catalyst immediately before use. This is then moulded to the shape of the ulcer and left in place for at least a week at a time. Its main use is for deep cavities (better for bed sores than straightforward venous ulcers) to enable them to granulate up from the bottom.

5 Activated charcoal dressings (Actisorb Plus, Carbonet, Denidor). These are applied over one of the other dressings if the ulcer is very smelly; the carbon absorbing some at least of the smell.

Overgranulation of ulcer

Healing of an ulcer can be delayed because too much granulation tissue is formed. A silver nitrate stick can be used on the overgranulated area before the dressing is applied. Patients usually find this very painful. Alternatively, a gauze swab soaked in 0.25%

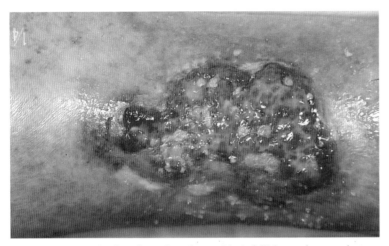

Figure 206 Ulcer healing from the edge and hair follicles and sweat ducts within it.

silver nitrate solution can be applied to the ulcer and covered with Jelonet.

Outer dressings

On top of all these dressings a 9″ × 9″ pad is usually applied to soak up any discharge. On top of this a cotton or crêpe bandage is applied to hold the dressings in place and on top of that the graduated compression bandage.

Analgesics for dressings

If applying a dressing or changing a dressing is painful, the patient should take two paracetamol or two co-proxamol tablets an hour before the dressing is done.

How does an ulcer heal?

Once any slough has been removed and the base of the ulcer is granulating, a new epidermis will grow in from the edge. If any skin appendages remain intact within the ulcer (if it has not been too deep) islands of epidermis will also appear within the ulcer and this will speed up the rate at which a new epidermis is formed (Figure 206).

Skin grafting for speeding up the healing process

Ulcers which are slow to heal but are clean can be grafted by applying pinch grafts or a split skin graft. A full thickness graft cannot be used, because the bacteria present on the ulcer will cause it to lift off. Instead small pieces of skin are scattered over the ulcer leaving open areas in between so that any exudate can escape.

Pinch grafts are simple to do but are time consuming if the ulcers are very large. Local anaesthetic is put into an area on the front of the patient's thigh (2–4 ml depending on the size of the ulcer(s) to be grafted). Small pinches of skin are removed from the anaesthetized area by sticking a No. 1 needle into the skin just past the bevel, and cutting off the skin with a No. 15 scalpel (Figure 207a). The pieces of skin removed are put into a sterile bowl containing lukewarm normal saline until sufficient pinches have been removed. The ulcer itself is cleaned with normal saline, and then the small pieces of skin are transferred to the surface of the ulcer with a pair of fine forceps (Figure 207c), taking care to put the skin on the ulcer with the epidermis uppermost (you can see which side has the needle hole in it). They are scattered over the surface moderately evenly. The whole is then covered with Jelonet upon which is spread a layer of 3% chlortetracycline hydrochloride ointment (Aureomycin). It is covered with a dry dressing,

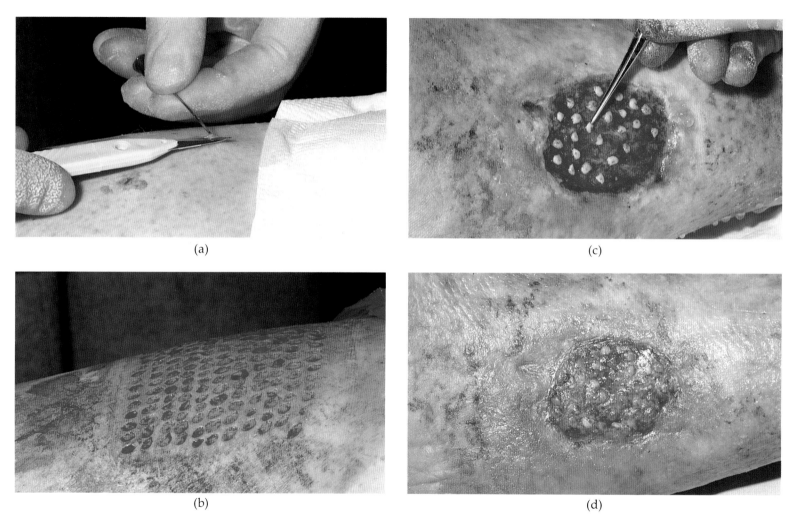

(a)

(b)

(c)

(d)

Figure 207 Pinch grafts. **(a)** Slicing off small pinches of skin from the donor thigh. **(b)** Thigh when all the pinches have been taken. **(c)** Putting the pinches on the ulcer with a pair of fine forceps. Notice the small hole in the centre of each pinch indicating that it is the outside of the skin. **(d)** Same ulcer as **(c)** 10 days later. When the dressing is removed, it is cleaned with normal saline and covered with Jelonet for a further 7 days.

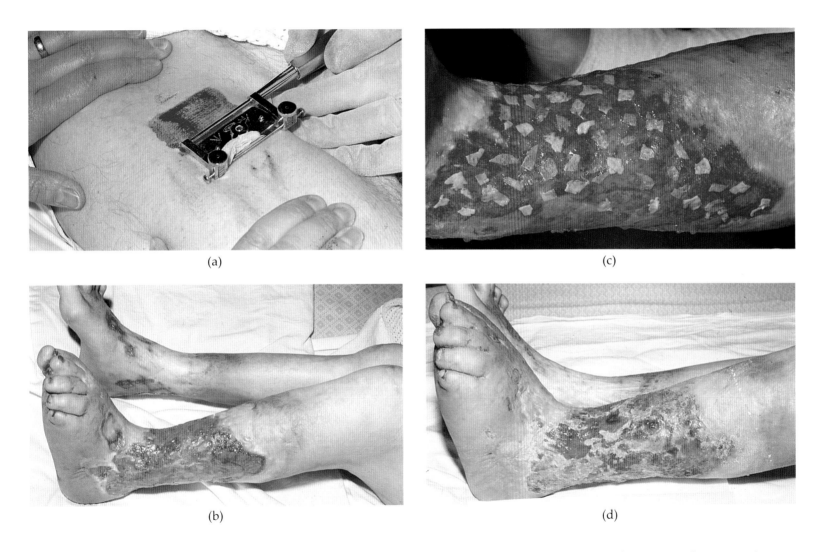

Figure 208 Split skin grafts. **(a)** Split skin being removed from donor thigh. **(b)** Large ulcer to be grafted. **(c)** Split skin graft cut into smaller pieces and applied over the large ulcer. **(d)** Same ulcer as **(c)** 1 month later.

a 9″ × 9″ pad, a Denidor (charcoal impregnated) pad, a cotton bandage, and a crêpe bandage if the patient is going to remain in bed, or a graduated compression bandage if the patient is going to be ambulant. The donor site is covered with Jelonet and a dry dressing. Both sites are left covered and untouched for 10 days. When the dressings are removed after 10 days the donor site is usually healed. The ulcer site should have the dressing soaked off with normal saline rather than just pulled off so that the grafts are not removed with the dressing. The grafted area is gently cleaned by pouring lukewarm saline over it and a fresh piece of Jelonet is applied to cover it for a further 7 days. At the end of that time the ulcer should be healed or nearly healed (*see* Figure 207d). Once it has healed the patient should wear graduated compression bandages for about 3 months; after this elastic stockings may be worn instead. These will need to be continued for the rest of her life so that the ulcer does not break down again.

Split skin grafts. The technique here is similar to pinch grafting except that the skin is removed as a single piece using a razor blade in a split skin knife to remove skin from the anterior thigh (*see* Figure 208a). The split skin then has to be cut up into smaller pieces to apply to the ulcer (*see* Figure 208c). This is much quicker to do than pinch grafting, but the patient often complains of a lot of pain from the donor site. Both the ulcer and the donor site are covered in the same way as for pinch grafts and left for 10 days.

A stubborn ulcer can be healed up in 3–4 weeks with grafting.

Treatment of complications of venous ulcers

1 Eczema around the ulcer. Some patients have eczema around their ulcers as part of their venous disease, others have a contact allergic eczema due to one of the dressings or bandages which have been applied as part of their treatment (*see* Figure 192, page 225).

The more common allergens are wool alcohols (lanolin), parabens, propylene glycol, antibiotics and rubber (Figure 209). If the leg is weeping, soak it in a dilute solution of potassium permanganate (so that it is a pale pink colour—*see* Figure 47, page 62) for 10 minutes and then apply a dilute topical steroid ointment which has white soft paraffin as its base rather than lanolin (1% hydrocortisone or 0.025% betamethasone 17 valerate [Betnovate RD]). Once the eczema has cleared the patient will need to be patch tested to find out exactly what the culprit is so that it can be avoided in the future.

Where are these allergens found?
- Wool alcohols (lanolin)—in many ointments, some paste bandages and in moisturizers that the patient may have used quite independently of her treatment.
- Parabens—a preservative in many creams and in all paste bandages.
- Propylene glycol—in many creams and ointments used on ulcers and some steroid preparations (*see* Mims for a complete list).
- Antibiotics—particularly neomycin, bacitracin, framycetin and fusidic acid used as ointments or as impregnated dressings used inappropriately on an ulcer.
- Rubber—this is the most difficult to cope with because the patient will need ongoing compression bandaging for the rest of her life. Red line bandages do not contain rubber and it is possible to get elastic stockings which do not contain rubber, but they need to be asked for specifically.

2 Soft tissue calcification (Figures 210 and 211). It is not uncommon for there to be calcification in the soft tissues of the lower leg in patients with venous disease. If this is in the base of an ulcer it can be mistaken for slough (Figure 210) and you can spend months wondering why you cannot get an ulcer clean! If it is stopping an ulcer healing it will need to be removed surgically.

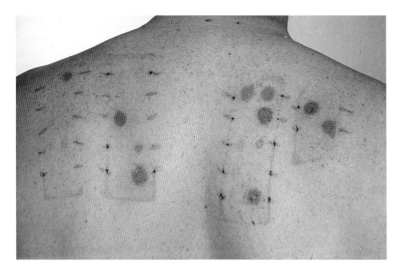

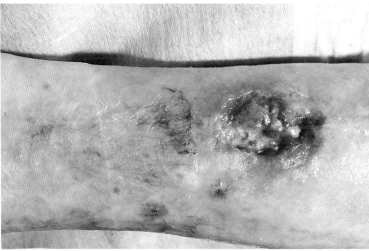

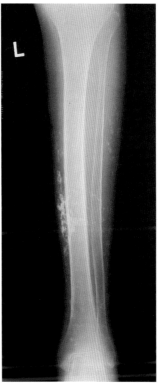

Figure 211 Same patient as Figure 210. Soft tissue calcification on X-ray.

Figure 209 (*above*) Patch testing result in a patient with long standing venous ulceration of the legs: many positive patch tests.

Figure 210 (*below*) Calcium in the base of an ulcer. It was thought to be adherent slough for several weeks!

3 Cellulitis (*see* Figure 198, page 228). Penicillin V or erythromycin, 500 mg every 6 hours will deal with this. If it does not respond, the patient will need to be admitted to hospital for treatment with intravenous benzyl penicillin.

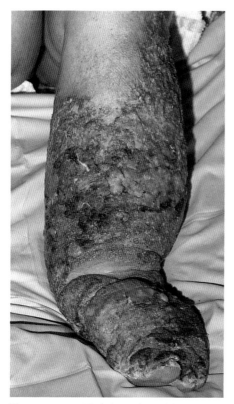

Figure 212 **(a)** Nodular polypoid hyperplasia.

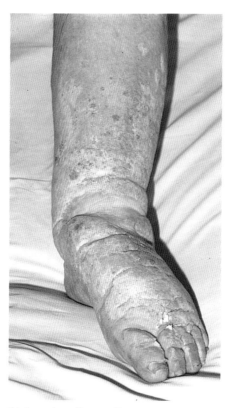

(b) Same leg after curettage.

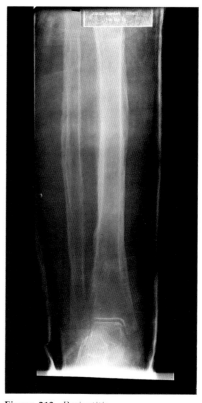

Figure 213 Periostitis.

4 Nodular polypoid hyperplasia. This can be extremely unpleasant for the patient, mainly because of the unpleasant smell that is generated within the thick keratin (Figure 212a). It is simple to remove with a curette; all the excess tissue is scraped off (Figure 212b). No anaesthetic is needed. If the patient will then wear graduated compression bandages or stockings, it will not recur.

5 Periostitis (Figure 213). The patient should rest in bed with the foot elevated and take adequate analgesics until the pain goes.

Do systemic drugs have any part to play in the healing of venous ulcers?

The simple answer is probably 'No'. Two drugs are promoted to improve the rate of healing but the evidence of any real benefit is so far lacking. The drugs are:

1 **Stanozolol**, an anabolic steroid. Because it is a fibrinolytic drug, it is meant to break down the fibrin cuff around capillaries and therefore improve perfusion through the capillary wall. By the time the patient has developed an ulcer it is probably too late to reduce the amount of fibrosis around the ankle. The dose is 10 mg daily; once started it should be continued for 6 months to see if it is going to do any good.

2 **Oxpentifylline**, a xanthine derivative which decreases blood viscosity, decreases platelet aggregation and alters the shape of red blood cells so that they are able to thread their way through the capillaries more easily. The dose is 400 mg daily and if started they should be continued for 6 months to see if there is any improvement.

Elevation of the leg, exercise, compression bandaging and, later, elastic stockings are the mainstays of treatment of venous ulcers.

Arterial ulcers

A patient with an arterial ulcer should be referred to a vascular surgeon in the first instance, because it is not a question of what kind of dressing or bandage should be put on the ulcer, but whether it is possible to improve the blood supply to the limb or not. Preliminary investigations include:

1 feeling the pulses and listening for bruits

2 measurement of the blood pressure in the arm and at the ankle with a Doppler probe (Figure 214).

$$\frac{\text{Systolic blood pressure ankle}}{\text{Systolic blood pressure arm}} = ?$$

This is called the resting ankle/brachial pressure index:

If it is >0.9 there is no arterial disease.

If it is <0.9 there is arterial disease.

If it is <0.7 there is clinically significant arterial disease.

If it is <0.5 the patient will be getting rest pain.

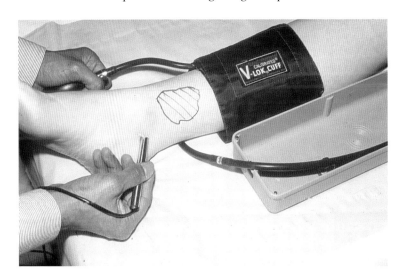

Figure 214 Measurement of the systolic blood pressure at the ankle using a Doppler probe. Courtesy of Dr Raj Mani.

3 duplex imaging Doppler. This combines the hand held continuous wave Doppler together with real time B-mode imaging to give picture images of the blood flow and measurement of blood flow.

4 arteriogram to find out where the problem is, how extensive it is and whether the disease is amenable to surgery. The surgical techniques which are available depend on where the atheroma is

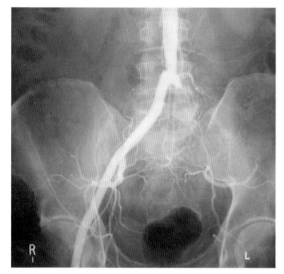

Figure 215 Major arterial block in iliac artery; suitable for treatment with a Teflon graft.

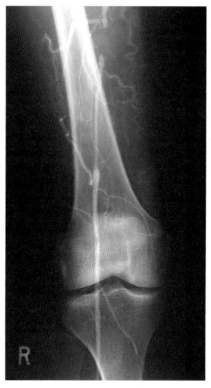

Figure 216 Block in superficial femoral artery which would be amenable to angioplasty.

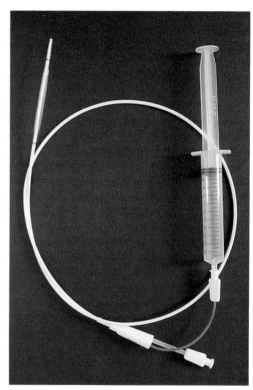

Figure 217 PCTL balloon dilation catheter used for angioplasty.

present. If there is a block high up in the aorto-iliac segment (Figure 215), a Teflon prosthesis can be used to replace it. Stenosis in the femoropopliteal segment can also be treated by reconstructive surgery, normally using the patient's own long saphenous vein for the bypass. If the stenosis is localized (Figure 216), percutaneous transluminal dilation angioplasty is much simpler and can be done under local anaesthetic. If the disease is distal to the popliteal artery, the blood supply can still be improved by lumbar sympathectomy; this can be done either surgically or with phenol. Whatever is done, the patient must stop smoking and any associated hypertension must be treated to prevent further atheroma from developing.

If it is not possible to improve the arterial blood supply, it is very unlikely that the ulcer will heal and gangrene will be the inevitable outcome. Early rather than late amputation is advised before the pain becomes intolerable.

Treatment of the ulcer itself

If there is any slough present, it should be removed either with a pair of sharp scissors or a scalpel or with a desloughing agent such as Varidase (for the technique of using this and other desloughing agents *see* page 229). Once the ulcer is clean it should be covered with a non-adhesive dressing such as Jelonet, Melolin or N-A; this can be left in place for a week at a time so that any new epithelial cells will not be removed as soon as they have formed. The dressing is covered with a light bandage simply to keep it in place. Do not apply tight bandages or any kind of elastic support because they can impede the arterial supply further. Adequate analgesics must also be given during the healing process since these ulcers are always painful.

Neuropathic ulcers

Loss of sensation means that patients may not notice an injury to their anaesthetic feet or legs. Rubbing from shoes, treading on a nail, being bumped into by a supermarket trolley, having the toes accidentally trodden on, or burning by a hot water bottle are some of the common sources of injury. If the patient does not notice what has happened and does not protect the area from further damage an ulcer can form. On the sole of the foot a callous often builds up around the injury making an ulcer seem smaller than it really is or sometimes completely covering it. It is essential to remove the callous with a scalpel to see how big the ulcer is. If nothing is done at this stage repeated trauma will cause the ulcer to enlarge and secondary infection is likely to occur (sometimes leading to osteomyelitis). The foot should be X-rayed and bacteriology swabs taken. If osteomyelitis is present the patient should be admitted to hospital so that high doses of intravenous antibiotics can be given.

To get the ulcers healed, the patient must be stopped from weight bearing and any source of friction removed. Making the patient go to bed for weeks or sometimes months at a time in order to heal the ulcer(s) is not a very satisfactory solution from the patient's point of view. An alternative is to apply a below knee walking plaster for 2 months at a time. This removes any friction and allows the ulcer to heal. After 2 months, when the plaster of Paris is removed, the ulcer is usually healed; if it is not, it is put back on for a further 2 months. If the ulcer is very dirty and there is a lot of exudate, the plaster of Paris can have a window cut in it to allow the ulcer to be cleaned regularly and to minimize the unpleasant smell for the patient.

Removing the slough and applying non-adherent dressings is the same as for venous ulcers, *see* pages 229 and 233. There is no need for elastic support. The idea is simply to keep the ulcer clean and free of friction while it heals.

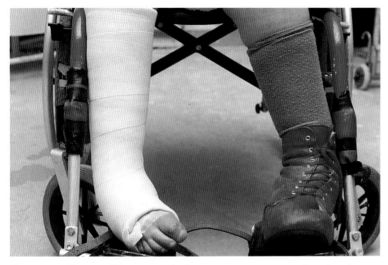

Figure 218 Plaster of Paris on right leg to protect a neuropathic ulcer from injury in a paraplegic girl.

When the ulcer is healed the patient must be taught to take care of his anaesthetized limbs:

1 The feet should be washed and dried carefully every day, particularly between the toes, and clean socks or tights put on.

2 The feet must be examined for signs of injury at least once a day for blisters, abrasions, cuts or just erythema. If the patient cannot do this himself he must get someone to do it for him. Any abnormality should be taken seriously; it should be carefully cleaned and protected from further injury. He will need to have a supply of non-adherent dressings, gauze swabs, 9″ × 9″ pads and soft bandages at home to use when necessary.

3 The patient should wear shoes that fit well, preferably made of soft leather without a seam and with Plastazote insoles so that they do not slip or rub. The shoes must be worn all the time the patient is not in bed, indoors as well as out of doors. He must not walk around bare footed.

4 Callosities on the soles should be soaked in warm water for 10–15 minutes each day and then rubbed down gently with a pumice stone to keep them flat. Regular chiropody is also essential.

5 The patient should be told not to use a hot water bottle and not to sit too close to a fire.

6 At the first sign of ulceration or an injury that is not healing, the patient should see his doctor for further advice.

Ulcers in a diabetic patient

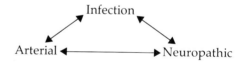

Patients with diabetes mellitus can have both arterial and neuropathic ulcers. It is important to sort out which of the two is the main culprit and to treat it as outlined under arterial ulcer (page 241) or neuropathic ulcer (page 243). The arterial disease can be arteriosclerosis of the major limb vessels or small vessel disease, in which case the treatment options may be severely limited. Either arterial or neuropathic ulcers (or both) can be complicated by bacterial infection and it is important to deal with this promptly with systemic antibiotics. Necrobiosis lipoidica can also ulcerate on occasion (*see* page 124).

URTICARIA

Acute urticaria

This is very often a type I allergic reaction to a food or a drug; it may just be urticaria or it may be part of a full blown anaphylactic reaction. If it is just the rash, give a short-acting antihistamine such as chlorpheniramine (Piriton), 4 mg every 4 hours until it settles. In a life threatening situation, where there is oedema of the larynx and/or the tongue and the patient is having difficulty in breathing, inject 0.5 ml of 1:1000 adrenaline intramuscularly immediately and repeat it every 10 minutes until the oedema settles. At the same time give chlorpheniramine 10 mg intramuscularly so that there will be a longer lasting effect. If it is due to food or a drug the patient should be warned not to take it again.

Chronic urticaria

This is not a type I allergic reaction and in most patients a cause will not be found. It is however always worth taking a thorough medical history and doing a general physical examination to exclude some general medical illness or a focus of infection as the cause. There is no need for routine blood tests.

Patients should be told not to take aspirin or codeine tablets because these have a direct effect on mast cells causing them to degranulate and will make urticaria worse. Since some food additives are chemically related to aspirin, it is sometimes worth putting the patient on a diet free of azo dyes and preservatives for a period of 6 weeks.

Azo dyes are used to artificially colour food; those which cause problems are:

tartrazine	-orange-yellow colour
sunset yellow	-yellow colour
new coccine	-red colour

Benzoic acid and its derivatives are food preservatives and are found mainly in peas and bananas. The diet involves the patient eating fresh food rather than ready-made meals, but avoiding peas and bananas. Anything that comes in a packet or tin should have the label checked to make sure there are no preservatives or artificial colouring materials in them.

The mainstay of treatment is for the patient to take a long acting, non-sedative, antihistamine until the urticaria gets better spontaneously. This means that they are taken regularly to prevent the urticaria from occurring, usually until the patient has been free of a rash for 4 weeks. The tablets are then stopped. If the rash recurs, the patient goes back on the antihistamines for a further 4 weeks, and so on, until when the tablets are stopped the rash does not reappear. They can be continued for months or years quite safely if necessary.

The antihistamines that work are those which selectively inhibit the peripheral H_1 receptors. The non-sedative ones either do not penetrate the blood/brain barrier well or they have less affinity for brain H_1 receptors than for peripheral H_1 receptors. The choice of drugs is between:

- terfenadine
- cetirizine dihydrochloride
- astemizole
- loratadine
- mequitazine.

If the first drug you try does not work, increase the dose (*see* Table 26) before trying one of the others. Patients often need higher doses of antihistamines than are normally recommended by the manufacturers to control their chronic urticaria. It is often a question of trial and error to find which drug suits which particular patient, but it is usually possible to find one that will work.

Table 26 Long acting non-sedative antihistamines and how they are used

Drug	Dosage and how to take it	How does it work, precautions and side effects

Terfenadine (Triludan)	Start with 60 mg twice a day. Double it to 120 mg twice a day if the lower dose does not work. For children it comes as a suspension (30 mg/5 ml); the dose is:
	  Children aged 3–6, 15 mg twice a day
	  Children aged 7–12, 30 mg twice a day.
		Selective H_1 blocker; >98% bound to plasma proteins so it does not easily cross the blood/brain barrier. Do not use during pregnancy. Do not exceed the recommended dose or use it in patients with liver disease or those taking ketaconazole or erythromycin because of the risk of ventricular arrhythmias (prolonged QT interval). Rarely can cause sedation or headaches.

Cetirizine 2HCl (Zirtek)	10 mg once a day, at night before the patient goes to bed. Dose can be doubled to 20 mg if 10 mg does not work.	Selective H_1 receptor blocker chemically related to hydroxyzine. Highly ionized at physiologic pH making it less likely to penetrate the blood/brain barrier. Rapid effect. Lasts 24 hours. Avoid in pregnancy. May cause slight fatigue, especially if dose increased.
Astemizole (Hismanal)	10 mg once a day. Take on an empty stomach because it is not absorbed well when given with food.	H_1, H_2 and 5-HT receptor antagonist. Slow to start working—takes 4–5 days to have maximum effect and stays in body for several weeks after drug has been stopped. Do not use during pregnancy or lactation. Increases appetite so can cause weight gain.
Loratadine (Clarityn)	10 mg once a day. If no effect dose can gradually be increased up to 40 mg/day as a single dose.	Selective H_1 blocker with low affinity for brain H_1 receptors; 97–98% protein bound so it does not easily cross the blood/brain barrier. Well absorbed by mouth with rapid action within 1–2 hours. Not affected by age or renal status but not as effective as terfenadine or cetirizine dihydrochloride. Do not use in pregnancy or during lactation. No sedation at 10 mg/day, but will cause it if the dose is increased. Occasionally causes headaches and nausea.
Mequitazine (Primalan)	Start with 5 mg twice a day. Gradually increase the dose until it works, up to 20 mg twice a day.	Has some effect on brain H_1 receptors so more likely to cause sedation than other drugs in this table. Also has some anti-cholinergic effects so can cause dry mouth and blurred vision. Do not use in pregnancy or in patients with epilepsy.

If the non-sedative antihistamines do not work:

1 add an H_2 blocker, eg cimetidine 200–400 mg four times a day, or

2 use an ordinary sedative antihistamine but warn the patient not to drive or handle moving machinery and not to drink alcohol while taking them, eg:

(i) brompheniramine LA 12 mg twice a day, increasing to 24 mg twice a day if necessary, *or*

(ii) hydroxyzine hydrochloride (Atarax) 10 mg three times a day and 25 mg at night, *or*

(iii) mebhydrolin (Fabahistin) 50 mg three times a day, increasing to 100 mg three times a day if necessary.

Topical steroids do not work in urticaria and systemic steroids (even short courses) should not be prescribed, in spite of their effectiveness, because on withdrawal the urticaria will be just as bad as before and there is a very high risk of long-term dependence.

Cholinergic urticaria

The options are for the patient to take a non-sedative long acting antihistamine on a regular basis to prevent it occurring (*see* Table 26) or to take a short acting antihistamine before exercise (eg chlorpheniramine 4–8 mg). Antihistamines do not work as well in this condition as they do in ordinary chronic urticaria.

Physical urticarias

Cold urticaria

It is possible to desensitize the patient to the cold but it is extremely tedious to do and is best done under supervision by a dermatologist. It is much easier for the patient to take a non-sedative antihistamine such as terfenadine 60–120 mg twice a day or cetirizine dihydrochloride 10 mg at night on a regular basis to prevent it occurring.

Pressure urticaria

Pressure urticaria is often associated with ordinary chronic urticaria and it is treated in the same way with non-sedative antihistamines which block the peripheral H_1 receptors, eg terfenadine 60–120 mg twice a day or cetirizine 2HCl 10 mg at night (*see* Table 26). If they do not work, hydroxyzine hydrochloride 10 mg three times a day and 25 mg at night, or cyproheptadine 4 mg three or four times a day, may be more effective.

Delayed pressure urticaria

Delayed pressure urticaria occurs mainly on the hands and feet, the effect being maximal after 6–8 hours. It responds best to dapsone. Start with a dose of 50 mg/day; the effective dose varies between 50 mg on alternate days and 150 mg/day. Patients on dapsone must have a full blood count measured regularly because of the risk of haemolysis (*see* page 40).

Solar urticaria

The alternatives here are to use a non-sedative antihistamine regularly through the summer months and on bright sunny days in the winter to prevent it occurring, or to protect the patient from exposure to the wavelength of light that is causing it. Almost certainly help will be needed from a dermatologist with an interest in light-induced problems. If the rash is caused by UVB, it will not occur on a sunny day if the patient is indoors (because window glass cuts out UVB) and a high protective factor non-opaque sunscreen (*see* page 141) should prevent it. If it is due to UVA the patient will need a sunscreen containing titanium dioxide (*see* pages 140 and 141) or possibly a course of PUVA (*see* page 164).

Urticarial vasculitis

Urticarial vasculitis does not usually respond to systemic antihistamines. The patient should be referred to a dermatologist to look for a cause and to supervise treatment. Systemic steroids or dapsone may be needed.

VASCULITIS

Vasculitis is a pathological rather than a clinical diagnosis and often a skin biopsy is needed to sort out what is going on. There are several different patterns dependent on the size and site of the vessels involved.

1 Capillaries in the superficial and mid-dermis (**leucocytoclastic vasculitis; Henoch-Schönlein purpura**). Clinically there will be a polymorphic rash with some palpable purpura.
2 Arteries at the junction of the dermis and subcutaneous fat (**cutaneous polyarteritis nodosa**). There will be livedo reticularis and nodules and/or ulceration on the lower legs.
3 Arteries and veins in the subcutaneous fat (**nodular vasculitis; erythema nodosum**). There will be red nodules or plaques deep in the skin (in the subcutaneous fat).

Leucocytoclastic vasculitis

The first thing is to look for a cause and treat if possible:
- an infection somewhere
- a drug (thiazide diuretics, antibiotics, non-steroidal anti-inflammatory drugs, thioureas and many others)
- a connective tissue disease
- cryoglobulinaemia or other plasma protein abnormality.

If no cause can be found the patient can be reassured that it is a self-limiting condition which gets better after 3–6 weeks. Bed rest will stop new lesions from developing on the skin. Otherwise treatment is symptomatic, with analgesics for pain. It is worth checking the urine for protein, blood and casts and the blood urea and creatinine to make sure that the kidneys are not involved. If there is renal damage specialist help should be sought because treatment with cyclophosphamide may be needed. There is no evidence that systemic steroids help.

The skin lesions themselves do not need any treatment unless there are necrotic lesions which are weeping and crusted. Non-stick dressings (Melolin or N-A) can be applied to necrotic lesions until they heal. It is not usually necessary to apply a topical debriding agent.

Henoch-Schönlein purpura

This diagnosis should be thought of in any child with purpura who has a normal platelet count. If there has been a preceding streptococcal throat infection, oral phenoxymethylpenicillin should be given as for tonsillitis:
- child aged <5years   125 mg every 6 hours for 7 days
- child aged >5years   250 mg every 6 hours for 7 days
- adult   500 mg every 6 hours for 7 days.

More often there will be no obvious cause for it. It gets better spontaneously in 3–6 weeks and treatment is largely symptomatic. Bed rest will stop new lesions from occurring on the skin; the joint pains and abdominal pain will need to be treated with analgesics. Renal involvement may be more serious. Proteinuria or microscopic haematuria without impairment of renal function will normally get better spontaneously in less than 4 weeks. If acute nephritis or progressive renal failure occur, the patient should be referred urgently to a renal physician.

Cutaneous polyarteritis nodosa

Most patients will require treatment with systemic steroids; they should be referred to a dermatologist, rheumatologist or general physician so that the diagnosis can be confirmed and the best treatment sorted out (this disease is not the same as systemic polyarteritis nodosa—it affects only the skin, muscles and nerves).

Nodular vasculitis

A focus of infection should be looked for and treated if found. There are a small minority of patients in whom the cause is tuberculosis; treatment of this will cure the vasculitis. If no infective cause is found, treatment is symptomatic. Sometimes immunosuppressive drugs are helpful. It is often a case of trial and error to find something that will work for a particular individual.

Erythema nodosum (*see* page 73)

VENOUS LAKE

Most patients do not seem to mind having these lesions on their lips. If they want them removed there are various ways of doing it.
1 Surgical excision under a local anaesthetic is simple to do and produces a good cosmetic result. The lip will heal well if the excision line is sited perpendicularly across the lip.
2 Infrared coagulator. This is used in the same way as for removing tattoos, *see* pages 207 and 208.

3 The argon or tuneable dye laser can be used without any anaesthetic and gives excellent cosmetic results. This is the treatment of choice if there is one in use near where the patient lives (*see* inside front cover).

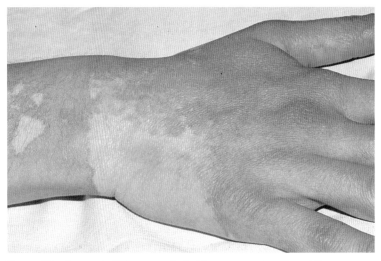

Figure 219 Areas of vitiligo unprotected by a sunscreen: the white areas have burnt in the sun.

VITILIGO

Always check the urine for sugar and send blood for an autoimmune profile because patients with vitiligo have a higher incidence of diabetes, thyroid disease, pernicious anaemia and Addison's disease.

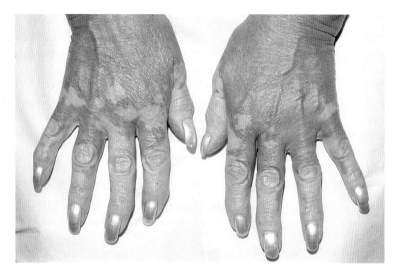

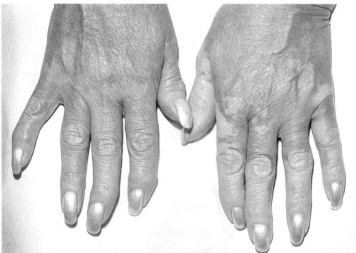

Figure 220 **(a)** (*above*) Vitiligo on the dorsum of both hands. **(b)** (*below*) Cosmetic camouflage on the right hand; left hand untreated for comparison.

The white areas of skin burn in the sun (Figure 219), so patients should be advised to protect affected skin by keeping covered up in the sun and using a high protective factor sunscreen on the white areas (*see* page 141).

If the face or hands are involved, cosmetic camouflage can successfully hide it (Figure 220). This service is provided free by the British Red Cross in many local hospitals and is particularly useful for patients with pigmented skins in whom vitiligo can be very disfiguring. An alternative method of disguise is to use dihydroxyacetone to colour the white areas; this is available 'over the counter' in artificial suntan lotions or creams. It is not as good as cosmetic camouflage because it is more difficult to get a good colour match, and if it is accidentally applied to the surrounding normal skin, that will become darker, highlighting the difference which the patient had hoped to hide. Some patients will prefer it because it does not have to be applied every day like the cosmetic camouflage and it is not like make-up.

There is no easy way to get the white areas to repigment. In some patients the skin will repigment spontaneously, but there is no way of knowing which ones will do so. PUVA can be used but it does not always work. If started it needs to be continued for at least 6 months to see if there is going to be any effect. Tablets of 8-methoxypsoralen, 0.6 mg/kg body weight, are given 2 hours before exposure to UVA twice a week (*see* page 166 for side effects).

If the vitiligo is very extensive (Figure 221), it is often better to get rid of the remaining normal pigment by using 20% monobenzyl ether of hydroquinone cream twice a day to the normal skin so that the skin becomes a uniform white colour. This chemical causes an initial inflammatory reaction but this is followed by permanent depigmentation. A high protective factor sunscreen will then be needed all over the skin when the patient is out in the sun (*see* page 141).

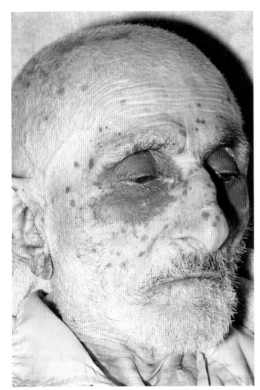

Figure 221 Very
extensive vitiligo. The
only normal skin left is
the brown discolouration
around the eyes. This
patient would be suitable
for treatment with the
monobenzyl ether of
hydroquinone.

Patients may want to get in touch with others who are similarly affected or to receive information from a self-help group:

> THE VITILIGO SOCIETY
> PO Box 919
> London, SE21 8AW
> Tel: 081 776 7022

WARTS

Although there are approximately 70 different human papilloma viruses (HPVs) only six commonly cause warts in man:

HPV-1 causes deep painful plantar warts which are usually solitary and found over pressure areas such as the heel or the metatarsal heads.

HPV-2 causes common warts on the hands and feet, filiform warts on the face, mosaic warts on the feet and some genital warts.

HPV-3 causes plane warts on the hands and face.

HPV-4 causes multiple, small, endophytic warts on the palms and soles, which are flat or have a slightly depressed rough surface.

HPV-6 and **HPV-11** cause most genital warts.

The vast majority of other HPV types have only been found in patients with epidermodysplasia verruciformis, in which there is an inherited abnormality of the host response to HPVs. These patients also have an increased risk of cutaneous malignancy.

HPV-5 and **HPV-8** have been found in patients who have received organ transplants; they are also at risk of cutaneous malignancy.

HPV-7 seems to be almost unique to butchers and fish-handlers, although it has also been found in a small number of patients with AIDS.

There is no single treatment for warts which can be guaranteed to work. Indeed the large number of treatments which are available means that none of them is particularly effective and most of the remedies that we think of as 'old wives' tales' work as well as anything the doctor has to offer. There is no point in referring the patient to a dermatologist unless the appropriate treatment is liquid nitrogen and that is not available in the surgery. Referral for other reasons is likely to result in disappointment when the patient discovers that there is no magic cure available at the hospital.

Warts clear spontaneously when the patient has built up enough cell-mediated immunity to the wart virus, so if they are not causing symptoms they can be left alone. The average life of a wart is 27 months, but this varies in an individual patient from a few months to several years; 35% of warts disappear within 6 months.

Generally speaking, warts in children respond to treatment better than those in adults; single warts and those which have not been present for long do better than multiple warts or those which have been present for years. On the feet, single warts respond readily to treatment but mosaic warts do not.

Types of treatment available

1   Keratolytic agents. Salicylic acid and lactic acid are found in many proprietary wart paints and gels. These are applied once a day, usually with an applicator supplied with the bottle or tube, and left to dry. Any hard skin on the surface of the wart should first be removed by rubbing down the surface with a pumice stone or emery board. Examples of keratolytic paints and gels are:

Duofilm paint	16.7% salicylic acid 16.7% lactic acid	Cuplex gel	16% salicylic acid 4% lactic acid
Salactol paint	16.7% salicylic acid 16.7% lactic acid	Salatac gel	12% salicylic acid 4% lactic acid

Salicylic acid can also be made up as an ointment, 5% or 10% in white soft paraffin, as a paint, any concentration you like in flexible collodion, or as 20% or 40% plasters.

2   Formaldehyde and glutaraldehyde. 5% formalin solution or 10% glutaraldehyde solution can be used to soak plantar warts in once a day for about 10 minutes. 10% glutaraldehyde in aqueous ethanol can be used as a wart paint. It stains the warts brown so is not suitable for treating warts on the hands.

3   Cytotoxic drugs   Podophyllin
5-Fluorouracil
Bleomycin.

Podophyllin comes as a 10%, 15%, 20% and 25% solution in tinc. benz. co. or spirit. It is dark brown in colour so is not suitable for warts on the face and hands. It is applied to plantar warts every night by the patient, and to genital warts once a week by a nurse or doctor (for instructions *see* genital warts, page 260). Podophyllotoxin is a highly purified form of podophyllin; it is available as a 0.5% solution and cream for use by the patient himself on penile warts.

5% 5-fluorouracil cream can be applied daily to warts around the nails.

Bleomycin can be injected directly into warts, preferably with a bifurcated needle. This is rather unpleasant for the patient, but it is a useful treatment for stubborn mosaic warts on the feet.

4   Antiviral agents. These are theoretically a good idea, but none of the antiviral agents currently available work for warts.

5   Freezing with liquid nitrogen or carbon dioxide
(i) Liquid nitrogen   Temperature $-195.6°C$
This can be obtained direct from British Oxygen if you have a large enough container to put it in, or from your local hospital pharmacy where it can be supplied in small amounts (enough for a morning or evening surgery) into a vacuum flask with a hole in the lid or into a Dewar flask.
(ii) Carbon dioxide   Temperature $-56.6°C$
Carbon dioxide snow (dry ice) is obtained by releasing carbon dioxide gas rapidly into a chamois leather bag. It then has to be compressed to form a stick the same diameter as the wart through a wooden or plastic funnel.

Carbon dioxide slush is made by mixing a few drops of acetone with carbon dioxide snow. The amount required is then picked up on an orange stick with a tiny amount of cotton wool on the end; it is very useful for small filiform warts on the face or beard area.

The idea behind freezing warts is to produce a blister at the dermo–epidermal junction; since the wart is entirely within the epidermis (Figure 222), it should lift off with the blister.

6 Cautery. This works in the same way as freezing with liquid nitrogen, the heat causing a blister to form at the dermo–epidermal junction. It is not very practical to use because patients cannot tolerate it without a local anaesthetic. A machine which uses a very low current (Hyfrecator) can be used for patients with very numerous tiny warts in the beard area.

7 Surgical removal. It is not usually a good idea to excise warts because it is difficult to tell with a scalpel whether you have removed the whole wart or not; consequently the recurrence rate is high and the patient is left with a scar. Because of the shape of a wart (Figure 222), they can be scooped out easily with a curette and any bleeding stopped with a silver nitrate stick or with a cautery. An alternative is to burn the surface with the cautery first, which separates the wart from the surrounding dermis, making it easier to curette out.

Treatment of warts at different sites

Warts on the hands

Treatment of warts on the hands depends on the age of the patient and how many warts are present. In young children if there are lots of warts (*see* Figure 225), the best thing is to leave well alone until the warts clear spontaneously. If the child's mother insists on

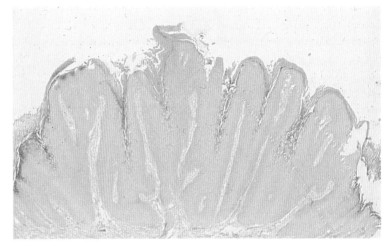

Figure 222 Histology of viral wart: the wart is entirely within the epidermis.

treatment, then get her to paint on one of the salicylic acid/lactic acid wart paints or gels (Duofilm or Salactol paint, or Cuplex or Salatac gel) carefully onto each wart at night before the child goes to bed. It should be left to dry before the child goes to bed. The next night the paint or gel which is still present is rubbed off with an emery board and further paint or gel applied. This is done each night until the warts disappear. Most warts will be gone in 3 months; it is not worth changing the treatment or giving up on the treatment in less than 12 weeks.

In older children and adults the choice of treatment basically depends on how many warts are present. If there is a single wart or a small number of large warts, the treatment of choice is to freeze them with liquid nitrogen. Pare down any hyperkeratosis on the surface before freezing (Figure 223). Mould a piece of cotton wool around the end of an orange stick so that it is just smaller in

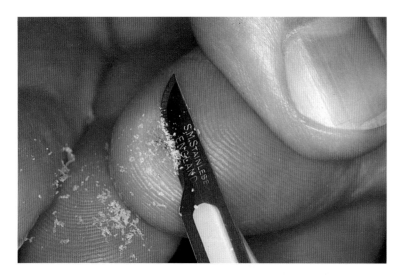

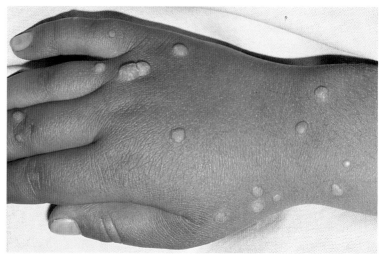

Figure 225 Multiple warts on the back of a 4-year-old girl's hand. Leave alone or use one of the keratolytic wart paints topically.

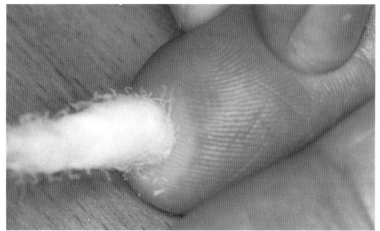

Figure 223 (*above*) Pare down the hyperkeratosis on the surface of a wart before freezing.

Figure 224 (*below*) Freezing a single wart on the finger with liquid nitrogen on a cotton wool bud.

diameter than the wart itself (this is better than using a liquid nitrogen spray gun because you can make your cotton wool bud any size you want and therefore you can localize the freezing accurately). Dip it into the liquid nitrogen and apply firmly and vertically onto the wart (Figure 224). Continue freezing until a 1 mm white halo appears around the wart—this can take anything from 10–30 seconds to occur. While you are freezing it, the patient experiences a burning sensation; afterwards it may throb. A blister should occur within 48 hours—warn the patient that this will happen and tell them to leave it alone. If the blister is very large they can puncture it with a sterile needle. After 7–10 days the

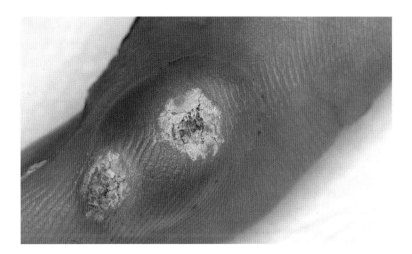

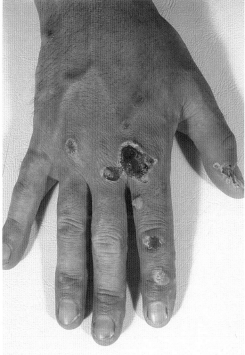

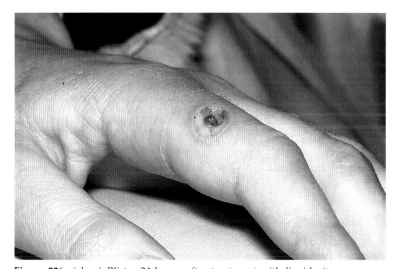

Figure 228 One week after warts frozen with liquid nitrogen: crusts beginning to separate.

Figure 226 (*above*) Blister 24 hours after treatment with liquid nitrogen.

Figure 227 (*below*) Ulcer on finger because liquid nitrogen applied for too long.

blister will dry out and the scab should drop off within a few days (Figure 228). If the wart has not gone the treatment can be repeated every 2–3 weeks until it does so.

Do not do several freeze/thaw cycles or you may cause necrosis of the skin and the patient will end up with an ulcer which can take several weeks to heal (Figure 227) and leave a permanent scar; rarely it can also cause damage to the cutaneous nerves or rupture an underlying tendon.

If large numbers of warts are present, liquid nitrogen is not a practical option because it will be too painful. The options now are to leave alone or to apply one of the salicylic acid/lactic acid wart paints or gels each night until they go. If the patient is going to use a wart paint, tell him to first pare down any hyperkeratosis and to clean off any previous wart paint. The paint or gel is then carefully applied to the warts and allowed to dry. It is repeated every night until the wart goes. Most warts will be gone after 3 months; do not think of changing the treatment until the patient has been using the present one for 12 weeks.

Since most patients want treatment for the warts on their hands because they do not like the look of them, podophyllin and glutaraldehyde paints are unsuitable because they stain the warts brown (Figure 229).

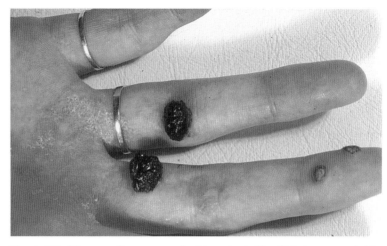

Figure 229 Warts on fingers treated with podophyllin. This is not a suitable treatment on the hands because it stains the warts brown making them more unsightly than they were before.

Warts on the feet

There are two reasons why patients complain of warts on their feet; either they are painful or, particularly in children, they are not allowed to go swimming. A wart is usually painful because there is a build-up of hard skin (callous) around it (Figure 230), not because the wart is growing in rather than sticking out. If the hard skin is pared down regularly with a scalpel or rubbed down with a pumice stone to keep it flat, it will not be painful. The other reason why a wart can be painful is if the blood vessels within it thrombose causing the wart to go black (Figure 231) and become exquisitely painful. Treatment of this is to use analgesics for a few days until the wart falls out.

If a child is not allowed to go swimming because of warts on the feet, he or she can wear a sock with a plastic sole while at the swimming baths*. The only problem with them is that they tend to balloon out making it less easy for the child to swim, but this is a small price to pay for being able to go swimming.

Treatment of the warts themselves depends on whether they are single or few in number or whether they are mosaic (compare Figures 230 and 232).

*Two kinds are available commercially.
Plastosoks available from Carita House, Stapely, Nantwich, Cheshire, CW5 7CJ, and **Britmarine Olympic Socks** available from Haffenden-Richborough Ltd, Sandwich, Kent, CT13 9NH. Both are also available from local sports shops.

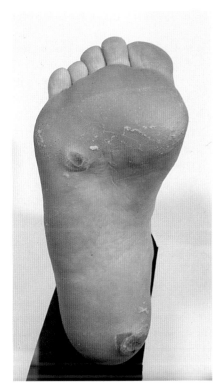

Figure 230 Deep painful plantar warts due to HPV-1. Notice the thick hyperkeratosis around each wart—this is what causes the pain.

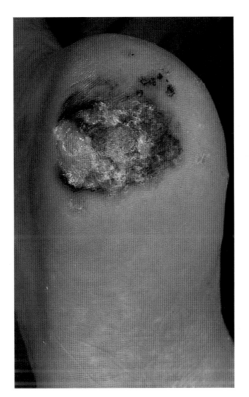

Figure 231 Thrombosed warts on the heel. These cause severe pain, but it is short lived because with the blood supply cut off the warts will soon fall out.

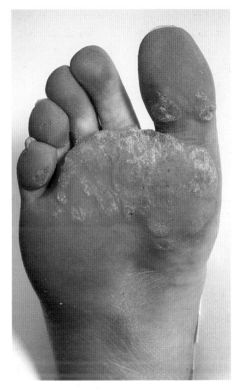

Figure 232 Mosaic warts on the ball of the foot and the plantar aspect of the toes. This type of wart does not respond well to any kind of treatment.

Treatment of single/few plantar warts (Figure 230)

The most important thing is for the patient to pare down the hard skin every night with a scalpel or to rub it down flat with a pumice stone so that it does not hurt. A wart paint or gel is then applied carefully just to the wart; it is left to dry and the wart covered with an Elastoplast overnight. In the morning the plaster is removed to allow the wart to harden up again before the wart is pared down the next night. If the plaster is left on for too long the wart becomes soggy and painful. If this occurs, treatment will have to be left off

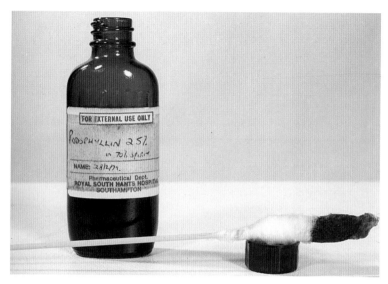

Figure 233 Podophyllin paint is brown. It can be used on the feet or the genitalia where the appearance of the warts does not matter, but it is not suitable for use on the hands.

for a few days. One of the reasons why the treatment does not work is that the patient stops using it if the foot becomes sore.

Preparations suitable for use on the feet
1 Salicylic acid/lactic acid mixtures Duofilm or Salactol paint, Cuplex or Salatac gel.
2 Podophyllin 20% or 25% in tinc. benz. co. or spirit. Although this preparation is brown (Figure 233) it does not matter on the sole of the foot.
3 Glutaraldehyde 10% solution.
Whichever paint (or gel) is chosen, it should be used each night before the patient goes to bed until the wart is gone. A fair trial of

a treatment is to use it for 12–16 weeks before giving up and changing to something else.

Freezing with liquid nitrogen is not a good treatment for plantar warts, because you need to freeze for quite a long time to produce a blister (because of the thick layer of keratin on the sole of the foot) and this will be painful for the patient. It certainly should not be used to treat plantar warts in young children.

Any kind of surgery is contraindicated on the feet. The most likely outcome is recurrence of the wart, and there is always the risk that scarring will lead to the formation of permanent callosities, especially over pressure points.

Treatment of mosaic warts (Figure 232)
These do not respond well to any kind of treatment. The simplest thing to do is to get the patient to soak the affected part of the foot in a 5% solution of formalin once a day. First apply a thickish layer of white soft paraffin (Vaseline) around the warts and between the toes, if the warts are on the ball of the foot or on the plantar aspect of the toes, so that the formalin does not make the normal skin sore. Then pour the formalin into a saucer or shallow bowl and soak the warts in it for 10 minutes each day. The next day rub down any hard skin on the surface with a pumice stone or foot scraper before repeating the treatment. Alternatives are:
1 Paint on one of the wart paints, containing salicylic acid and lactic acid or podophyllin as described for solitary warts (*see* left), *or*
2 Apply 40% salicylic acid plasters cut to the same size as the warts. These are stuck onto the warts shiny side down, taped securely in place with Hyperfix (or something similar), and left for a week at a time. When they are removed the soggy keratin is removed with a sharp scalpel blade before putting on a new plaster. This can be done once a week by the nurse or chiropodist until no wart is left, *or*

3 If you are really stuck, inject bleomycin into the warts using a bifurcated needle. This is a painful procedure and will require a local anaesthetic injection first or even a regional nerve block.

Plane warts

These need no treatment because they are generally asymptomatic. The problem is more often one of diagnosis. Once you reassure the patient that they are just warts, they are usually happy to leave well alone. If treatment is insisted upon, give the patient 5% salicylic acid ointment to rub onto the warts twice a day until they go. Another alternative is to lightly freeze them with liquid nitrogen (5 second freeze time).

Warts on the trunk and limbs

Solitary warts on the trunk or limbs can be frozen with liquid nitrogen or curetted off under local anaesthetic. If multiple warts are present, one of the salicylic acid/lactic acid wart paints can be applied each night (*see* page 252) until they clear. Always check the hands and feet too; most patients with warts in unusual places will also have warts at more common sites.

Warts around the nails (periungual warts)

Warts around the nails are difficult to treat because:
1 They can be sited over the nail matrix (proximal nail fold). Freezing with liquid nitrogen can damage the underlying matrix and cause a nail dystrophy (permanent distortion of the nail plate).
2 They can destroy the cuticle (Figure 234). If this occurs, a wart paint may run down between the wart and the nail causing a painful paronychia.

Ideally you would want to leave well alone but patients often want treatment. A complication is that they tend to pick or chew

warts around the nails and as a consequence sometimes get warts on their lips (Figure 235). Probably the simplest thing to do is to give the patient 5% or 10% salicylic acid ointment to apply twice a day. Freezing very cautiously with liquid nitrogen can be tried if the patient becomes desperate for something to be done. Applying 5% 5-fluorouracil cream twice a day would be another alternative.

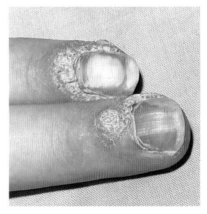

Figure 234 Periungual warts. On the index finger the warts are situated over the nail matrix and the cuticle is almost completely destroyed.

Warts on the face and beard

Warts on the face can be treated by freezing with liquid nitrogen or by curettage and cautery. Single filiform warts (Figure 235) are probably best curetted off under a local anaesthetic and the base cauterized to stop any bleeding. They usually curette out very easily and should heal without leaving a scar.

Multiple warts in the beard area (Figure 236) can be hidden by the patient growing a beard! If treatment is required they can be frozen with carbon dioxide slush if you have access to a cylinder of carbon dioxide gas from which to make it (*see* page 253). Collect a small

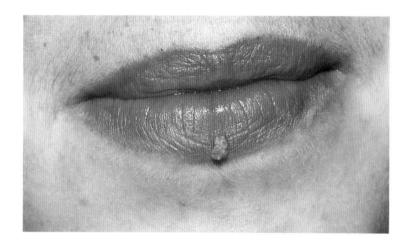

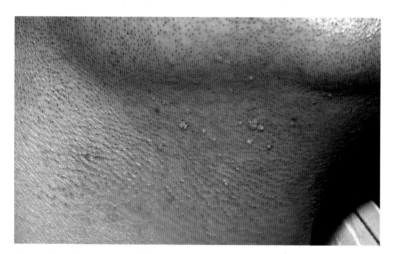

Figure 235 (*above*) Single filiform wart on the lower lip. The patient also has periungual warts.

Figure 236 (*below*) Multiple tiny filiform warts in the beard area spread by shaving.

amount of carbon dioxide slush on the end of an orange stick and fashion it into a fine point so that you can be very accurate in touching each wart. Apply it to the warts individually until they go white. An alternative would be to cauterize them using a Hyfrecator. The end is placed near to the wart and the current switched on; a spark will flash onto the wart causing electro-desiccation. Because this machine runs on a very low current the patient can usually tolerate it without a local anaesthetic so all the warts can be treated in a single go.

Genital and perianal warts

The most important part of the treatment for genital warts is to screen the patient for other sexually transmitted diseases so referral to the local department of genitourinary medicine is required.

It is not easy for patients to treat their own genital warts because of the difficulty in applying topical treatments accurately. Most treatments are therefore done by a nurse or doctor. Three modalities of treatment are commonly used.

1 Podophyllin or podophyllotoxin paint.
2 Freezing with liquid nitrogen or nitrous oxide.
3 Surgical removal.

1 Podophyllin or podophyllotoxin. Until recently podophyllin was only available in a relatively crude form and it was made up as a 10%, 15%, 20% or 25% solution in tinc. benz. co. First apply white soft paraffin (Vaseline) to the normal skin around the warts to protect it from the burning effects of podophyllin. Then, starting with 10% podophyllin, the nurse applies the solution on a cotton wool bud to each individual wart (Figure 237). The patient is instructed to leave it in place for 4 hours and then to wash it off with soap and water. One week later the treatment is repeated, but this time the paint is left on the warts for 6 hours. Treatment is only done once a week, otherwise the patient will become very sore.

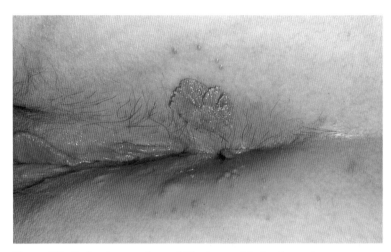

Figure 237 Perianal warts. It would be impossible for the patient to see these well enough to be able to apply podophyllin herself.

Each week the paint is left in place longer:

First week	4 hours
Second week	6 hours
Third week	8 hours
Fourth week	10 hours
Fifth week	12 hours.

On the sixth week, if the warts are not gone, the concentration of podophyllin is increased to 15% and the time goes back to 4 hours. 15% podophyllin is then used for 5 weeks, leaving it on the skin for 2 hours longer each week. If the warts still are still present by week 11, the podophyllin strength is increased to 20%, and after another 5 weeks to 25%. Most warts will be gone before this.

Podophyllotoxin is a highly purified form of the active principle of podophyllin and it can be used by the patient himself on penile warts. A 0.5% alcohol based solution is applied to each wart twice a day for 3 consecutive days. If the warts are not gone 7 days later the treatment is repeated. This substance has two advantages over ordinary podophyllin:

- it works more quickly
- it can be done by the patient himself.

Disadvantages are:

- it can only be used by the patient on penile warts because it still has to be applied accurately to the individual warts
- it can cause erythema, oedema, a burning sensation and erosions on the penis
- it is more expensive.

2 Freezing with liquid nitrogen or nitrous oxide. Liquid nitrogen is a suitable treatment if there is a single wart or only a few warts present. The skin around the wart is put on the stretch so that the liquid nitrogen can be applied accurately to the wart and not to the adjacent normal skin. It is applied with a hand made cotton wool bud (so that it can be the same size as the wart) until the whole wart goes white. Treatment can be repeated every 3 weeks until the wart is gone.

If you have a nitrous oxide cryoprobe this is very suitable for genital warts. The end of the probe is dipped in KY jelly and then applied to the wart. The probe is switched on and the wart frozen until a 1 mm white halo appears around it. Cryoprobes come with varying sized ends, so one that is the same size as the wart can be used.

3 Surgical removal. Surgical removal under a general anaesthetic is a useful treatment if there are very extensive warts, particularly if the anal canal is involved as well as the skin. 50–75 ml of 1:30,000 adrenaline in physiological saline is injected subcutaneously underneath the warts. This causes the skin to swell up like a balloon so that the warts are separated from each other and stick out like fingers. Taking hold of the warts with a pair of fine-toothed forceps they are then snipped off with a pair of sharp pointed scissors. The adrenaline means that there is very little bleeding; any persistent bleeding points can be diathermied.

Warts in patients who are immunosuppressed

Patients who have had renal or heart and lung transplants and are on immunosuppressive therapy are often covered in viral warts. Treatment at any one site will be the same as for any other patient (*see* pages 252–262), but the response is likely to be poor. Some of these patients will end up having interferon, etretinate or become sensitized to dinitrochlorobenzene and having that painted on their warts. These treatments should only be attempted by those who are familiar with their use and all the side effects that can occur.

XANTHOMAS

Patients presenting with xanthomas should have their fasting lipids measured. Apart from total cholesterol and triglycerides you may also get a figure for low density lipoprotein (LDL) and high density lipoprotein (HDL). Most of the cholesterol in normal patients is carried by LDL; smaller proportions are carried by HDL and very low density lipoprotein (VLDL). Most triglyceride in fasting serum

is carried by VLDL. Chylomicrons transport dietary triglycerides and will be found in the serum after a fatty meal; they should not be present in fasting serum. If lipid levels are high the main reason for lowering them is to decrease the incidence of, and mortality from, coronary artery disease and to prevent acute pancreatitis rather than to get rid of the xanthomas.

Table 27 Desirable and abnormal lipid levels

	Desirable level	Abnormal level
Total cholesterol (TC)	<5.2 mmol/l	>6.5 mmol/l
LDL cholesterol (LDLC)*	<4.0 mmol/l	>5.0 mmol/l
HDL cholesterol (HDLC)	>1.0 mmol/l	<0.9 mmol/l
Triglyceride (TG)	<2.0 mmol/l	>2.5 mmol/l

$$*LDLC = TC - HDLC - \frac{TG}{2.2}$$

Treatment of hyperlipoproteinaemia

Secondary causes of hyperlipidaemia such as hypothyroidism, diabetes or excess alcohol intake should be excluded or treated. If there is a primary hyperlipidaemia, treatment can be initiated with a low fat diet (less than 30% of the daily calories from fat and only 10% from saturated fat) and weight reduction before thinking of introducing lipid-lowering drugs. If hyperlipidaemic patients with xanthomas do not respond to dietary measures it is worth referring them to a physician with an interest in lipid disorders so that the most appropriate lipid-lowering drugs can be instituted (*see* Table 28).

Table 28 Fredrickson/WHO classification of hyperlipoproteinaemia

Type	Main biochemical features		Xanthomas	Other problems	Frequency of occurrence
I	Cholesterol ↑ TG ↑↑	Chylomicrons ↑ LDL ↓ VLDL →	Eruptive xanthomas		Rare (children)
IIa	Cholesterol ↑↑	LDL ↑ VLDL →	Xanthelasma, tendon and tuberose xanthomas	↑ Coronary heart disease	Common
IIb	Cholesterol ↑↑ TG ↑	LDL ↑ VLDL ↑	Xanthelasma, tendon and tuberose xanthomas	↑ Coronary heart disease ↑ Peripheral vascular disease	Common
III	Cholesterol ↑ TG ↑↑	LDL ↓	Plane xanthomas along palmar creases, tuberose and tendon xanthomas and occasionally eruptive xanthomas	↑ Coronary artery disease	Uncommon
IV	Cholesterol ↑ TG ↑↑	LDL → VLDL ↑	Eruptive xanthomas	Diabetes and alcoholism	Common
V	Cholesterol ↑ TG ↑↑	Chylomicrons ↑ LDL ↓ VLDL ↑↑	Eruptive xanthomas	Diabetes and obesity If TG >10–12 mmol/l ↑ risk of pancreatitis	Uncommon

Table 29 Lipid-lowering drugs

Group of drugs	Dose	Precautions and side effects	Effect on cholesterol	Effect on triglycerides
Fibric acid derivatives Gemfibrozil* Bezafibrate Fenofibrate	600 mg twice a day 200 mg three times a day, or 400 mg of the long-acting preparation once a day 100 mg three times a day	Can cause myositis especially in patients with poor renal function	↓↓	↓↓↓
Anion exchange resins Cholestyramine* Colestipol*	8–12 g twice a day 10 g twice a day	Because they act by binding bile salts within the gut, interfering with their reabsorption and increasing their faecal excretion, they should be taken at least 2 hours before or after digoxin, thyroxine and warfarin (to avoid binding to these drugs in the gut). They commonly cause gastrointestinal upsets	↓↓↓	↑
HMGCoA reductase inhibitors (β-**hydroxy-**β-**methylglutaryl-Co A reductase inhibitors)** [*statins*] Simvastatin Pravastatin	10–40 mg at night 20 mg twice a day	They may cause a myositis. Do not use in renal transplant patients or those with hepatic dysfunction	↓↓↓	↓↓
Nicotinic acid derivatives Nicotinic acid* Acipimox	20 mg twice a day 250 mg twice or three times a day	They cause headaches and flushing (less marked if taken with food or aspirin). They can also cause rashes, gastrointestinal upsets, hyperuricaemia, hyperglycaemia and abnormal LFTs	↓	↓↓↓

*Trial evidence for decreased risk of coronary artery disease.

Eruptive xanthomas begin to disappear after 2 weeks of treatment and should have disappeared after 6 weeks. Tendon and tuberose xanthomas take months rather than weeks to disappear.

Xanthelasma

If the patient has xanthelasmas rather than eruptive, tendon or tuberose xanthomas, the lipid levels may all be normal. If they are abnormal, treatment is the same as for other xanthomas, *see* page 262. If they are normal, or if the cholesterol level has been brought back down to normal with a low-fat diet or one of the lipid-lowering drugs, the xanthelasmas themselves can be treated either by:

1 **surgical excision** by a dermatologist or a plastic surgeon, *or*

2 **painting on a supersaturated solution of trichloroacetic acid (TCA).** Before starting treatment, take two orange sticks and on the end of one put a tiny wisp of cotton wool, on the end of the other a large bud of cotton wool. You will also require a saturated solution of trichloroacetic acid and a bottle of surgical spirit. Dip the tiny wisp of cotton wool into the trichloroacetic acid, and the large bud of cotton wool into the surgical spirit. You are now ready to start treatment. Paint the trichloroacetic acid onto the xanthelasma being careful not to get it onto the normal skin (Figure 238), and as soon as the skin goes white (a few seconds, Figure 239), smother it with the surgical spirit (Figure 240). It stings quite a lot and the patient will need a tissue to wipe away the tears which form. This passes off in a few minutes. A week later the treated area will scab over (Figure 241) and the area should be back to normal in about 6 weeks.

Either of these methods of treatment can be repeated if further xanthelasma occur.

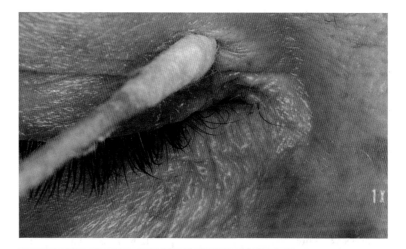

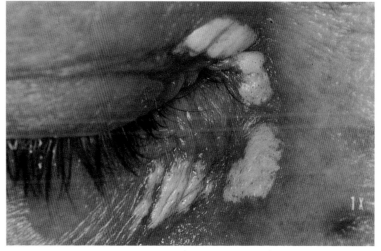

Figure 238 (*above*) Applying trichloroacetic acid with a very fine cotton wool swab accurately on top of the xanthelasmas.

Figure 239 (*below*) The skin goes white almost immediately after painting with trichloroacetic acid.

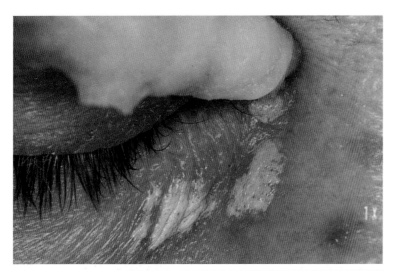

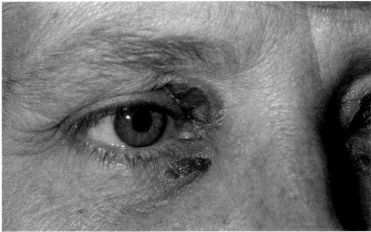

YELLOW NAIL SYNDROME

There is nothing that can be done to make the nails go back to their normal colour or to speed up their rate of growth. If onycholysis is a problem, it is probably best to remove the affected nail by pulling it off with a pair of artery forceps, having first anaesthetized the end of the finger with a ring block. Some patients will have bilateral pleural effusions due to poor lymphatic drainage of the pleural cavity. If so they should be referred to a thoracic surgeon so that the fluid can be drained off and the two layers of pleura stuck together with some talcum powder to stop the fluid reaccumulating.

Figure 240 (*above*) Applying surgical spirit liberally as soon as the skin over the xanthelasmas goes white.

Figure 241 (*below*) Five days after treatment with trichloroacetic acid: the treated areas are crusted over.

Index

List of drugs and associated drug reactions

ACTH	Acne
Allopurinol	Erythrodermic
	Purpura
	Toxic epidermal necrolysis
	Vasculitis
Ampicillin	Erythrodermic
	Exanthematous
	Vasculitis
Aminophylline	Eczema (cross-reacts with ethylene diamine)
Amiodarone	Hyperpigmentation
	Phototoxic
Androgens	Acne
Aspirin	Histamine release (urticaria)
Barbiturates	Acne
	Erythrodermic
	Fixed drug reaction
	Purpura
	Toxic epidermal necrolysis
β-blockers	Lichenoid
β-carotene	Orange discolouration
Benzodiazepines	Exanthematous
	Fixed drug eruption
Bromides	Acne
Busulphan	Hyperpigmentation
Captopril	Erythrodermic lichenoid
	Exanthematous
	Pemphigus
Carbamazepine	Erythrodermic
	Exanthematous
Carbimazole	Hair loss
	Purpura
	Toxic epidermal necrolysis

Chloroquine	Erythrodermic
	Lichenoid
	Hyperpigmentation of skin/bleaching of hair
Chlorpromazine	Erythrodermic
	Photoallergic
	Purpura (thrombocytopenia)
Chlorpropamide	Eczematous (cross-reacts with PPD and benzocaine)
	Lichenoid
Cimetidine	Erythrodermic
Clofazimine	Pigmentation—red/pink
Codeine	Histamine release (urticaria)
Contraceptives	Erythema nodosum
	Pigmentation of face (chloasma)
Co-trimoxazole	Purpura (thrombocytopenia) (*see* also sulphonamides)
Coumarins	Skin necrosis
Cyclosporin A	Hypertrichosis
Cytotoxics	Hair loss
	Purpura (thrombocytopenia)
Dapsone	Pigmentation—blue/grey
Diazoxide	Hypertrichosis
Diclofenac	Pemphigoid
Diphenylhydantoin	Hypertrichosis
Frusemide	Pemphigoid
	Phototoxic
Gold	Erythrodermic
	Lichenoid
	Pigmentation of face—blue/grey
	Purpura (thrombocytopenia)
	Vasculitis
Heparin	Hair loss
	Vasculitis